NUTRITIONAL ANEMIAS

CRC SERIES IN
MODERN NUTRITION
Edited by Ira Wolinsky and James F. Hickson, Jr.

Published Titles

Manganese in Health and Disease, Dorothy J. Klimis-Tavantzis

Nutrition and AIDS: Effects and Treatments, Ronald R. Watson

Nutrition Care for HIV-Positive Persons: A Manual for Individuals and Their Caregivers,
   Saroj M. Bahl and James F. Hickson, Jr.

Calcium and Phosphorus in Health and Disease, John J.B. Anderson and
   Sanford C. Garner

Edited by Ira Wolinsky

Published Titles

Practical Handbook of Nutrition in Clinical Practice, Donald F. Kirby
   and Stanley J. Dudrick

Handbook of Dairy Foods and Nutrition, Gregory D. Miller, Judith K. Jarvis,
   and Lois D. McBean

Advanced Nutrition: Macronutrients, Carolyn D. Berdanier

Childhood Nutrition, Fima Lifschitz

Nutrition and Health: Topics and Controversies, Felix Bronner

Nutrition and Cancer Prevention, Ronald R. Watson and Siraj I. Mufti

Nutritional Concerns of Women, Ira Wolinsky and Dorothy J. Klimis-Tavantzis

Nutrients and Gene Expression: Clinical Aspects, Carolyn D. Berdanier

Antioxidants and Disease Prevention, Harinda S. Garewal

Advanced Nutrition: Micronutrients, Carolyn D. Berdanier

Nutrition and Women's Cancers, Barbara Pence and Dale M. Dunn

Nutrients and Foods in AIDS, Ronald R. Watson

Nutrition: Chemistry and Biology, Second Edition, Julian E. Spallholz,
   L. Mallory Boylan, and Judy A. Driskell

Melatonin in the Promotion of Health, Ronald R. Watson

Nutritional and Environmental Influences on the Eye, Allen Taylor

Laboratory Tests for the Assessment of Nutritional Status, Second Edition,
   H.E. Sauberlich

Advanced Human Nutrition, Robert E.C. Wildman and Denis M. Medeiros

Handbook of Dairy Foods and Nutrition, Second Edition, Gregory D. Miller,
   Judith K. Jarvis, and Lois D. McBean

Nutrition in Space Flight and Weightlessness Models, Helen W. Lane
   and Dale A. Schoeller

Eating Disorders in Women and Children: Prevention, Stress Management, and Treatment, Jacalyn J. Robert-McComb
Childhood Obesity: Prevention and Treatment, Jana Pařízková and Andrew Hills
Alcohol and Coffee Use in the Aging, Ronald R. Watson
Handbook of Nutrition and the Aged, Third Edition, Ronald R. Watson
Vegetables, Fruits, and Herbs in Health Promotion, Ronald R. Watson
Nutrition and AIDS, Second Edition, Ronald R. Watson
Advances in Isotope Methods for the Analysis of Trace Elements in Man, Nicola Lowe and Malcolm Jackson
Nutritional Anemias, Usha Ramakrishnan

Forthcoming Titles

Nutrition for Vegetarians, Joan Sabate
Tryptophan: Biochemicals and Health Implications, Herschel Sidransky
Handbook of Nutraceuticals and Functional Foods, Robert E. C. Wildman
The Mediterranean Diet, Antonia L. Matalas, Antonios Zampelas, Vasilis Stavrinos, and Ira Wolinsky
Handbook of Nutraceuticals and Nutritional Supplements and Pharmaceuticals, Robert E. C. Wildman
Insulin and Oligofructose: Functional Food Ingredients, Marcel B. Roberfroid
Micronutrients and HIV Infection, Henrik Friis
Nutrition Gene Interactions in Health and Disease, Niama M. Moussa and Carolyn D. Berdanier

NUTRITIONAL ANEMIAS

Edited by

Usha Ramakrishnan

CRC Press

Boca Raton   London   New York   Washington, D.C.

Library of Congress Cataloging-in-Publication Data

Nutritional anemias / edited by Usha Ramakrishnan.
    p. cm.
Includes bibliographical references and index.
ISBN 0-8493-8569-5
    1. Anemia--Nutritional aspects. I. Ramakrishnan, Usha. II. Modern Nutrition (Boca Raton, Fla.)

RC641.N836 2000
616.1′52—dc21

00-045504

Series Preface
for Modern Nutrition

The CRC Series in Modern Nutrition is dedicated to providing the widest possible coverage of topics in nutrition. Nutrition is an interdisciplinary, interprofessional field noted by its broad range and diversity. The titles and authorship in this series reflect that range and diversity.

Published for a scholarly audience, the volumes in the CRC Series in Modern Nutrition are designed to review and explore recent trends, developments, and advances in nutrition. As such, they will also appeal to the educated general reader. The format for the series will vary with the needs of the author and the topic, including, but not limited to, edited volumes, monographs, handbooks, and texts.

Contributors from any bona fide area of nutrition, including the controversial, are welcome.

The Series welcomes the timely and authoritative contribution, *Nutritional Anemias*, edited by Dr. Usha Ramakrishnan. This book will be of interest to a cross section of life scientists. It contains a wealth of information, authoritatively written and edited.

Ira Wolinsky, Ph.D.
University of Houston
Series Editor

Preface

Nutritional anemias constitute the largest nutrition and health problem that affects populations in both developed and developing countries. While iron deficiency is the major cause of nutritional anemias in most settings, the roles of other nutrients (folic acid, vitamins B_{12} and C) and infections have received attention recently. The prevalence of nutritional anemia is very high among young children and women of reproductive age in many developing countries, especially in South Asia, and is associated with a range of functional consequences such as adverse pregnancy outcomes, limited school performance, and reduced work productivity. Considerable strides have been made in our knowledge of this important topic in the past 20 years in terms of research as well as experience in the planning and implementation of strategies for the prevention and control of nutritional anemias. However, much remains to be done.

It is hoped that this comprehensive book will serve as a timely and valuable resource for those working in the fields of public health and nutrition. Academics in university settings, practitioners in program implementation, and policy makers could use it in teaching and/or training activities. A balanced approach that combines knowledge of the etiology and consequences of nutritional anemias through the lifecycle with a discussion of current strategies, namely supplementation, fortification, food based strategies, and control of helminth infection in the prevention and control of nutritional anemias has been used. Special attention is paid to relevant research, controversies, and lessons learned from previous worldwide efforts toward finding solutions to eliminate this preventable condition.

As editor, I would like to acknowledge my contributors, leading experts in their fields, for the time they spent in preparing their thoughtful and well-written chapters despite their hectic schedules and other responsibilities. A debt of gratitude is owed to my mentor, Dr. Reynaldo Martorell, Chair, Department of International Health and Robert W. Woodruff Professor of International Nutrition, Rollins School of Public Health, Emory University, for his support, constant encouragement, and valuable guidance at various stages of this project. Last but not least, this book would not have been possible without the support of my family and the faculty, staff, and students at the Department of International Health, especially Nancy Sterk, Linda King, and Khaleelah Muwwakkil for their patience and understanding. Funding from the National Institutes of Health (NIH-HD34531-02) is acknowledged.

Usha Ramakrishnan

About the Editor

Dr. Usha Ramakrishnan earned her master's degree in foods and nutrition from the University of Madras, India. She participated in the evaluation of the "Integrated Child Development Services Scheme," a large national program for pregnant, and lactating women, and young children at the National Institute of Public Development and Child Development in New Delhi, India. Her interest in maternal and child nutrition led her to join Cornell University where she earned her Ph.D. in international nutrition. Her doctoral dissertation described a randomized clinical trial on the impact of vitamin A supplementation on growth and morbidity of preschool children in south India. Dr. Ramakrishnan received the Young Investigator Award from the Society of International Research (SINR), American Society of Nutritional Sciences.

Dr. Ramakrishnan is an assistant professor in the Department of International Health at Rollins School of Public Health at Emory University and is actively involved in several research projects. She teaches graduate level courses on maternal and child nutrition assessment for epidemiology. She also advises masters and doctoral students.

Dr. Ramakrishnan's research interests are maternal and child nutrition and micronutrient malnutrition. She is currently involved in collaborative research projects with the Instituto Nacional de Salud Pública in Cuernavaca, Mexico. One project is a randomized controlled trial of the effects of multiple micronutrient supplements during pregnancy and early childhood on birth outcomes and child growth and development funded by the Thrasher Research Fund, UNICEF, Micronutrient Initiative, and Conacyt (Mexico).

Dr. Ramakrishnan is the principal investigator on an investigation funded by a grant from the National Institutes of Health to study iron status of women of reproductive age in the U.S. Her other research interests include the intergenerational effects of malnutrition and childcare practices. She is part of a large NIH study that examines the intergenerational effects of malnutrition in Guatemala, and has co-authored papers on the impact of early childhood nutrition on pregnancy outcomes and intergenerational effects of birth size.

In sum, Dr. Ramakrishnan is committed to the betterment of the lives of women and young children and has pursued this goal since the days of her undergraduate training in nutrition. She is interested in conducting applied research to identify effective strategies that will reduce the high rates of nutritional anemia during pregnancy and early childhood, low birth weight, and poor child growth and development in developing countries as well as at-risk populations in developed countries. She has served as consultant for several non-governmental organizations (Mothercare, UNICEF, BASICS), has given presentations at international and national meetings, and is an active member of the American Society for Nutritional Sciences, American Society for Public Health, Delta Omega Society, and other professional societies.

Contributors

Lindsay Allen, Ph.D., R.D.
Department of Nutrition
University of California – Davis
Davis, California

John L. Beard, Ph.D.
Nutritional Programs and Human
  Development
Pennsylvania State University
University Park, Pennsylvania

Don Bundy, Ph.D.
The World Bank
Washington, D.C.

Jennifer Casterline-Sabel, Ph.D.
Department of Nutrition
University of California – Davis
Davis, California

Lesley Drake, Ph.D.
Department of Zoology
Oxford University
Oxford, U.K.

Eva-Charlotte Ekström, Ph.D.
International Center for Diarrhoeal
  Disease Research
Dhaka, Bangladesh

Ralph Green, Ph.D.
School of Medicine
University of California – Davis
Davis, California

Andrew Hall, Ph.D.
Helen Keller International
Dhaka, Bangladesh

Eva Hertrampf, M.D.
Department of Hematology
University of Chile
Santiago, Chile

Carol E. Levin, Ph.D.
International Food Policy Research
  Institute
Washington, D.C.

Mahshid Lotfi, Ph.D.
The Micronutrient Initiative
Ottawa, Ontario

Betsy Lozoff, Ph.D.
Center for Human Growth and
  Development
University of Michigan
Ann Arbor, Michigan

Sean Lynch, M.D.
Hampton Veterans Affairs Medical Center
Eastern Virginia Medical School
Hampton, Virginia

Manuel Olivares, M.D.
Department of Hematology
University of Chile
Santiago, Chile

Santosh Jain Passi, Ph.D.
Department of Nutrition and Dietetics
University of Delhi
New Delhi, India

Fernando Pizarro, M.T.
Department of Hematology
University of Chile
Santiago, Chile

Usha Ramakrishnan, Ph.D.
Department of International Health
Emory University
Atlanta, Georgia

Marie T. Ruel, Ph.D.
International Food Policy Research
  Institute
Washington, D.C.

Barbara Underwood, Ph.D.
National Academy of Sciences
Washington, D.C.

Sheila C. Vir, Ph.D.
UNICEF
New Delhi, India

Theodore D. Wachs, Ph.D.
Department of Psychological Sciences
Purdue University
West Lafayette, Indiana

Tomás Walter, M.D.
Department of Hematology
University of Chile
Santiago, Chile

Table of Contents

1 Nutritional Anemias Worldwide: A Historical Overview

Barbara Underwood

CONTENTS

1.1 INTRODUCTION

Anemias of nutritional origin are acquired problems caused by diets that lack sufficient quantity of bioavailable essential hematopoietic nutrients to meet the need for hemoglobin and red blood cell synthesis. Need is influenced by environmental factors that cause excessive blood loss or hemolysis. Nutritional anemias are unlikely to be inherent to man's existence, but evolved as ancient man's lifestyle turned from hunting animals and foraging for wild berries fruits and green leaves, to growing cereal crops and cultivating vegetables to provide energy and nutrient needs. This caused his primary menu to shift toward foods containing less bioavailable hematopoietic nutrients (iron and vitamin B_{12}) or those that enhance their utilization (vitamins C and A), and a shift of his culinary practices to those that exposed food to longer heat exposure that was potentially destructive for certain nutrients (folates). Furthermore, he acquired a taste for spices and teas to enhance dining pleasures, and they further render hematopoietic nutrients (iron) less bioavailable.

Not all nutritional anemias are attributable to diet and changing lifestyles. Physiological factors may contribute to a decline in normal functions associated with aging, such as low stomach acidity which decreases the bioavailability of vitamin B_{12} from food. This factor in the etiology of nutritional anemia that results from atrophic gastritis may be a more recent development in man's evolution associated with increased longevity.

0-8493-8569-5/01/$0.00+$.50

Environmental factors that expose humans to infections, such as hookworm, schistosomiasis, and other parasites that can lead to excessive loss or competition for hematopoietic nutrients, are also of concern, particularly among populations exposed to poverty and deprived living conditions. Obviously, the acquired nature of nutritional anemias is complex and requires multiple considerations in finding the appropriate mix of remedial measures. From a global public health perspective, however, iron is by far the most significant hematopoietic nutrient lacking in quantity or availability from diets. Nevertheless, to restrict the consequences to those from anemia far understates the health impact of iron deficiency that occur, before hematopoiesis is affected, e.g., compromised immunity, cognitive functions, and work performance.

1.2 THE EVOLUTION OF NUTRITIONAL ANEMIAS

1.2.1 CHANGES IN ENVIRONMENT, LIFESTYLES, AND FOOD SOURCES

The earth's crust contains about 4.7% iron. It was largely unavailable until plants evolved chelators (phytates and polyphenols) to trap iron and other minerals essential to their survival. Magnesium is another mineral which was critical for the evolution of the protoporphyrin compound (chlorophyll) needed to trap radiant energy and transform it into energy for support of metabolic processes critical to plant survival. Furthermore, the appearance and evolution of aquatic and animal life required efficient transfer of oxygen to support energy needs for metabolism and mobility. Hence protoporphyrin compounds to facilitate efficient uptake, binding, and transport of oxygen to tissues evolved (e.g., iron protoporphyrin compounds in the form of hemoglobin and myoglobin).

Man's evolution, relevant to the dietary origin of nutritional anemias, can be presumed from fossil evidence, such as tooth structures dating from 1.8 million years ago to modern times. Evidence of progressively decreasing tooth size suggests that man's diet evolved from predominantly flesh based, for which large tearing canine teeth were required, to diets that required the grinding surfaces of molars to facilitate mastication of fruits, vegetables, and cereal grains. Nutritional anemias could be presumed to be rare during the hunting phase of man's evolution and probably surfaced when modern man emerged some 40,000 years ago — the late Pleistocene period — when anthropological evidence indicates increased consumption of wild fruits, leaves, grains, and nuts.[1] Cultivated cereal grains and vegetables became prominent dietary constituents with the onset of agriculture, which began about 10,000 years ago.[2] They introduced significant problems due to the increased consumption of inhibitors of iron absorption, e.g., phytates and polyphenols and decreased intakes of enhancers of iron absorption and utilization, e.g., vitamin C and preformed vitamin A. Today, the balance between animal, cereal, and vegetable foods in man's diet varies widely among cultures and so does the prevalence of anemias. Tracking the emergence of nutritional anemias based on primary food sources alone cannot fully account for the variability in prevalence because it does not account for the effects of food preparation and storage on bioavailability and infection related disease modifiers that also vary among cultures.

1.2.2 MEDICAL, ART, AND LITERATURE RECORDS

Ancient Greeks recognized the benefits of iron salts to improve muscular weakness in injured war veterans. The weakened sufferers hoped to assume some of the strength of this metal by drinking water in which a sword had rusted.[3] The pale hues of fatigued and fainting women were commonly portrayed in art — particularly by the Dutch school of painters — and are referred to in several Shakespearean plays and sonnets to describe lovesick women. Anemia symptoms were first identified by the term "chlorosis" — a Greek term meaning green. Historians are unsure when this identification first appeared but in the 16th century it was associated with a series of symptoms: pallor, fatigue, poor appetite, and gastrointestinal, neurological, and menstrual disturbances, common in adolescent girls.[4] Snydenham, a 17th century physician, prescribed iron salts for treatment of chlorosis. In the 18th century, blood was shown to contain iron, and from 1832 to 1843, chlorosis was noted to be associated with low levels of iron in the blood and a reduced number of red cells.[5] During this period, Blaud marketed his famous Blaud pills shown to cure chlorosis; they were made of ferrous sulfate and potassium carbonate and contained 24 mg iron. These reports appeared after the birth of modern hematology following the invention of the microscope in the 17th century. Although colleagues debated the etiology of chlorosis even during the 20th century, tracking the evolution of nutritional anemias through symptoms and signs, such as chlorosis, paleness, spoon shaped nails, obviously is qualitative and inadequate for determining the changing global prevalence of nutritional anemias.

The merging of knowledge of the chemical composition of blood with the description of the morphologic characteristics of red cells in health and disease made possible by modern hematology[6] have allowed significant advances in our understanding of the etiology of nutritional anemias in modern times. Hemoglobin was discovered in the 19th century by Hoppe-Seylers who showed that the blood pigment was composed of hematin, which contained iron, and protein. A means of estimating its concentration in blood by color comparison to a standard (the first hemoglobin-ometer) was described by Gowers about 1880, and was followed quickly by a more accurate methodology, i.e., the Sahli hemoglobinometer, modifications of which are still used today. Progress in understanding anemia was enhanced further around the 1890s when Hüfner, Haldane, and Smith demonstrated stoichiometric relationships between hemoglobin and its iron content, iron, and oxygen, and hemoglobin and oxygen carrying capacity.[7] Although a merging of anemia symptomatology and hematology occurred in the first half of the 19th century when chlorosis was associated with a decrease in the quantity and size of the red cell and a reduction in iron content, microscopic examination revealed there were other anemias in which, although hemoglobin was reduced, red cell size was not. The presence of enlarged red cells suggested that nutritional anemia had multiple etiologies.

Many scientists in the 20th century have made significant contributions to our knowledge of nutritional anemias, both from the fields of nutritional biochemistry and hematology. Dr. Whipple and colleagues at the University of Rochester developed a dog model in which they maintained a uniform anemia level over time, allowing systematic study of blood regeneration in response to dietary factors.[8] Carl

Moore and his students at St. Louis University and Clement Finch and his students at the University of Washington added much to our knowledge of iron absorption, metabolism, and assessment of status of hemopoietic nutrients. Max Wintrobe at the University of Utah provided standardization in hematology through his exhaustive textbook which is a seminal reference. Minot and Murphy at the Thorndike Laboratory in Boston shocked the medical world with the report that giving liver to pernicious anemia patients relieved the symptoms. Castle, from the same institution, provided the explanation with the discovery of intrinsic factor. They, together with Lucy Wills from the U.K., whose discovery of the beneficial effects of brewer's yeast in the treatment of the macrocytic anemia observed in Indian women, introduced us to macrocytic, megaloblastic anemias from deficiencies of vitamin B_{12} and folate.

1.3   HISTORICAL ACCOUNTING
OF PREVALENCE ESTIMATES

Unfortunately, we are unable to retrospectively apply the currently available armory of biochemical yardsticks to ancient reports and quantitatively track global prevalence through the centuries. The importance of the problem was recognized by WHO and FAO at the first meeting of the Joint Advisory Committee in 1949, and at each subsequent meeting through the late 1950s. Between 1955 and 1958, WHO sponsored a national survey of anemia in Mauritius, identifying a prevalence of 15 to 64% for anemia, with a hypochromic microcytic variety prevailing and associated with hookworm infection. The anemia subsequently was shown to respond to bread enrichment with iron. WHO followed up with investigations of nutritional anemia among pregnant women in India, 38% of whom were anemic; half of those who were severely anemic showed megaloblastic changes in their bone marrow, which were responsive to combined iron and folic acid prophylaxis. These studies prompted WHO to establish internationally acceptable standards for the study of anemia based on hemoglobin levels, but the standards set were general for age and sex categories.[9] WHO then recommended an agenda for field studies of anemia and a large multi-country collaborative study involving seven countries was set up in the early 1960s to fill in gaps in knowledge.[9]

WHO sponsored studies were greatly extended by 30 surveys between 1956 and 1970, sponsored by the International Committee on Nutrition for National Defense, later renamed the Interdepartmental Committee on Nutrition for National Defense (ICNND). These surveys, under the guiding hands of Harold Sandstead and Arnie Schaeffer, contributed in a major way to advancing knowledge of the prevalence of nutritional anemias by standardizing methodologies and establishing interpretive guidelines based on occidental populations composed mainly of men. *The Manual for Nutrition Surveys*[10,11] included procedures and interpretive guidelines for hemoglobin and hematocrit in very broad terms with a slide set that showed morphologic characteristics of blood cells associated with micro and macrocytic anemias. Latter surveys measured serum iron, folate, and vitamin B_{12}. Although data were not available from all countries, it was clear that on a global scale, lack of iron was by far the commonest nutritional cause of anemia, followed by folate deficiency, with lesser roles for vitamin B_{12} and protein. In the early 1960s, the ICNND surveys expanded the age and sex coverage of the interpretive guidelines, but these were still based on occidental populations. Finally, in 1968, WHO standardized the definition of anemia based on hemoglobin levels and established cutoffs that were age and sex specific. The criteria have changed little since then, except for the inclusion of correction factors established for altitude, smoking, and race[12] and recently, to further divide the criteria for the 6 to 11 and 12 to 14 year age groups. Attention to folate and vitamin B_{12} deficiencies as causes of anemia occurred as a result of the WHO collaborative trials in Indian women in the late 1960s and early 1970s; recommended assessment methods and interpretation guidelines emerged. However, few representative national surveys were conducted, particularly by developing countries, where these assessment procedures have been applied.

Consequently, hemoglobin has emerged as the fair weather surrogate in most national and regional surveys of nutritional anemias, particularly in developing countries, because of ease of measurement in comparison with other specific causative nutrients. The databank available at the WHO which estimates the global and regional prevalence of anemia, therefore, does not allow differentiation of nutritional etiology or that caused by nonnutritional factors.

1.3.1 CURRENT PREVALENCE ESTIMATES

WHO first attempted to assemble the available information about women from a global view in 1982,[13] and updated it in 1992.[14] In 1985, the available prevalence data were collected by WHO from published literature and consultant assignment and evaluated using WHO reference values for normal age/sex/altitude specific hemoglobin concentration. Information from 523 studies between 1960 and 1985 were analyzed, many of which suffered from deficient numbers and lack of representative study populations. Nonetheless, using this yardstick as a surrogate for nutritional anemia, WHO estimated that about 1300 million people, or about 30% of the world's population in 1980 suffered from anemia, about half (600 to 700 million) due to iron deficiency.[15] The prevalence was highest in young children and pregnant women, and varied from about 56% in young children in Africa and South Asia, and 20 to 26% in Latin America and East Asia, to about 8 to 18% in developed countries. This does not include the large group of individuals who are iron deficient and do not have anemia.

In the 1990s, the Nutrition Program at WHO established the Micronutrient Deficiency Information System, which continuously updates prevalence information for iron, iodine, and vitamin A deficiencies. These data indicate a worldwide prevalence of 34% in young children and adult men, and 56% in pregnant women, with broad regional variations up to 80% among pregnant women in Southeast Asia. The examination of trends indicates that anemia has a long way to go before control will be achieved, especially when compared to the progress made for deficiencies of other micronutrients, namely vitamin A and iodine that have been high on the global agenda for elimination and control as public health problems. There is an urgent need to accelerate progress because the functional consequences of iron deficiency even without anemia are estimated by WHO to affect another billion people. Today, although we may differ as to how to interpret degrees of public health significance or prevalence cutoffs and how they should be used to initiate and monitor intervention programs,[16] indisputably, anemia remains one of the most frequently observed and potentially controllable nutritional deficiency diseases. This book provides for the first time a synthesis of our experiences in addressing this public health problem with a view to the future. The first section is a comprehensive update on current knowledge and latest findings on the epidemiology of nutritional anemias including the prevalence and assessment of the problem and functional consequences during the lifecycle. The second part is a careful review of the different approaches, namely supplementation, fortification, food based, and disease control strategies that have been used in the prevention and control of nutritional anemias, followed by a synthesis in the last chapter.

REFERENCES

1. Eaton, S. B. and Konner, M., Paleolithic nutrition. A consideration of its nature and current implications, *New Engl. J. Med.,* 312, 283, 1985.
2. Newman, M. T., Nutritional adaptation in man, in *Physiological Anthropology,* Damon, A., Ed., Oxford University Press, London, 1975.
3. Hughes, E. R., Human iron metabolism, in *Metal Ions in Biological Systems: Iron in Model and Natural Compounds,* Vol. 7, Sigel, H., Ed., Marcel Dekker, New York, 1977, chap 9.
4. Patek, A. J. and Heath, C. W., Chlorosis, *J. Amer. Med. Assoc.,* 106, 1463, 1936.
5. Beard, J. L., Dawson, H., and Piñero, D. J., Iron metabolism: a comprehensive review, *Nutr. Rev.,* 54, 295, 1996.
6. Bowering, J., Sanchez, A. M., and Irwin, M. I., A conspectus of research on iron requirements of man, *J. Nutr.,* 106, 985, 1976.
7. Rybo, E., Diagnosis of iron deficiency, *Scand. J. Haematol.,* 43, 1, 1985.
8. Whipple, G. H. and Robscheit-Robbins, F. S., Blood regeneration in severe anemia, *Am. J. Physiol.,* 72, 395, 1926.
9. Patwardhan, V. N., Nutritional anemias — WHO research program. Early developments and progress report of collaborative studies, *Am. J. Clinical Nutr.,* 19, 63, 1966.
10. Interdepartmental Committee on Nutrition for National Defense, *Manual for Nutrition Surveys,* Superintendent of Documents, U.S. Government Printing Office, Washington, D.C., May 1957.
11. Interdepartmental Committee on Nutrition for National Defense, *Manual for Nutrition Surveys,* 2nd ed., National Institutes of Health, Bethesda, MD, 1963.
12. Iron Deficiency Anemia, Prevention, assessment and control, Report of a joint WHO/UNICEF/UNU consultation. World Health Organization, Geneva, 1988.
13. Royston, E., The prevalence of nutritional anaemia in women in developing countries: a critical review of available information, *World Health Statistics Q.,* 35, 52, 1982.
14. The prevalence of nutritional anaemia in women, WHO/MCH 92.2, World Health Organization, Geneva, 1992.
15. DeMaeyer, E. and Adiels-Tegman, M., The prevalence of anaemia in the world, *World Health Statistics Q.,* 38, 302, 1985.
16. Stoltzfus, R. J., Rethinking anaemia surveillance, *Lancet,* 349, 1764, 1997.

2 Prevalence and Causes of Nutritional Anemias

Lindsay Allen and Jennifer Casterline-Sabel

CONTENTS

2.1 INTRODUCTION

Anemia is defined as a low hemoglobin (Hb) concentration or low hematocrit. It is usually caused by iron deficiency, the most common nutrient deficiency in the world. However, several micronutrient deficiencies in addition to iron can cause anemia. For example, it is now recognized that vitamin A deficiency may be a common cause of impaired Hb synthesis and a contributor to anemia. Less is known about the global prevalence of riboflavin deficiency, but it also produces alterations in iron metabolism and Hb synthesis. Although the iron supplements supplied to women in developing countries usually contain folic acid, a deficiency of this vitamin — which can cause anemia if severe — is probably relatively uncommon in developing countries. Vitamin B_{12} deficiency can also cause or contribute to anemia, and may be more prevalent than is appreciated currently. Therefore, although iron deficiency anemia is the main topic of this review, information is presented on the prevalence and causes of vitamin A, riboflavin, folic acid, and vitamin B_{12} deficiencies and their possible contributions to the global prevalence of anemia. To the extent that they cause anemia, they should be included in multiple micronutrient supplements intended to prevent or treat this condition.

2.2 PREVALENCE OF ANEMIA

The World Health Organization (WHO) estimates that about 2 billion individuals, or about 40% of the world's population, suffer from anemia.[1-3] The population groups with the highest prevalence of anemia are: pregnant women and the elderly (about 50%), infants and children 1 to 2 years (48%), school children (40%), nonpregnant women (35%), and preschoolers (25%). In four out of six studies on adolescents, the prevalence was 32 to 55% in both genders.[4] These estimates of the prevalence of anemia in different regions and population groups are generally not representative because few countries have reported data to WHO on their anemia situation; much of the information comes from hospital records or isolated reports, and there are few data on groups other than pregnant women.

Anemia affects 3 to 4 times more people in nonindustrialized regions than in wealthier areas (Table 2.1). For nonindustrialized and industrialized countries, respectively, the percent of individuals with anemia is: pregnant women, 56 and 18%; schoolers, 53 and 9%; preschoolers, 42 and 17%; and men, 33 and 5%.[1] In Europe, the anemia prevalence is about 10% which is about one-fourth the prevalence in most other regions of the world. The prevalence in Southeastern Asia is particularly high, at 53%.

TABLE 2.1
Global Prevalence of Anemia and Iron Deficiency[1]

WHO Region	Anemia		Iron Deficiency Anemia[a]		Iron Deficiency[b]	
	Million	%	Million	%	Million	%
Africa	237	39	175	29	438	73
Americas	142	18	106	14	266	34
S.E. Asia	765	53	574	39	1435	99
Europe	80	9	60	7	150	17
E. Med.	179	38	135	29	337	72
W. Pacific	578	38	434	29	1084	72
TOTAL	1981	34	1484	26	3710	64

[a] Assuming that 75% of the anemia population is also iron deficient.

[b] Estimated as 2.5 times the prevalence of iron deficiency anemia in regions with up to 40% prevalence of iron deficiency anemia. When prevalence is >40%, virtually the entire population is iron deficient.

There are also substantial differences in the prevalence of anemia among developing countries, with the poorest zones affected most (Table 2.1). Among pregnant women the problem is worst in Africa (47% in east central Africa to 56% in west central Africa) and Asia (63% in southeastern Asia to 75% in south central Asia). The same is true for preschoolers: 42 to 53% in regions of Africa and 47 to 64% in south central and southeastern Asia respectively. Reports indicate that anemia is highly prevalent in Kazakhstan, Uzbekistan, and other countries in the former Soviet Union. About half the total number of anemic women live in the Indian subcontinent where about 88% of pregnant women are affected.[5]

Little progress has been made in reducing the global prevalence of anemia. Among adult women, for example, the prevalence has increased in all regions except South America, the Near East, and North Africa.[6] In an attempt to increase the awareness of policy makers to the seriousness of the problem, it has been proposed that countries be classified with respect to the degree of public health significance of anemia. An anemia prevalence of >40% is high; 15 to 40% is medium; and <15% is low.[7] One criticism of these cut-offs is that virtually everyone in a population group would be considered iron deficient where anemia prevalence is judged to be high.

Although iron deficiency is recognized as the major cause of nutritional anemia, there are even fewer data on iron deficiency than on anemia; assessment of iron status is generally more expensive than measurement of Hb, can require a larger blood sample, and is often confounded by infections. Assuming that 75% of anemia is due to iron deficiency, the prevalence of iron deficiency anemia (IDA) in different regions of the world varies from <10% in industrialized nations to almost 40% in Southeast Asia (Table 2.1). More cases of iron deficiency than anemia exist because anemia generally occurs after iron stores have been depleted. As shown in Table 2.1, the prevalence of iron deficiency is estimated to be between 2 and 2.5 times that of iron deficiency anemia. There are about 4 billion iron deficient individuals in the world.[1,3]

2.3   CAUSES OF NUTRITIONAL ANEMIAS

The nature of these nutrient deficiencies, especially iron, and their role in the etiology of nutritional anemias is described in this section.

2.3.1   IRON DEFICIENCY

Iron deficiency can result from a failure to consume high amounts of iron required for growth and failure to replace losses during menstruation and pregnancy; a low intake of either total iron or absorbable (bioavailable) iron; or excessive iron losses due to parasitic infections.

2.3.1.1   Increased Iron Requirements

Estimated daily iron requirements vary greatly with age, gender, and physiological status. The approximate amount of iron required, expressed as mg per day per 1,000 kcal, is: for infants, 1; preschoolers and schoolers, 0.4; adolescent girls 0.8

and boys, 0.6; adult men, 0.3; nonpregnant women, 0.6; pregnant women, 1.9 in the second trimester, and 2.7 in the third; and lactating and postmenopausal women, 0.4.[8] Unless they have access to more iron rich foods or supplements, in a household where meals contain inadequate amounts of absorbable iron, individuals with the highest iron requirements — especially pregnant women and infants — are at greatest risk of developing iron deficiency. In some regions a cultural bias toward males means they consume a disproportionate amount of a household's animal products.

2.3.1.1.1   Pregnancy

Pregnant women have the highest prevalence of anemia. Iron requirements increase from 1.25 mg per day in the nonpregnant woman to about 6 mg per day during pregnancy because iron is transferred to the fetus and deposited in the placenta, and more maternal Hb is synthesized. Women who have low iron stores at the start of pregnancy — the normal situation, especially in developing countries — are at high risk of developing anemia during their second and third trimesters. They require iron supplements to reduce their risk of anemia.[2] However, even in industrialized countries, it is unlikely that women will consume enough iron from food alone to meet their recommended iron intakes and maintain iron stores during pregnancy. In the U.S., for example, the recommendation is for all pregnant women to consume an additional 30 mg of iron daily as a supplement, or 60 mg daily if they are anemic.[8] The current international recommendation is 60 mg iron with 400 µg folic acid daily for 6 months during pregnancy, continuing for 3 months postpartum in regions where the prevalence of anemia in pregnancy is >40%.[2] For severely anemic women, the recommended dose is 120 mg/day.

A short interval (less than 2 years) between pregnancies, adolescent pregnancy, and multiple births, are also risk factors for anemia. A woman's iron stores in late pregnancy predict her iron status postpartum.[9] Breastfeeding delays the onset of menstruation and helps to protect iron stores. In general, the prevalence of anemia is lower in the immediate postpartum months, unless blood loss during delivery was severe. After 2 to 3 months the additional Hb synthesized during pregnancy and iron stores fall, causing anemia to reappear. Iron needs in lactation depend on maternal iron status at delivery and the duration of postpartum amenorrhea. These considerations indicate that it is important to ensure adequate iron status prior to, during, and after pregnancy. The childbearing years are the times when most women in developing countries are at risk of iron deficiency anemia.

2.3.1.1.2   Menstruation

About half of the iron requirement of menstruating women is targeted to cover the loss of iron in menstrual blood. Menstruation explains why the iron requirements of women, expressed as mg/1,000 kcal, are almost twice those of men and why iron deficiency is much more common in women. The median amount of iron lost in menstrual flow averages about 0.48 mg per day over the month. There is a wide range in this value with 25% of women losing >0.8 mg iron per day, 10% losing >1.3 mg, and 5% losing as much as 1.6 mg per day. Women with heavier menstrual losses are therefore at considerably higher risk of developing anemia. Intrauterine devices can double menstrual losses.[10]

2.3.1.1.3   Infancy

Because of the large amounts of iron deposited during rapid growth, the iron requirements of infants per 1,000 kcal are particularly high. During the first 4 months of life the total body iron is fairly constant, and about half of the storage iron is mobilized for the production of Hb, myoglobin, and enzymes. The amount of iron in breast milk is quite low and recent reports suggest it might not be absorbed as efficiently as previously thought. After about 4 to 6 months of age it is believed that infants need more iron than can be supplied in breast milk alone. In industrialized countries, this situation is avoided by iron fortification of complementary foods, recommended for all infants starting at around 6 months. In developing countries, about half of the infants are anemic by one year of age.[11] Not only is complementary feeding often delayed beyond 6 months of age, but it is generally more difficult to supply the infants with iron fortified complementary foods, and the type of foods usually given (cereals, legumes, milk, fruits, and vegetables) tend to be particularly low in bioavailable iron. The inclusion of iron rich foods such as liver, meat, or dry fish could help in this situation but these foods tend to be consumed rarely and in small amounts.[12,13] This implies that some form of iron supplement is needed by most infants between 6 months and 2 years of age. After the age of 2 years, the prevalence of anemia tends to fall because iron requirements are lower and children start to consume a more varied diet. However, the high prevalence in many countries persists due to iron depletion in early years followed by an inadequate diet, often compounded by parasitic infections.

The usual age of onset of anemia is controversial. In a recent comparative study of infants exclusively breastfed to 6 months in Honduras and Sweden, the ferritin concentrations of the Honduran infants were about half those of the Swedish infants at 4 months of age, presumably reflecting less iron stores *in utero*.[14] Iron supplements after 4 months improved Hb and ferritin similarly in both groups, suggesting that the response to iron at 4 to 6 months is not indicative of iron deficiency. From 6 to 9 months, iron supplements improved Hb and ferritin in Honduran infants but only improved ferritin in Sweden. This study indicated that the Hb cut-off for anemia during infancy may be set too high and that the global prevalence of anemia in infants has been overestimated. There is a need for updated guidelines on assessment of iron status and iron supplementation of infants.

Low birthweight, which is especially common in some developing regions such as south central Asia, is clearly a risk factor for anemia early in infancy. Infants with low birth weight are born with reduced iron stores which are depleted by 2 to 3 months of age. The international recommendation for low birthweight infants is to provide them with supplemental iron in the form of drops starting at 3 months of age.[2] Premature clamping of the umbilical cord deprives infants of up to one third of their potential blood volume. The delay of clamping until one minute after the cord ceases to pulsate, and holding the infant at or below the level of the placenta can significantly improve the amount of blood and therefore the amount of iron delivered to the newborn infant.[15]

2.3.1.1.4   Adolescence

The prevalence of iron deficiency and subsequent anemia increases at the start of adolescence.[16] In girls, this is caused by increased requirements for growth, exacerbated a few years later by the onset of menstruation. In boys, the incremental amount of iron deposited in muscle mass is larger than that in girls. This explains why the prevalence of iron depletion is similar for both genders in many regions.

2.3.1.2   Low Intake and/or Bioavailability of Dietary Iron

The best sources of iron are meat, fish, and poultry because they are relatively high in iron, and the heme iron they contain has a high bioavailability so that about 20% is absorbed. In industrialized countries, daily iron intakes range from 8 to 18 mg for adults and vary little across socioeconomic status groups. In nonindustrialized countries, intakes are often higher, especially where legumes are consumed, and range from 15 to 30 mg. Estimates of daily intake include Bangladesh, 23 mg, the Philippines, 11 mg, and Latin America (maize eating areas), 16 mg. However, the average bioavailability of the nonheme iron in most plant sources, including cereals and legumes, is only about 2 to 5%.[17] Phytates, found in high amounts in undegermed maize, whole wheat, brown rice, and legumes, are strong inhibitors of iron absorption, as are polyphenols in legumes, tea, nuts, and coffee, and oxalate in spinach and other leafy greens. Fermentation, soaking, and germination can improve iron absorption from cereals and legumes and have been recommended as approaches to improve the iron availability in complementary foods. Leavening of bread by yeast releases some of the iron bound to phytate and the consumption of unleavened bread, in the Middle East for example, is a risk factor for iron deficiency.

Because the inclusion of ascorbic acid in a meal improves nonheme iron absorption by increasing iron solubility, a low ascorbic acid intake can add to the risk of anemia.[18] However, the influence of ascorbic acid in most diets is less than the influence of the type and amount of iron present. In a supervised community intervention trial in rural Mexico, the consumption of 25 mg of ascorbic acid, as limeade, with meals twice a day for 8 months failed to improve the iron status of iron deficient women.[19] Calcium can also impair iron absorption and the calcium salts used to prepare maize tortillas in some Latin American countries may contribute to iron deficiency.

The iron status of the individual is another major influence on the amount of iron absorbed; percent absorption is inversely related to iron status across a wide range of serum ferritin concentrations. To take into consideration the influence of both diet and iron status on iron absorption, FAO/WHO defined two levels of iron status that could be achieved (no anemia without iron stores, and no anemia with iron stores) and three different types of diets.[20] For diets based on cereals, roots, and tubers and containing almost no fish, poultry, meat, or ascorbic acid, dietary iron bioavailability is assumed to be only 5% for nonanemic individuals. Intermediate diets, with a bioavailability of about 10%, consist mainly of cereals, roots, or tubers and contain negligible amounts of animal products and ascorbic acid. High bioavailability diets (15%) contain generous amounts of meat, poultry, and fish and/or other foods high in ascorbic acid; these are the predominant diets in industrialized countries. These estimates of 5 to 15% iron absorption from the different types of diets are about 50% higher for individuals with iron deficiency anemia. To meet their iron requirements from a diet with intermediate iron bioavailability, men would have to absorb about 4%, preschool children 5 to 6%, and women 8%.[11]

2.3.1.3 Infections and Parasites

Infections and parasites contribute to anemia by increasing nutrient losses especially iron. Since they affect men and women equally, a high prevalence of anemia in men often indicates the extent to which anemia in the population is due to these conditions.[21]

2.3.1.3.1 Malaria

Plasmodium falciparum malaria is the primary cause of severe anemia in malarious areas of tropical Africa, where malaria, anemia, or both constitute the largest outpatient and admission health problems for many health centers. Malaria contributes to about 60% of all cases of severe anemia in infants in Tanzania, while iron deficiency accounts for about 30%.[22] The anemia, which occurs during and after acute infection, is caused by acute and chronic hemolysis, subsequent suppression of erythropoiesis, and possibly secondary folate deficiency.

Coexisting iron deficiency and malaria will exacerbate the anemia,[22] but do not affect the Hb response to antimalarial drugs. It is essential to detect and treat malaria if severe iron deficiency is to be reduced in regions of endemic *P. falciparum*. Integrated strategies to control iron deficiency and malaria are essential where these conditions co-exist.[2] Iron supplementation does not increase the risk or severity of malaria.[23] Malaria prophylaxis during pregnancy can improve Hb and birthweight.[23]

2.3.1.3.2 HIV Infection

HIV infection is strongly associated with anemia, particularly in Africa, and having one condition increases the risk of developing the other. Up to 70% of individuals who have AIDS are anemic. The anemia may be caused by chronic disease; nutrient deficiencies; anti-red cell antibodies; an imbalance of growth factors resulting from HIV actions on macrophages, fibroblasts, and T-cells; uncontrolled parvovirus B_{19} infection; and overdosage with medications.[24] Those who receive blood transfusions to treat anemia risk infection with HIV from donors' blood. In the past decade, this risk has been greatly reduced through the screening strategies adopted by hospitals.

2.3.1.3.3 Helminth Infections

Hookworms (*Necator americanus* and *Ancyclostoma duodenale*) infect approximately 1 billion individuals and cause blood loss from the intestinal mucosa.[25] The amount of blood and iron lost is proportional to the number of worms.[2] Blood loss from hookworm infestation is a significant contributor to moderate and severe anemia in affected populations.[26,27] A moderate hookworm load can double iron losses and induce a fecal iron loss of 3.4 mg per day.[28] Older children and adults tend to be infected more than infants and young children.[25]

Schistosomiasis, especially *S. haemotobium*, causes urinary iron loss through damage to the urinary tract. This schistosome is limited to Africa and the Middle East. Mean iron losses in heavily infected children can be 0.7 mg per day, and a strong association between iron status and urinary schistosomiasis has been reported in sub-Saharan Africa.[29] Trichuriasis and ascaris infection can affect iron status adversely by provoking gastric and intestinal ulceration and blood loss, although blood loss is less severe than in schistosomiasis or hookworm infection.

Clearly, in areas where these parasites are highly prevalent, attempts to control the infestations are critical for anemia prevention (see Chapter 11 for details). The infections will limit the effectiveness of other interventions including iron fortification and supplementation. Detailed recommendations have been published for helminthic control as a complement to iron supplementation.[2]

2.3.2 ANEMIA RESULTING FROM OTHER MICRONUTRIENT DEFICIENCIES

Iron deficiency is very often associated with deficiencies of other micronutrients, which are less often evaluated. Diets that are low in animal products are low in absorbable iron as well as retinol, riboflavin, folic acid, vitamin B_{12}, and other micronutrients. In very poor regions, fruit and vegetable intake may also be inadequate and subsequently low amounts of folic acid and ascorbic acid will be consumed. Intestinal parasites can cause the simultaneous malabsorption of iron, retinol, folic acid, and vitamin B_{12}, as can blood losses due to hookworm infestation.

2.3.2.1 Vitamin A Deficiency

According to WHO, approximately 2.8 million or about 0.1% of children under 5 years of age have clinical signs of xerophthalmia.[1] Approximately 1 million are in Africa and 1 million are in Southeast Asia. Subclinical vitamin A deficiency affects about 256 million, or 40%, of children under 5 years.[1] Night blindness prevalence in pregnant and lactating women is as high as 20% in some countries in Southeast Asia. The main causes of deficiency are low dietary intake, especially of preformed vitamin A in animal products and β-carotene in fruits, and parasites including *Ascaris lumbricoides*, and *Shigella* dysentery. Children under 5 years of age and lactating women have the highest requirements for the vitamin and most often suffer from deficiency symptoms. Although vitamin A requirements are not substantially increased by pregnancy, there is an increase in clinical symptoms such as night blindness in pregnant women with low vitamin A stores.

Vitamin A deficiency causes anemia. Vitamin A depletion in adult male volunteers in the U.S. caused a marked fall in Hb, from about 160 to <110 g per liter in a year.[30] This was reversible with iron plus vitamin A supplements, but not with iron alone. While the exact mechanisms remain to be determined, they include impaired mobilization of iron stores, possibly due to an effect of vitamin A deficiency on transferrin receptors. Supplementation of vitamin A deficient individuals with vitamin A alone increases Hb concentrations by about 10 g per liter.[31] In several studies, the addition of vitamin A improved the Hb response to iron supplements.[32,33] Weekly supplementation with 23,000 IU of vitamin A as retinol or β-carotene reduced the prevalence of anemia by 45% among women free of hookworm infection.[34] The extent to which vitamin A deficiency contributes to the global prevalence of pregnancy anemia remains to be determined, but could be substantial.

2.3.2.2 Riboflavin Deficiency

Riboflavin deficiency tends to both co-exist and interact with iron deficiency. The intake of riboflavin and absorbable iron is usually low when animal product consumption, including milk, is limited. The global prevalence of riboflavin deficiency is unknown, but is probably quite high where animal product intake is low. Reported prevalences of deficiency include: 77% of lactating women[35] and over 50% of elderly[36] in Guatemala; over 90% of adults in China[37]; and almost all pregnant and lactating women in The Gambia.[38] Pregnant and lactating women are thought to be at highest risk of riboflavin deficiency because of their high requirements.

Riboflavin deficiency may exacerbate iron deficiency by increasing intestinal iron loss, reducing iron absorption, impairing mobilization of intracellular iron, and increasing crypt cell proliferation.[39-41] Deficiency may impair the synthesis of globin, and reduce the activity of NADH-FMN oxidoreductase so that iron becomes trapped in ferritin. Supplementation of riboflavin deficient individuals with the vitamin caused an increase in Hb concentrations and an improved hematological response to iron supplements in iron deficient Gambian men and lactating women.[42,43] Similarly, supplements containing both iron and riboflavin increased the serum ferritin concentrations of anemic lactating Guatemalan women more than iron supplements alone.[35] Hemoglobin concentrations were not improved significantly although this could have been due to the relatively short duration of the intervention (60 days). A study in Europe reported improvements in Hb levels when riboflavin was added to iron supplements for anemic pregnant women,[44] as did a study of Thai children.[45]

2.3.2.3   Folic Acid Deficiency

Folic acid deficiency can produce a megaloblastic, macrocytic anemia because this nutrient is required for the synthesis of erythrocytes. Changes in red blood cell morphology and the number of cells occur later than the drop in serum and red blood cell folate concentrations. New data are needed on the global prevalence of folate deficiency. In the U.S., prior to folic acid supplementation of flour, about 15% of women had suboptimal folate status assessed by low serum and erythrocyte folate concentrations.[46] The prevalence has been reported to be higher in Africa and Asia[47,48] but few data are available. No abnormal values for folic acid in serum and/or red blood cells were observed in studies in Thailand,[49] Guatemala,[50] or Mexico.[51] The folate content of foods such as legumes, leafy greens, and fruits is considerable and in some poor regions these may be consumed in larger amounts than in industrialized countries. Clearly the prevalence of folic acid deficiency is uncertain.

For many years, folic acid has been included in the iron supplements usually supplied to pregnant women in developing countries, on the assumption that many have folic acid deficiency that contributes to anemia. A recent meta-analysis was conducted on 22 studies in which nonanemic pregnant women had been supplemented with folate for at least 16 weeks, with and without iron.[52] Folic acid treatment was associated with a 40% reduction in risk of anemia in late pregnancy and a 35% reduction in risk of megaloblastosis. However, the current global impact of folic acid on anemia is less clear. Almost half of the studies in the meta-analysis took place in the U.K. over 30 years ago and only four were done in the last 20 years. The most significant effects were seen in Africa, where folic acid deficiency and megaloblastosis may have been caused by malaria. A WHO collaborative study in Burma and Thailand found no incremental benefit of folate on the Hb concentrations of pregnant women or nonpregnant women,[53] but these countries are not known to have a high prevalence of deficiency. Small, nonsignificant increases in Hb — usually compared to iron alone — have been reported in pregnant women in Australia,[54] Burma,[55] India,[56-57] Liberia,[58] Nigeria,[59] and Thailand.[60] In south Benin, folate deficiency was associated with (but was not necessarily the cause of) anemia in 20% of adults.[64] A significant increase in Hb was found only in South Africa.[62] Increasingly, the main rationale for including folate in iron supplements for anemic women is reduction of risk of neural tube defects.

Malabsorption of folate has been observed secondary to infection with *Giardia lamblia*, and bacterial overgrowth. For example, in 10 to 20% Swedish children with chronic giardiasis, the fractional absorption of both folate and vitamin B_{12} was subnormal.[63] Folate requirements are increased as a result of the hemolysis that occurs with malaria. In pregnant women in northern Nigeria, chemoprophylaxis slowed the rate of fall in serum folate[64] and prevented severe anemia and megaloblastosis even without the use of folate supplements.[65] Low birthweight and premature infants develop folic acid deficiency and megaloblastic anemia in the first 2 months of life.[66] In a British study, adding folate to iron supplements improved Hb of low birthweight infants at 6 to 9 months compared to iron alone.[67]

2.3.2.4 Vitamin B_{12} Deficiency

There are few data on the global prevalence of vitamin B_{12} deficiency, which can result in megaloblastic anemia. Even less is known about its global contribution to anemia. Because this vitamin is found only in animal products, and it is actively reabsorbed from bile, deficiency has been traditionally associated with long term consumption of strict vegetarian diets. Pernicious anemia, an autoimmune disorder involving a defect in the synthesis of gastric intrinsic factor needed for vitamin B_{12} absorption, only explains about 2% of the prevalence of deficiency in U.S. adults. In an international survey of anemia conducted between 1973 and 1982, the prevalence of serum vitamin B_{12} concentrations indicating deficiency was low in the 21 countries that made this assessment.[68] One exception was rural India, where animal product intake is especially low. However, the methods used may have overestimated serum concentrations of the vitamin by 40 to 50%.[69] More recent studies in rural Mexico, for example, indicate that between one fifth and one third of individuals ranging from preschoolers to adult men and women have some degree of vitamin B_{12} deficiency.[51,70] Almost half of lactating women in peri-urban Guatemala City had marginal or deficient plasma vitamin B_{12} concentrations; their infants were at risk of deficiency of the vitamin as early as 3 months of age; and there were low concentrations of the vitamin in breast milk.[71] We have also observed that about one third of Kenyan schoolers have vitamin B_{12} deficiency (unpublished data). The elderly have an especially high prevalence of this vitamin deficiency. For example, we have reported that about 7% of elderly (age >65 years) Hispanics in northern California have deficient (<200 µg per liter) concentrations of the vitamin in plasma and an additional 16% have marginal concentrations (200 to 220 µg per liter).[72] Other studies in the U.S.[73] and Europe[74] show similarly high prevalences of deficiency in the elderly. The cause is probably gastric atrophy, in which reduced secretion of gastric acid causes malabsorption of food bound vitamin B_{12}.[75] Crystalline vitamin

B_{12} in supplements or in fortified foods can still be absorbed by individuals with gastric atrophy. In developing countries, the prevalence of vitamin B_{12} deficiency at all ages, would be expected to be substantially higher than in developed countries. Intakes and stores of the vitamin will be lower because smaller quantities of animal products are consumed. Few if any sources of crystalline vitamin B_{12} exist in developing countries and gastric atrophy (which is possibly caused by infection with *Helicobacter pylori*) is expected to be even more common. Infection with *Giardia lamblia*,[76] bacterial overgrowth subsequent to *Giardia* infection,[77] and the fish tapeworm, *Diphyllobothrium latum*,[78] can also cause malabsorption of the vitamin. The risk of vitamin B_{12} deficiency is likely to be highest when impaired absorption and low intakes co–exist.

Even though vitamin B_{12} deficiency may emerge as a relatively common problem on a global scale, its contribution to anemia is uncertain. Anemia does not usually appear until an individual has a relatively severe state of depletion of the vitamin. Infants born to and breastfed by strict vegetarian mothers develop anemia and hematological abnormalities that are reversible by vitamin B_{12}. A few studies of pregnant women tested the benefit of adding vitamin B_{12} to folate and iron supplements. The additional B_{12} failed to improve Hb further in two Indian studies,[56,57] one of which was of very short duration. Premature, low birthweight infants treated with iron, vitamin E, and folic acid showed an improvement in Hb concentrations when they were also given parenteral vitamin B_{12}.[66] Additional studies are needed to examine the prevalence, causes, and consequences of vitamin B_{12} deficiency — including anemia — in other regions of the world.

2.4 CONCLUSIONS

In a recent meta-analysis of the effects of iron supplementation on anemia in developing countries, the authors conclude that "there is a suggestion in the data, not well documented except in a couple of studies, that something other than iron may be operating to limit hemoglobin response and anemia control."[79] While the majority of anemia in the world is caused by iron deficiency, it is important to consider, prevent, and treat other micronutrient deficiencies that could limit Hb response to iron supplementation.

REFERENCES

1. Malnutrition, The Global Picture, World Health Organization, Geneva, 2000.
2. Guidelines for the Use of Iron Supplements to Prevent and Treat Iron Deficiency Anemia, International Nutritional Anemia Advisory Group, Washington, D.C., 1988.
3. Fourth Report on the World Nutrition Situation, ACC/SCN/IFPRI, Geneva, 2000.
4. Kurz, K. M. and Johnson-Welch, C., The Nutrition and Lives of Adolescents in Developing Countries: Findings from the Nutrition of Adolescent Girls Research Program, International Center for Research on Women, Washington, D.C., 1994.
5. Evaluation of the National Nutritional Anaemia Prophylaxis Programme, Indian Council of Medical Research, New Delhi, India, 1989.

6. United Nations Administrative Committee on Coordination/Sub-Committee on Nutrition, Statement on iron deficiency control, June, 1990, Dublin, in *Controlling Iron Deficiency,* Gillespie, S. R., Mason, J. R., and Kevany, J., Eds., World Health Organization, Geneva, State-of-the-Art Series, 1991.

7. Indicators for Assessing Iron Deficiency and Strategies for its Prevention, World Health Organization, Geneva, 1996.

8. Gillespie, S., *Major Issues in the Control of Iron Deficiency,* The Micronutrient Initiative, Ottawa, 1998.

9. Allen, L. H., Anemia and iron deficiency: effects on pregnancy outcome, *Am. J. Clinical Nutr.,* 71(55), 1280S, 2000.

10. Gillebaud, J., Bonnar, J., Morehead, J., and Matthews, A., Menstrual blood loss and iron deficiency, *Lancet,* 1, 387, 1976.

11. Institute of Medicine, *Nutrition during Pregnancy,* National Academy Press, Washington, D.C., 1990.

12. National Strategies for Overcoming Micronutrient Malnutrition, World Health Organization, Geneva, Doc. EB89/27, 1991.

13. Brown, K. H., Dewey, K. G., and Allen, L. H., *Complementary Feeding of Young Children in Developing Countries: A Review of Current Scientific Knowledge,* World Health Organization, Geneva, 1998.

14. Domellöf, M., Cohen, R. J., Dewey, K. G., Hernell, O., Landa Rivera, L., and Lonnerdal, B., Hematologic responses to iron supplementation in Swedish and Honduran breast fed infants, *FASEB J.* 14(4):A561, abs. 406.4, 2000.

15. Grajeda, R., Perez-Escamilla, R., and Dewey, K. G., Delayed clamping of the umbilical cord improves hematological status of Guatemalan infants at 2 months of age, *Am. J. Clinical Nutr.,* 65, 425, 1997.

16. Dallman, P. R., Changing iron needs from birth through adolescence, in *Nutr. Anemias,* Fomon, S. J., and Zlotkin, S., Eds., Nestlé Nutrition Workshop Series, Vevey-Raven Press, New York, 30, 1992, 29.

17. Allen, L. H. and Ahluwalia, N., *Improving Iron Status through Diet,* John Snow, Inc., Washington, D.C., 1997.

18. Layrisse, M., Martinez-Torres, C., Mendez-Castillo, H., et al., Relationship between iron bioavailability from diets and the prevalence of iron deficiency, *Food Nutr. Bull.,* 12, 301, 1990.

19. Garcia, O. P., Dias, M., Rosado, J. L., and Allen, L. H., Ascorbic acid from lime juice does not improve iron status of iron deficient women in rural Mexico, *FASEB J.,* 13(4):A207, abs. 190.4, 1999.

20. Requirements of vitamin A, iron, folate and vitamin B_{12}, Food and Agriculture Organization/World Health Organization, Rome, 1988.

21. Yip, R., Iron deficiency: contemporary scientific issue and international programmatic approaches, *J. Nutr.,* 124, 1479S, 1994.

22. Menendez, C., Kahigwa, E., Hirt, R., et al., Randomised placebo controlled trial of iron supplementation and malaria chemoprophylaxis for prevention of severe anemia and malaria in Tanzanian infants, *Lancet,* 350, 844, 1997.

23. Menendez, C., Todd, J., Alonso, P. L., Francis, N., Lulat, S., Ceesay, S., M'Boge, B., and Greenwood, B. M., The effects of iron supplementation during pregnancy, given by traditional birth attendants, on the prevalence of anaemia and malaria, *Trans. Royal Soc. Trop. Med. Hyg.,* 88, 590, 1994.

24. Bain, B. J., The hematological features of HIV infection, *Br. J. Haema.,* 99, 1, 1997.

25. Stephenson, L. S., *Impact of Helminth Infections on Human Nutrition,* Taylor and Francis, New York, 1987.

26. Gillespie, S. and Johnston, J. L., *Expert Consultation on Anemia Determinants and Interventions,* The Micronutrient Initiative, Ottawa, 1998.

27. Srinivasan, V., Radhakrishna, S., Ramanathan, A. M., and Jabbar, S., Hookworm infection in a rural community in South India and its association with haemoglobin levels, *Trans. Roy Soc. Trop. Med. Hyg.,* 81, 973, 1987.

28. Stoltzfus, R. J., Albonico, M., Chwaya, H. M., Schulze, K., Tielsch, J., and Savioli, L., Effects of the Zanzibar school based deworming program on iron status of children, *Am. J. Clinical Nutr.,* 68, 179, 1998.

29. Stephenson, L. S., Latham, M. C., Kurz, K. M., Kinoti, S. N., Oduori, M. L., and Crompton, D. W., Relationships of *Schistosoma haematobium,* hookworm and malarial infections and metrifonate treatment to hemoglobin level in Kenyan school children, *Am. J. Trop. Med. Hyg.,* 34, 519, 1985.

30. Hodges, R. E., Sauberlich, H. E., Canham, J. E., Wallace, D. L., Rucker, R. B., Mejia, L. A., and Mohanram, M., Hematopoietic studies in vitamin A deficiency, *Am. J. Clinical Nutr.,* 31, 876, 1978.

31. Sommer, A. and West, K. P., *Vitamin A Deficiency: Health, Survival and Vision,* Oxford University Press, New York, 1996.

32. Mejia, L. and Chew, F., Hematological effect of supplementing anemic children with vitamin A alone and in combination with iron, *Am. J. Clinical Nutr.,* 48, 595, 1988.

33. Suharno, D., West, C. E., Karyodi, D., and Hautvast, J. G. A. J., Not only supplementation with iron but also with vitamin A is necessary to combat nutritional anaemia in pregnant women in West Java, Indonesia, *Lancet* 342, 2315, 1993.

34. Stoltzfus. R. J., Dreyfuss, M., Shrestha, J. B., Khatry, S. K., Schultz, K., and West, K. P. Jr., Effect of maternal vitamin A or beta-carotene supplementation on iron-deficiency anemia in Nepalese pregnant women, post partum mothers, and infants, Abstracts XVIII, IVACG Meeting, Cairo, 1997.

35. Allen, L. H. and Ruel, M., Supplementation of anemic lactating Guatemalan women with riboflavin improves erythrocyte riboflavin concentrations and ferritin response to iron treatment, *FASEB J.,* 11(3):A654, abs. 3772, 1997.

36. Boisvert, W.A., Castenada, C., Mendoza, I., Langeloh, G., Solomons, N. W., Gershoff, S. N., and Russell, R.M., Prevalence of riboflavin deficiency among Guatemalan people and its relationship to milk intake, *Am. J. Clinical Nutr.,* 58, 85, 1993.

37. Campbell, T. C., Brun, T., Junshi, C., Zulin, F., and Parpia, B., Questioning riboflavin recommendations on the basis of a survey in China, *Am. J. Clinical Nutr.,* 51, 436, 1990.

38. Bates, C. J., Prentice, A. M., Paul, A. A., Sutcliffe, B. A., Watkinson, M., and Whitehead, R. G., Riboflavin status in Gambian pregnant and lactating women and its implications for RDAs, *Am. J. Clinical Nutr.,* 34, 928, 1981.

39. Bates, C. J., Human riboflavin requirements and metabolic consequences of deficiency in man and animals, *World Rev. Nutr. Diet,* 50, 215, 1987.

40. Powers, H. J., Weaver, L. T., Austin, S., Wright, A. J. A., and Fairweather-Tait, S. J., Riboflavin deficiency in the rat: effects on iron utilization and loss, *Br. J. Nutr.,* 65, 487, 1991.

41. Fairweather-Tait, S. J., Powers, H. J., Minski, M. J., Whitehead, J., and Bownes, R., Riboflavin deficiency and iron absorption in adult Gambian men, *Annu. Nutr. Metab.,* 36, 34, 1992.

42. Powers, H. J., Bates, C. J., Prentice, A. M., Lamb, W. H., Jepson, M., and Bowman, H., The relative effectiveness of iron and iron with riboflavin in correcting a microcytic anemia in men and children in rural Gambia, *Hum. Nutr. Clinical Nutr.,* 37C, 413, 1983.

43. Powers, H. J., Bates, C. J., and Lamb, W. H., Hematological response to supplements of iron and riboflavin by pregnant and lactating women in rural Gambia, *Hum. Nutr. Clinical Nutr.*, 39C, 117, 1984.

44. Decker, K., Dotis, B., Glatzle, D, and Hinselmann, M., Riboflavin status and anaemia in pregnant women, *Nutr. Metab.*, 21, 17, 1977.

45. Buzina, R., Jusic, M., Milanovic, N., Sapunar, J., and Brubacher, G. The effects of riboflavin administration on iron metabolism parameters in a school going population, *Int. J. Vitam. Nutr. Res.*, 49, 136, 1979.

46. Senti, F. R. and Pilch, S. M., Analysis of folate data from the 2nd Health and Nutrition Examination Survey, *J. Nutr.*, 115, 1398, 1985.

47. Fleming, A. F., Tropical obstetrics and gynaecology. I: Anaemia in pregnancy in Tropical Africa, *Trans. Royal. Soc. Trop. Med. Hyg.*, 83, 441, 1989.

48. Baker, S. J., Nutritional anemias. Part 2: Tropical Asia., *Clinical Haemat.*, 10, 843, 1981.

49. Areekul, S., Folic acid deficiency in Thailand, *J. Med. Assoc. Thailand*, 65, 1, 1982.

50. Franzetti, S., Mejia, L. A., Viteri, F. E., and Alvarez, E., Body iron reserves of rural and urban Guatemalan women of reproductive age, *Arch. Latinoamer. Nutr.*, 34, 69, 1984.

51. Allen, L. H., Rosado, J. L., Casterline, J. E., Martinez, H., Lopez, P., Muñoz, E., and Black, A. K., Vitamin B_{12} deficiency and malabsorption are highly prevalent in rural Mexican communities, *Am. J. Clinical Nutr.*, 62, 1013, 1995.

52. Mahomed, K., Folate supplementation in pregnancy, *Cochrane Database of Systematic Reviews*, 1997.

53. Charoenlarp, P. et al., A WHO collaborative study on iron supplementation in Burma and in Thailand, *Am. J. Clinical Nutr.*, 47, 280, 1988.

54. Fleming, A. F., Martin, J. D., Hahnel, R., and Westlake, A. J., Effects of iron and folic acid antenatal supplements on maternal haematology and fetal wellbeing, *Med. J. Aust.*, 2, 429, 1974.

55. Batu, A. T., Toe, T., Pe, H., and Nyunt, K. K., A prophylactic trial of iron and folic acid supplements in pregnant Burmese women, *Isr. J. Med. Sci.*, 12, 1410, 1976.

56. Sood, S. K., Ramachandran, K., Mathur, M., et al., WHO sponsored collaborative studies on nutritional anaemia in India: 1. The effects of supplemental oral iron administration to pregnant women, *Q. Med. J.*, 44, 241, 1975.

57. Iyengar, L. and Apte, S. V., Prophylaxis of anemia of pregnancy, *Am. J. Clinical Nutr.*, 23, 725, 1970.

58. Jackson, R. T. and Latham, M. C., Anemia of pregnancy in Liberia, West Africa: a therapeutic trial, *Am. J. Clinical Nutr.*, 35, 710, 1982.

59. Osifo, B., The effect of folic acid and iron in the prevention of nutritional anaemias in pregnancy in Nigeria, *Br. J. Nutr.*, 24, 689, 1970.

60. Sirisupandit, S. et al., A prophylactic supplementation of iron and folate in pregnancy, *Southeast Asian J. Trop. Med. Public Health*, 14, 317, 1983.

61. Hoffbrand, A. V., Folate deficiency in premature infants, *Arch. Diseases Child.*, 45, 441, 1970.

62. Hercberg, S. et al., Relationship between anaemia, iron and folacin deficiency, haemoglobinopathies and parasitic infection, *Hum. Nutr. Clinical Nutr.*, 40, 371, 1986.

63. Hjelt, K., Pærregaard, A., and Krasilnikoff, P. A., Giardiasis: haematological status and the absorption of vitamin B_{12} and folic acid, *Acta Paediatr.*, 81, 29, 1992.

64. Fleming, A. F., Hendrickse, J. P. de V., and Allan, N. C., The prevention of megaloblastic anemia in pregnancy in Nigeria, *J. Obstet. Gynaecol. Br. Commonw.*, 75, 425, 1968.

65. Fleming, A. F., Ghatoura, G. B. S., Harrison, K. A., Briggs, N. D., and Dunn, D. T., The prevention of anaemia in pregnancy in primigravidae in the guinea savanna of Nigeria, *Ann. Trop. Med. Parasitol.,* 80, 211, 1986.

66. Worthington-White, D. A., Behnke, M., and Gross, S., Premature infants require additional folate and vitamin B_{12} to reduce the severity of the anemia of prematurity, *Am. J. Clinical Nutr.,* 60, 930, 1994.

67. Stevens, D., Burman, D., Strelling, M. K., and Morris, A., Folic acid supplementation in low birthweight infants, *Pediatrics,* 64, 333, 1979.

68. DeMaeyer, E. and Adiels-Tegman, M., The prevalence of anaemia in the world, *World Health Stat. Q.,* 38:302, 1985.

69. Kanazawa, S. and Herbert, V., Noncobalamin vitamin B_{12} analogues in human red cells, liver, and brain, *Am. J. Clinical Nutr.,* 37, 774, 1983.

70. Casterline, J. E., Allen, L. H., and Ruel, M. T., Vitamin B_{12} deficiency is very prevalent in lactating Guatemalan women and their infants at three months postpartum, *J. Nutr.,* 127, 1966, 1997.

71. Miller, J. W., Green, R., Allen, L. H., Mungas, D., M., and Haan, M. N., Homocysteine correlates with cognitive function in the Sacramento Area Latino Study on Aging, *FASEB J.,* 13, A374, 1999.

72. Pennypacker, L., Allen, R. H., Kelly, J. P., Matthews, L. M., Grigsby, J., Kaye, K., Lindenbaum, J., and Stabler, S. P., High prevalence of cobalamin deficiency in elderly outpatients, *J. Am. Geriatr. Soc.,* 39, 1155, 1991.

73. Joosten, E., van den Berg, A., Riezler, R., Naurath, H. J., Lindenbaum, J., Stabler, S. P., and Allen, R.H., Metabolic evidence that deficiencies of vitamin B_{12} (cobalamin), folate, and vitamin B_6 occur commonly in elderly people, *Am. J. Clinical Nutr.,* 58, 468, 1993.

74. Carmel, R., Sinow, R. M., Siegel, M. E., and Samloff, I. M., Food cobalamin malabsorption occurs frequently in patients with unexplained low serum cobalamin levels, *Arch. Int. Med.,* 148, 1715, 1988.

75. Cowen, A. E. and Campbell, C. B., Giardiasis — a cause of vitamin B_{12} malabsorption, *Dig. Dis.,* 18, 384, 1973.

76. Tandon, B. N., Tandon, R. K., Satpathy, B. K., and Shriniwas, Mechanism of malabsorption in giardiasis: a study of bacterial flora and bile salt deconjugation in upper jejunum, *Gut,* 18, 176, 1977.

77. Van Henshroek, M. B., Morris-Jones, S., Meisner, S., Jaffar, S., Bayo, L., Dackour, R., Phillips, C., and Greenwood, M. P., Iron, but not folic acid, combined with effective antimalarial therapy promotes haematological recovery in African children after acute falciparum malaria, *Trans. Roy. Soc. Trop. Med. Hyg.,* 89, 672, 1995.

78. Nyberg, W., The influence of *Diphyllobothrium latum* on the vitamin B_{12} intrinsic factor complex. I. *In vivo* studies with Schilling test technique, *Acta Med. Scand.,* 167, 185, 1960.

79. Beaton, G. H. and McCabe, G. P., *Efficacy of Intermittent Iron Supplementation in the Control of Iron Deficiency Anemia in Developing Countries: An Analysis of Experience,* The Micronutrient Initiative, Ottawa, 1999.

3 Assessment of Nutritional Anemias

Sean Lynch and Ralph Green

CONTENTS

0-8493-8569-5/01/$0.00+$.50
© 2001 by CRC Press LLC

3.1 INTRODUCTION

The World Health Organization estimates that more than one third of the world's population is anemic. Nutritional deficiencies are the primary cause. Over 500 million suffer from iron deficiency anemia.[1] An inadequate intake or impaired absorption of vitamin A, folic acid, or vitamin B_{12} accounts for a smaller but significant number of cases. The detection, prevention, and treatment of nutritional anemia is complicated by the high prevalence of infectious diseases that cause anemia in many tropical countries. The most important are malaria and hookworm.

Programs designed to control anemia can have numerous public health benefits including reduced mortality among pregnant women and their infant children, improved developmental and cognitive performance in childhood, and increased productivity in adults. Successful intervention, however, depends on accurate identification of the causative factors. It is therefore important to establish accurate and reliable criteria for both identifying the specific nutritional causes of anemia and evaluating the impact of intervention strategies.

3.2 IRON DEFICIENCY

Iron is essential for metabolic processes that are concerned with oxygen transport, oxidative metabolism, and cellular growth.[2,3] Most functional iron is present in the form of heme in hemoglobin, myoglobin, cytochromes, catalase, and peroxidase. Nonheme iron compounds include the metalloflavoproteins, the iron sulfur proteins, and ribonucleotide reductase. Anemia is the most easily identifiable manifestation of functional iron deficiency although it is important to note that the suboptimal iron supply affects all tissues. Functional consequences are the result of inadequate oxygen delivery because of the reduced circulating hemoglobin level and diminished functional activity of iron containing tissue enzymes.[2,3] The most important are impaired mental development and physical coordination in infants, poor school achievement in later childhood, and a limited ability to perform tasks requiring physical activity at all ages. The neurological and cognitive abnormalities are thought to result from the effect of iron deficiency on brain neurotransmitters. The precise biochemical basis is poorly understood. The limitation in the ability to perform prolonged physical activity is due primarily to compromised oxidative metabolism in skeletal muscles. There are many other consequences of iron deficiency including impaired immunity, abnormalities of the mucosa of the mouth and esophagus, koilonychia (spoon nail), impaired temperature regulation, and perversions of taste leading to the consumption of nonfood items (pica) or a craving for ice (pagophagia).

TABLE 3.1
Indicators of Iron Deficiency[a]

Indicator	Normal	Storage Iron Depletion	Early Functional Iron Deficiency	Iron Deficiency Anemia
Serum ferritin (µg/l)	130 (M) 35 (F)	<12	<12	<12
TIBC (µg/dl)	330	360	390	410
Transferrin saturation (%)	35	30	<15	<15
EP (µg/dl rbc)	30	30	100	200
STfR (mg/l)	5.5	5.5	10	14
Erythrocytes (hemoglobin, hematocrit, rbc indices)	Normal	Normal	Normal	Microcytic, hypochromic anemia[b]

[a] Data from Bothwell et al.,[2] Brittenham,[3] Looker et al.[6]

[b] Critical levels for the diagnosis of anemia (hemoglobin concentration, g/dl): 6 months to 5 yrs, 11.0; 5 to 11 yrs, 11.5; 12 to 13 yrs, 12.0; menstruating women, 12.0; pregnancy, 11.0; men, 13.0.[85] Critical hemoglobin values are for individuals living at sea level. Values should be corrected for the effect of altitude at elevations over 1000 meters above sea level.[86,87]

Healthy iron replete individuals maintain a body iron store that is available for any increase in the requirement of the functional compartment. An individual with an iron store of 1000 mg can use 40 mg per day from the store to meet increased needs. If iron stores are inadequate and the replacement of functional iron depends on increased dietary absorption, the functional compartment can only be replenished at a rate of 2 to 4 mg per day unless therapeutic or supplementary iron is provided.[4]

When impaired iron balance leads to the gradual development of iron deficiency anemia, a sequence of well defined changes occurs in iron storage, iron transport, and eventually the metabolic functions that are dependent on iron. The earliest evidence of iron deficiency is the absence of iron stores (stage of storage iron depletion). There are no functional consequences, but there are no iron reserves to meet future physiological or pathological requirements. At the next stage, laboratory testing reveals evidence of a suboptimal rate of iron delivery to the bone marrow and other tissues although there is no detectable anemia (early functional iron deficiency — traditionally called iron deficient erythropoiesis). The third and final stage is characterized by a decrease in functional iron with the onset of anemia and its associated clinical symptoms (iron deficiency anemia). A series of laboratory investigations can be used to characterize these three stages of iron deficiency (Table 3.1).

3.2.1 STORAGE IRON DEPLETION

Storage iron depletion is characterized by the absence of iron stores. This is evident in bone marrow biopsy material stained for iron. However, less invasive techniques are available to evaluate storage iron status.

3.2.1.1 Serum Ferritin

The serum ferritin concentration provides a quantitative estimate of the size of the iron store in healthy individuals and those with uncomplicated iron deficiency.[5] In an adult, 1 µg/L in the serum ferritin indicates the presence of approximately 8 mg of storage iron.[2] The average serum ferritin concentration, for menstruating women living in the U.S. is 36 µg/L (approximately 300 mg storage iron) and for men 137µg/L (approximately 1000 mg storage iron).[6] A similar relationship is present in children; 1 µg/L in serum ferritin indicates an iron store of about 0.14 µg/kg. When the serum ferritin concentration falls below approximately 12 µg/L, the iron store is totally depleted. Low serum ferritin concentrations are highly specific for iron deficiency. However, the serum ferritin may be affected by factors other than iron stores. Levels are increased by the presence of infections, inflammatory disorders, cancer, and liver disease. For this reason, individuals with depleted iron stores who also suffer from an infectious, inflammatory, or neoplastic disorder may have ferritin values that fall within the normal range.

3.2.1.2 Total Iron Binding Capacity

The total iron binding capacity (TIBC) is a measure of the plasma transferrin concentration. The transferrin level rises in response to iron storage depletion before there is evidence of an inadequate iron supply to functional tissues.[2] A raised TIBC is a less precise indicator of iron storage depletion than is the serum ferritin. The TIBC is also affected by inflammatory and neoplastic disorders that may reduce the level.

3.2.2 EARLY FUNCTIONAL IRON DEFICIENCY (IRON DEFICIENT ERYTHROPOIESIS)

Early functional iron deficiency is signaled by the presence of laboratory evidence indicating that the iron supply to the bone marrow and other tissues is marginally inadequate. At this stage there is no measurable decrease in hemoglobin synthesis. There is no anemia.

3.2.2.1 Serum Transferrin Saturation

Serum transferrin is normally about 30 to 35% saturated with iron. As the iron supply decreases the serum iron (SI) concentration falls. There is a concomitant rise in the transferrin concentration or TIBC. When the transferrin saturation (SI × 100/TIBC) is reduced to levels below 15%, the rate of iron delivery is insufficient to maintain normal hemoglobin synthesis.[2] The association of a low transferrin saturation with an increased total iron binding capacity is highly suggestive of the presence of iron deficiency. However, low transferrin saturation levels are also encountered in other conditions. Inflammatory disorders associated with the anemia of chronic disease (ACD) lead to an impairment of the release of iron from stores with resultant low serum iron levels and decreased serum transferrin saturation. Under these circumstances the TIBC is also characteristically reduced.

3.2.2.2   Erythrocyte Protoporphyrin Concentration

Once the iron supply is insufficient for optimal hemoglobin synthesis, the formation of heme from protoporphyrin IX is impaired. Red cells accumulate the excess protoporphyrin IX which remains in the cell for the duration of its lifespan and is measurable as the erythrocyte protoporphyrin (EP).[2,7] Increased EP levels are indicative of red cell maturation under conditions of suboptimal iron supply. However, EP levels can be increased in ACD and in other conditions that lead to impaired hemoglobin synthesis such as chronic lead intoxication.

3.2.2.3   Soluble Transferrin Receptor Concentration

The surfaces of all cells express transferrin receptors in proportion to their need for iron.[8] A truncated form of the extracellular domain of the receptor (serum or soluble transferrin receptor, STfR) is produced by proteolytic cleavage and is present in the plasma in direct proportion to the number of receptors expressed on the surfaces of all body tissues. As functional iron depletion occurs, more receptors appear on cell surfaces. The plasma soluble transferrin receptor level rises concomitantly.

Assays for STfRs have become available recently.[8,9] Levels are increased in iron deficiency and in the presence of increased hematopoiesis, but appear to be normal in ACD. The latter finding is very important since it suggests that this indicator will be useful in distinguishing iron deficient individuals from those with infectious, inflammatory, or neoplastic disorders. Iron deficiency and ACD are the two most important causes of anemia in the developing world. A laboratory test that differentiates the two conditions will have important implications for the design of appropriate intervention strategies in developing countries.

3.2.3   IRON DEFICIENCY ANEMIA

Tissue iron deficiency and its effect on cellular biochemical processes are as important as suboptimal oxygen delivery in determining the clinical consequences of iron deficiency. Unlike deficiencies of vitamin A, folic acid, and vitamin B_{12} which are discussed later, functionally significant tissue iron deficiency does not appear to occur in the absence of anemia. Anemia may therefore be used as the indicator for both functionally significant tissue iron deficiency and impaired oxygen delivery.

3.2.3.1   Hemoglobin and Hematocrit

Iron deficiency anemia is diagnosed on the basis of a reduced hemoglobin concentration or hematocrit in association with abnormal values for the indicators for iron deficiency. Low hemoglobin concentrations or hematocrit levels are not specific for iron deficiency and occur in many other conditions. There is a significant overlap between hemoglobin values found in iron deficient individuals and those in the normal population.[10,11] No single value can separate the anemic and nonanemic subjects. Iron deficient red blood cells are hypochromic and microcytic. The mean cell volume (MCV) and mean cell hemoglobin (MCH) is reduced. Cells also tend to vary in size and the red cell distribution width (RDW) is increased. Decreased MCV and MCH values are not specific for iron deficiency and occur in all conditions that cause impaired hemoglobin synthesis (e.g., thalassemias, ACD).

3.2.4 LABORATORY METHODS

3.2.4.1 Serum Ferritin

Serum ferritin assays are usually performed on serum from a venous blood sample using an enzyme linked immunoabsorbent assay (ELISA).[12] Samples are separated shortly after the blood clots and refrigerated or frozen for transport to a central facility. Capillary blood gives comparable results. Accurate values can be obtained from samples that are spotted onto filter paper and transported without refrigeration.[13] It is necessary to separate the plasma from the red blood cells before spotting the sample because hemolysis of the red cells causes the release of cellular ferritin resulting in spuriously high values.[14] Fortunately, it appears that separation can be accomplished at room temperature under nonrigorous conditions.

3.2.4.2 Serum Iron and Total Iron Binding Capacity (TIBC)

Serum Iron and TIBC are usually measured using chromogenic techniques.[12] The assay presents special difficulties in the field setting because of the high probability of sample contamination with iron.

3.2.4.3 Erythrocyte Protoporphyrin

Erythrocyte protoporphyrin is most easily measured by using a hematoflurometer to determine the protoporphyrin concentration in a drop of blood.[12] No processing is required. Erythrocyte protoporphyrin assays have been applied successfully in field studies by using a dedicated portable instrument.

3.2.4.4 Soluble Transferrin Receptor

Soluble transferrin receptor assays are customarily performed using an ELISA method[9] on serum that has been separated from venous blood shortly after obtaining the sample. Samples are refrigerated or frozen for transport to a central facility. A recent report indicates that accurate soluble transferrin receptor assays can be performed on blood samples spotted onto filter paper and transferred to the laboratory without refrigeration.[13] It is not necessary to separate the serum from the whole blood.

3.2.4.5 Hemoglobin

There are several methods for measuring hemoglobin. The photometric method is the standard technique in automated central laboratories. Portable battery operated devices are available for field use and are precise.[15-19] It is important to note that rigorous training of the operators and careful standardization and quality control of the assays are essential for reliable results. Capillary samples can be used, but the accuracy is far lower unless the method for obtaining the capillary samples is meticulously standardized.

The copper sulfate specific gravity method is used extensively in the U.S. for screening blood donors. It is cheap, rapid, and can be very reliable if the conditions of testing are carefully standardized. With few exceptions[20] it has not proven useful in developing countries mainly because of the difficulty in obtaining and maintaining standardized copper sulfate solutions.

The sensitivity of the filter paper method has, in the past, been too low to make it useful for surveys. Accuracy increases in the presence of severe anemia. A new color scale (WHO Colour Scale) may improve the sensitivity of this technique. Preliminary studies have shown it to be a reliable method for detecting anemia, especially severe anemia, when a venous blood sample is available.[21]

3.2.4.6   Hematocrit

The hematocrit is determined by centrifugation of a fresh blood sample.[12] Measurements carried out in the field using portable battery operated instruments have been difficult to standardize presumably because of the difficulty in obtaining controlled centrifugation speeds. Hemoglobin measurement is the preferred method of detecting anemia in field surveys.

3.3   VITAMIN A DEFICIENCY

Vitamin A is essential for normal vision. It is required both for the transduction of light into neural signals by the retina[22] and for the maintenance of normal differentiation of the cells forming the cornea and conjunctival membranes.[23] Adequate vitamin A levels are also required for the preservation of the integrity of epithelial surfaces throughout the body[22] and for normal immune function.[24-26] Anemia is not the most significant consequence of vitamin A deficiency from the clinical point of view, but several surveys have shown a direct correlation between serum retinol and hemoglobin levels.[27] While this could result from an inadequate dietary intake of both vitamin A and iron, vitamin A deficiency can lead to impaired mobilization of iron from stores, and supplementation with vitamin A alone can improve hemoglobin levels.

3.3.1   EVALUATION OF VITAMIN A STATUS

3.3.1.1   Dark Adaptation Test

The ability of the retina to adapt to low light levels depends on an adequate supply of vitamin A. A change in threshold of light perception with time can be used as a sensitive measure of vitamin A status.[28] The test is time consuming and not suitable for epidemiological surveys.

3.3.1.2   Pupillary Response Test

This test measures the threshold of light at which pupillary contraction occurs under dark adapted conditions.[29] Two recent studies suggest that it can be a reliable measure of vitamin A deficiency if the appropriate instrumentation is available.[29,30]

3.3.1.3   Conjunctival Impression Cytology

Epithelial conjunctival cells can be obtained by briefly applying cellulose acetate filter paper to the conjunctiva. The detached epithelial cells are then examined under a microscope after staining with PAS-hematoxylin.[31,32] This method has been used widely for determining vitamin A status in field studies.

3.3.1.4   Plasma Retinol Concentration

Plasma retinol concentrations are highly regulated and insensitive to the size of normal or moderately reduced liver vitamin A stores. However, the plasma retinol concentration falls when liver vitamin A reserves fall below a critical level of about 20 µg/g.[33] Plasma retinol concentrations below 0.70 µmol/L are considered to be indicative of vitamin A deficiency in population surveys.[23] Plasma retinol levels have been used to identify vitamin A deficiency in most epidemiological surveys designed to evaluate its role in the pathogenesis of nutritional anemia. Venous blood samples must be protected from light. Assays are performed by high pressure liquid chromatography on serum stored at –20°C.

3.3.1.5   Modified Relative Dose Response (MRDR)

The MRDR test permits the indirect assessment of the adequacy of hepatic vitamin A stores.[34,35] Retinol binding protein (RBP) accumulates in the liver in Vitamin A deficiency. It is rapidly released into the circulation after the administration of retinol. A rise in the plasma retinol level after the administration of a small dose of vitamin A is therefore a measure of liver vitamin A reserves. The use of a test dose of dehydroretinol, which is not naturally present in plasma, allows the evaluation of vitamin A stores to be based on the analysis of a single blood sample. Dehydroretinol combines with RBP in the same manner as retinol. A plasma dehydroretinol:retinol ratio >0.60, five hours after the administration of an oral dose of 3,4-didehydroretinyl acetate is used to identify marginal vitamin A deficiency.[34,35] This test has been used to evaluate vitamin A status in several field studies.[36]

3.4   FOLIC ACID AND VITAMIN B$_{12}$ DEFICIENCY

Both folate and vitamin B$_{12}$ are essential for normal DNA replication, a prerequisite for hematopoiesis. Specifically, methylenetetrahydrofolate is required for the conversion of deoxyuridine to thymidine. Formation of this form of folate requires an adequate vitamin B$_{12}$ status.[37] Consequently, either in folate or vitamin B$_{12}$ deficiency, thymidine is in short supply and deoxyuridine is misincorporated into DNA in place of thymidine.[38] This causes defective DNA synthesis, secondary strand breaks, and deranged growth and maturation of hematopoietic and other rapidly dividing cells. The net result is dyssynchrony between abnormal nuclear and apparently normal cytoplasmic development. This gives rise to anemia, which is characterized by larger than normal red cells (macrocytic anemia), as well as abnormal neutrophil leukocytes that contain increased numbers of nuclear segments (hypersegmentation of polymorphonuclear leukocytes).[39] In addition to the lowered red cell count, there may also be decreased numbers of neutrophilic white cells and platelets.

Apart from the more conspicuous and well recognized hematological effects of folate and vitamin B_{12} deficiency, there is increasing evidence that deficiencies of these vitamins can also result in a variety of complications affecting other organs. These nonhematological manifestations frequently precede and may occur without hematological abnormalities.[40,41] Folate deficiency is a major cause of raised levels of homocysteine in the blood. Homocysteine has been implicated as an independent risk factor for cardiovascular disease.[42-45] Another morbid effect of folate deficiency is an increased risk of neural and other developmental defects in infants born to folate deficient mothers.[46] Additionally, the association of folate deficiency with several neurological, gastrointestinal, and immunological disorders as well as an increased risk of certain cancers has been reviewed recently.[40]

Vitamin B_{12} deficiency can also result in nonhematological complications, the most important of which are neurological. They may precede or even occur in the absence of anemia.[47] Furthermore, there is some evidence to suggest that neurological complications occur more frequently in those vitamin B_{12} deficient individuals who are the least anemic.[48] The precise mechanism whereby vitamin B_{12} deficiency results in neurological damage is unknown. The uncommon occurrence of these complications in folate deficiency makes it unlikely that neurological damage is caused by disruption of the biochemical pathway that is implicated in anemia.[49] Other less common and less well characterized nonhematological complications of Vitamin B_{12} deficiency include gastrointestinal, immunological, and integumentary changes,[50] in addition to a possible link to vascular occlusive disease through the homocysteine mechanism.[51] Recently, reports have linked elevated homocysteine levels found in folate and vitamin B_{12} deficiency to Alzheimer-type neurodegenerative disease in the elderly.[52]

A number of demographic factors influence the prevalence of folate and vitamin B_{12} deficiency. In general, folate deficiency is more often the result of inadequate intake of the vitamin, whereas vitamin B_{12} deficiency usually arises from malabsorption. Evidence is mounting that genetic mutations of enzymes concerned with folate and vitamin B_{12} metabolism and particularly the common polymorphisms of those enzymes, play a significant role in determining vitamin needs.[53] In addition, population based food folate fortification programs designed to lower the risk of neural tube defects is changing the prevalence of folate deficiency, as well as potentially altering the clinical spectrum of vitamin B_{12} deficiency. There are reports that in certain geographic areas there may be a high prevalence of vitamin B_{12} deficiency in children who were not previously considered to be at risk for deficiency of this nutrient.[54]

The growing awareness that complications of folate and vitamin B_{12} deficiency extend beyond anemia is a direct consequence of the availability of more sensitive and specific laboratory tests for metabolites that accumulate in these deficiencies.[55,56]

3.4.1 STAGES IN THE DEVELOPMENT OF VITAMIN B_{12} OR FOLATE DEFICIENCY

Unlike iron in which progressive stages of storage depletion, early functional iron deficiency, and eventual anemia have been well characterized, information on the

TABLE 3.2
Indicators of Folate Deficiency[a]

Indicator	Normal	Folate Stores Depletion	Early Functional Folate Deficiency	Folate Deficiency Anemia
Plasma homocysteine (μmol/l)	<10	10–15	>15	>15
Serum folate (ng/ml)	>6	Unknown	3–6	<3
Red cell folate (ng/ml)	>200	<170	<170	<170
Deoxyuridine suppression test (%)	<10	10–20	20–30	30–50
Erythrocytes (hemoglobin, hematocrit, rbc indices)[b]	Normal	Normal	Normal	Macrocytic anemia
Other	Normal	Normal	Normal	Hypersegmentation of neutrophil nuclei[c]

[a] Adapted from Herbert.[60]

[b] For normal values see Table 3.1.

[c] Hypersegmentation of neutrophil nuclei is reported to be the earliest morphological change in the blood in megaloblastic macrocytic anemia.[75]

sequence of events in developing folate or vitamin B_{12} deficiency is incomplete and somewhat speculative. Shown in Tables 3.2 and 3.3 are arbitrary stages of deficiency for folate and vitamin B_{12} demarcated using the same template developed for iron deficiency[2] proposed by Herbert.[58]

Human studies of experimental deficiency have only been carried out for folic acid, and are limited to observations of a single individual conducted almost 30 years ago, before assays were available to measure homocysteine levels in the blood.[57] Under the conditions of this study, time to onset of folate deficiency was 4 to 5 months. In clinical situations, the rate would be influenced by the size of the body store, factors affecting the daily requirement, and the degree of dietary insufficiency or malabsorption.[40] Homocysteine levels rise when there is insufficient tissue folate to support folate dependent biochemical pathways. Based on Herbert's observations[58] as well as on inferences from other studies,[59] it can be assumed that in the face of a negative folate balance, plasma homocysteine levels will rise to detectably abnormal levels before the serum folate falls below the reference range. If the negative folate balance persists, serum folate levels fall below the reference range. It takes longer for the red cell folate concentrations to decrease to levels below the normal range. This is because of the 120 day life span of normal red cells and the inability of folate to enter or leave mature red cells.[50] Intracellular folate concentrations reach critically low levels for DNA synthesis somewhat sooner. Thus, the deoxyuridine suppression test, which can detect disruption of thymidine synthesis that leads to megaloblastic hematopoiesis,[60] becomes abnormal at an earlier time point.

TABLE 3.3
Indicators of Vitamin B$_{12}$ Deficiency

Indicator	Normal	Vitamin B$_{12}$ Depletion	Early Functional Vitamin B$_{12}$ Deficiency	Vitamin B$_{12}$ Deficiency Anemia
Serum methylmalonic acid (nmol/l)	<380	Unknown	>380	>380
Plasma homocysteine (μmol/l)	<10	10–15	>15	>15
Serum vitamin B$_{12}$ (pg/ml)[a]	>190	190–350	190–350	<190
Serum holotranscobalamin II (pg/ml)[b]	>50	30–50	<30	<30
Deoxyuridine suppression test (%)	<10	10–20	20–30	30–50
Erythrocytes (hemoglobin, hematocrit, rbc indices)[c]	Normal	Normal	Normal	Macrocytic anemia
Other	None	Normal	Normal	Hypersegmentation of neutrophil nuclei[d]

[a] Intervals for serum vitamin B$_{12}$ are based on published observations that the specificity of this measurement is poor, particularly in the 190–350 pg/ml range.[55,56]

[b] Reference intervals for holotranscobalamin II are based on two literature citations.[73,74]

[c] For normal values see Table 3.1.

[d] Hypersegmentation of neutrophil nuclei was found to be an insensitive indication of early vitamin B$_{12}$ deficiency.[65]

The time to onset of vitamin B$_{12}$ deficiency is more prolonged than that for folic acid because of the larger body store of vitamin B$_{12}$ in relation to the daily requirement. Following total gastrectomy, for example, the time to onset of megaloblastic anemia varied from 2 to 7 years.[61] If the cause of vitamin B$_{12}$ were dietary lack alone, the time to the onset of deficiency would be expected to be significantly longer since the vitamin B$_{12}$ excreted in the bile would be reabsorbed efficiently. Our understanding of the actual sequence of changes that occur in the evolution of clinically detectable vitamin B$_{12}$ deficiency is limited to speculation and extrapolation from various clinical observations.[53,56,61,62] Serum concentrations of vitamin B$_{12}$ would be expected to fall first, particularly the fraction attached to the plasma vitamin B$_{12}$ binding protein termed transcobalamin II (TCII). This fraction, termed holoTCII, is the form in which vitamin B$_{12}$ is taken up by cells.[63] Eventually, vitamin B$_{12}$ stores would be depleted, as the total serum vitamin B$_{12}$ concentrations fall below "normal." Normalcy with respect to serum vitamin B$_{12}$ is difficult to define precisely, because of the distribution of the vitamin between three binding proteins, transcobalamins, I, II, and III. When cellular B$_{12}$ stores fall below the levels required to maintain normal metabolism, concentrations of several metabolites begin to rise in the serum. Of these, methylmalonic acid (MMA) and homocysteine are the most useful for clinical screening purposes.[55,56] (Table 3.3)

3.4.2 LABORATORY METHODS

Direct measurement of vitamin levels in the blood remain the mainstay for establishing folate and vitamin B_{12} status and in screening for deficiencies of either nutrient. Both serum and red cell folate concentrations may be useful, whereas only serum vitamin B_{12} is clinically informative.[39] Beyond these assays, which constitute the standard test repertoire for diagnosing folate and vitamin B_{12} deficiency, measurements of homocysteine and MMA have come into vogue. These metabolite assays offer more sensitive and specific tests for identifying and differentiating folate and B_{12} deficiencies.[55,56] Replacement of the standard vitamin assays by these newer biochemical indices of vitamin status are limited only by cost and complexity of the assay methods, as well as some unanswered questions regarding the specificity of the tests.[53] Until recently, both tests required sophisticated equipment (high pressure liquid chromatography (HPLC) for homocysteine, and gas chromatography-mass spectrometry (GCMS) for MMA).[55,56]

Tests for folate and vitamin B_{12} deficiency are usually undertaken simultaneously in the clinical setting, because these investigations typically are prompted by the finding of macrocytic anemia.[39] However, since deficiency of one or other vitamin is more likely in certain target groups, testing in nutritional surveys may be focused on one particular vitamin only.

3.4.2.1 Hemoglobin and Hematocrit and Peripheral Blood Smear

Folate and vitamin B_{12} deficiency anemia is suspected on the basis of abnormally low hemoglobin concentration or hematocrit, associated with the typical red cell indices, i.e., macrocytic red cells (raised MCV) that vary in size (increased RDW). The raised MCV is not specific for folate and vitamin B_{12} deficiency. Several other conditions associated with marrow failure and other systemic diseases may also result in larger red cells.[39] Examination of a stained blood smear confirms the presence of large, often oval, red cells, as well as neutrophil leukocytes with increased numbers of nuclear lobes. Hypersegmented neutrophil leukocytes may be the earliest morphological change to appear in the blood.[64] However, the reliability of this finding in early vitamin B_{12} deficiency has been brought into question.[65] Neutrophil hypersegmentation may also be observed in iron deficiency.[66,67] It is important to note that macrocytic anemia is a late and inconsistent manifestation of folate and vitamin B_{12} deficiencies.[40,41,58,62,68]

3.4.2.2 Serum and Red Cell Folate Concentration

The serum folate concentration, still widely used as the screening test for folate deficiency, has a number of drawbacks. Serum folate concentration may not accurately reflect folate status and may be influenced, transiently, by recent dietary intake of folate. Plasma folate is in a constant state of flux. Spuriously normal serum levels may be observed in folate deficient individuals.[50] Red cell folate provides a more stable reflection of folate status because of the absence of folate transfer across the red cell membrane and the longevity of red cells. Both assays, however, are somewhat unreliable.[69] This is partially due to methodological problems, as evidenced by a recent interlaboratory comparison study among 20 research laboratories in which the overall coefficient of variation for serum folate was 27.6%, with the greatest variation at critically low folate concentrations. In this study, 2 to 9-fold differences were found between methods on the same samples.

A number of techniques have been used to measure folate. They have evolved from microbiological, using *Lactobacillus casei*, to competitive binding assays, using a folate binding protein obtained from milk, and a variety of detection systems including radioisotopic, enzyme linked, and chemiluminescent tags. Potential sources of variability in measured serum and red cell folate levels have been reviewed extensively.[56] Although red cell folate is generally more sensitive than serum folate for detection of folate deficiency, the measurement lacks specificity because red cell folate is subnormal in over half of individuals with vitamin B_{12} deficiency.[50] Folate is unstable, being susceptible to degradation by temperature, light, and oxidation.[50] Suitable freezing or refrigeration of specimens, light protection, and addition of ascorbate or other reducing agents are necessary to preserve activity in the assay. This renders collection of specimens in the field problematic. Recently, a method using dried blood spots on filter paper has been described for measurement of whole blood folate.[70] It offers a promising and inexpensive means of assessing folate status in field studies.

3.4.2.3 Serum Vitamin B_{12}

Assays for serum vitamin B_{12} are the standard screening tests for vitamin B_{12} deficiency. The methods used generally parallel those for folate. They include microbiological (using *Lactobacillus leichmannii* or *Euglena gracilis*), radioligand, enzyme linked, and chemiluminescent assays (using highly specific intrinsic factors as well as less specific vitamin B_{12} binding proteins from a variety of sources).[56] Both the sensitivity and specificity of the serum vitamin B_{12} assay have been questioned due to evidence of functional vitamin B_{12} deficiency in individuals with low normal serum vitamin B_{12} concentrations.[56,71] This evidence is based on the observation of elevated levels of serum metabolites that are indicative of vitamin B_{12} deficiency in individuals whose hematological and clinical findings respond to treatment with vitamin B_{12}. Although technical factors play a role in the lack of predictability of the serum vitamin B_{12} for identifying or excluding vitamin B_{12} deficiency, the major problem may relate to the distribution of the vitamin among several binding proteins, the transcobalamins in the plasma.[50,56] Of the three transcobalamins (TC I, II, and III), it is TCII that is concerned with cell uptake of vitamin B_{12}.[63,72] Attempts have been made to measure the fraction of the serum vitamin B_{12} that is attached to TCII.[73,74] The methods employed are technically difficult and the usefulness of currently available methods has limitations.[75] Until more sensitive methods are developed, the place of this test in the approach to diagnosis of vitamin B_{12} deficiency must remain in question.

3.4.2.4   Plasma Homocysteine Concentration

Folate and vitamin B_{12} are required as cosubstrate and cofactor, respectively, in the conversion of homocysteine to methionine. Consequently, blood levels of homocysteine, rise in deficiencies of either of the vitamins. Measurements of homocysteine have gained increasing acceptance in screening for or confirming the presence of these deficiencies.[55,56] An extensive literature on the measurement and clinical significance of homocysteine has accumulated as a result of the implication of this sulfur containing amino acid as a risk factor for atherothrombosis.[76]

There are several causes of an increased level of homocysteine in the plasma, and the test for plasma homocysteine does not distinguish between folate and vitamin B_{12} deficiency. Nevertheless, because of its sensitivity to the status of these vitamins, and because it is possible to further distinguish the two deficiencies by measurement of serum MMA levels, plasma homocysteine is an important screening and adjunctive test, most particularly for folate deficiency. A description and comparison of the various methods for measuring homocysteine lies beyond the scope of this review. Most methods require access to expensive equipment. However, an immunoassay based automated method that has been validated against standard methodology is now available in a microtiter plate format.[77]

3.4.2.5   Serum Methylmalonic Acid Concentration

Vitamin B_{12} is required for conversion of methylmalonate to succinate. Serum methylmalonic acid (MMA) levels therefore rise in vitamin B_{12} deficiency.[50] The test is highly specific and sensitive and can detect early functional vitamin B_{12} deficiency[55,56] under most circumstances although conditions, such as chronic renal failure, are associated with raised serum MMA levels.[56] At this time, the test remains technically challenging and expensive. The place for serum MMA measurement in the detection of vitamin B_{12} deficiency has been reviewed in detail elsewhere.[56,68]

3.4.2.6   Deoxyuridine (dU) Suppression Test

A test that directly measures the integrity of the DNA synthetic pathway dependent on folate and vitamin B_{12} is the dU suppression test, which may be carried out on either bone marrow cells or mitogen stimulated peripheral blood lymphocytes.[53] The test is highly specific. It can be used to discriminate between the two vitamin deficiencies and is capable of identifying early functional deficiency states. However, it is technically difficult to carry out, and therefore not suited to use in standard laboratory settings.

3.5   APPROACHES TO THE DIAGNOSIS
OF NUTRITIONAL ANEMIA

Since iron deficiency is the most prevalent cause of nutritional anemia, it is first necessary to evaluate iron status. No single laboratory value has yet been shown to be satisfactory as a sole criterion for determining the prevalence of iron deficiency in population surveys. The identification of iron deficiency anemia in population surveys has been based on the detection of anemia in association with a combination of laboratory tests providing evidence of low iron stores and suboptimal iron delivery to developing red blood cells. Cook and coworkers were the first to demonstrate that the use of several indicators of iron deficiency in combination significantly increases the accuracy with which the presence of iron deficiency anemia can be predicted.[78] They measured SF, serum transferrin saturation, and EP in over 1500 individuals living in the northwestern U.S. If only one indicator of iron deficiency was abnormal, the prevalence of anemia was 10.9%, only slightly higher than that for the whole population (8.3%). However, anemia was found in 28% of those with two abnormal values and 63% of those with three. This Ferritin Model (employing the SF, transferrin saturation, and EP) has been applied to the analysis of data from the National Health and Nutrition Examination Survey in the U.S. (NHANES II, NHANES III). The presence of two or more abnormal indicators was considered indicative of an impaired iron status.[79,80] Modifications of the model have been used successfully in the field in developing countries including populations in which malaria is holoendemic.[81] A second model, termed the MCV model, has results similar to the ferritin model. It uses the MCV, transferrin saturation, and EP as indicators.

Several field studies suggest that the recently perfected soluble transferrin receptor assay will prove to be a very useful and relatively specific indicator of iron deficiency in developing countries.[82] Its potential value resides in the ability to recognize early iron deficiency even in the presence of the anemia of chronic disease. It is possible that the use of the soluble transferrin receptor assay may be even more sensitive and specific if combined with the serum ferritin concentration and expressed as a ratio.

One other approach has been used to evaluate the iron status in population surveys. The indicators of iron status have been used in combination to estimate the body iron status of each individual in the survey sample.[83] A frequency distribution for iron status in the population is then calculated.

The choice of indicator(s) will depend on the setting in which iron deficiency is identified and the resources available. The use of multiple indicators provides the most reliable information. It has been shown repeatedly that in pregnancy, young children, and premenopausal women, anemia is almost always the result of iron deficiency unless malaria is an important factor. Hemoglobin values may be a sufficient reason to institute monitored iron fortification or supplementation interventions in this setting. As Yip[84] has pointed out, the prevalence of anemia in a sample of children and women can serve as an index of the severity of iron deficiency in areas where a low bioavailable iron intake is the predominant cause of anemia. Hemoglobin distribution curves in targeted population samples may be used to detect factors other than iron if men are included in the survey. When poor iron intake is the main etiological factor, children and women are disproportionately affected. Other causes such as other nutrient deficiencies and hookworm infections are less gender specific. Collateral health information, e.g., the prevalence of malaria and hookworm infection may provide supporting data. If further testing for iron deficiency is needed, the SF and EP assays are likely to be the most accessible laboratory tests. The STfR concentration is a very promising new test that may replace some of the older indicators.

The decision to search for other nutritional deficiencies depends on the setting in which the anemia is encountered. Vitamin A deficiency has serious health consequences that are unrelated to anemia. Considerable effort is being expended on the eradication of vitamin A deficiency on a worldwide basis at the present time. The dietary factors responsible and the population groups at risk are relatively well characterized. If vitamin A deficiency is considered to be a contributory factor to anemia, consideration should be given to measuring serum retinol levels in a subsample of the affected population group.

Folic acid and vitamin B_{12} deficiency should be considered whenever the initial evaluation of the anemia indicates the presence of macrocytosis. Folic acid deficiency may occur because of seasonal or social factors that limit the supply of fresh fruits and vegetables as well as in situations in which requirements are increased. The latter include pregnancy, lactation, prematurity, and diseases that cause increased cell turnover such as malaria and chronic hemolytic states. Vitamin B_{12} deficiency usually results from malabsorption rather than from an inadequate dietary intake alone. Ongoing research suggests that malabsorption of vitamin B_{12} may be important in old age and also in children in certain geographic areas. Despite their limitations, assays for red blood cell folate and serum vitamin B_{12} remain the most reliable screening tests for folic acid and vitamin B_{12} deficiencies.

REFERENCES

1. Cook, J. D., Skikne, B. S., and Baynes. R. D., Iron deficiency: the global perspective, *Adv. Experimental Biol. Med.*, 356, 219, 1994.
2. Bothwell, T. H., Charlton, R. W., Cook, J. D., and Finch, C. A., *Iron Metabolism in Man,* World Health Organization, Blackwell Scientific Publications, Oxford, 1979.
3. Brittenham, G. M., Disorders of iron metabolism: iron deficiency and overload, in *Hematology: Basic Principles and Practice*, Hoffman, R., Benz, E. J. Jr., Sharttil, S. J., Furie, B., Cohen H. J., Silberstein, L. E., and McGlave P., Eds., Churchill Livingstone, New York, 2000, 397.
4. Finch, C. A. and Huebers, H., Perspectives in iron metabolism, *New Engl. J. Med.,* 306, 1520, 1982.
5. Cook, J. D., Lipschitz, D. A., Miles, L. E. M., and Finch, C. A., Serum ferritin as a measure of iron stores in normal subjects, *Am. J. Clinical Nutr.,* 27, 681, 1974.
6. Looker, A. C., Gunter, E. W., Cook, J. D., Green, R., and Harris, J. W., Comparing serum ferritin values from different population surveys, *Vital Health Statistics*, 2, 111, 1991.
7. Garrett, S. and Worwood, M., Zinc protoporphyrin and iron-deficient erythropoiesis, *Acta Haematologica*, 91, 21, 1994.
8. Cook, J. D., Baynes, R. D., and Skikne, B. S., The physiological significance of circulating transferrin receptors, *Annu. Rev. Med.*, 44, 63, 1993.
9. Flowers, C. H., Skikne, B. S., Covell, A. M., and Cook, J. D., The clinical measurement of serum transferrin receptor, *J. Lab. Clinical Med.,* 114, 368, 1989.
10. Garby, L., Irnell, L., and Werner, I., Iron deficiency in women of fertile age in a Swedish community, II. Efficiency of several laboratory tests to predict the response to iron supplementation, *Acta Medica Scandinavica*, 185, 107, 1969.

11. Garby, L., Irnell, L., and Werner, I., Iron deficiency in women of fertile age in a Swedish community, III. Estimation of prevalence based on response to iron supplementation, *Acta Medica Scandinavica,* 185, 113, 1969.

12. International Nutritional Anemia Consultative Group, *Measurements of Iron Status,* The Nutrition Foundation, Inc., Washington, D.C., 1985.

13. Ahluwalia, N., Lonnerdal, B., Lorenz, S. G., and Allen, L. H., Spot ferritin assay for serum samples dried on filter paper, *Am. J. Clinical Nutr.,* 67, 88, 1998.

14. Cook, J. D., Flowers, C. H., and Skikne, B. S., An assessment of dried-spot technology for identifying iron deficiency, *Blood,* 92, 1807, 1998.

15. Stone, J. E., Simmons, W. K., Jutsum, P. J., and Gurney, J. M., An evaluation of methods of screening for anaemia, *Bull. World Health Organ.,* 62, 115, 1984.

16. von Schenk, H., Falkensson, M., and Lundberg, B., Evaluation of "HemoCue", a new device for determining hemoglobin, *Clinical Chem.,* 32, 526, 1986.

17. Neville, R.G., Evaluation of portable haemoglobinometer in general practice, *Br. Med. J.,* 294, 1263, 1987.

18. Cohen, A. R. and Seidl-Friedman, J., HemoCue system for hemoglobin measurement, *Am. J. Clinical Pathol.,* 90, 302, 1988.

19. Hudson-Thomas, M., Bingham, K. C., and Simmons, W. K., An evaluation of the HemoCue for measuring haemoglobin in field studies in Jamaica, *Bull. World Health Organ.,* 72, 423, 1994.

20. Pistorius, L. R., Funk, M., Pattinson, R. C., and Howarth, G. R., Screening for anaemia in pregnancy with copper sulfate densitometry, *Int. J. Gynecol. Obstet.,* 52, 33, 1996.

21. Lewis, S. M., Stott, G. J., and Wynn, K. J., An inexpensive and reliable new haemoglobin colour scale for assessing anaemia, *J. Clinical Pathol.,* 51, 21, 1998.

22. Spron, M. B., Roberts, A. B., and Goodman, D. S., Eds., The Retinoids: Biology, Chemistry, and Medicine, Raven Press, New York, 1994, 351.

23. Sommer, A. and West, K. P., *Vitamin A Deficiency: Health, Survival, and Vision,* Oxford University Press, New York, 1996.

24. Katz, D., R., Drzymala, M., Turton, J. A., Hicks, R. M., Hunt, R., Palmer, L., and Malkovsky, M., Regulation of accessory cell function by retinoids in murine immune responses, *Br. J. Experimental Pathol.,* 68, 343, 1987.

25. Blomhoff, H. K., Smeland, E. B., Erikstein, B., Rasmussen, A. M., Skrede, B., Skjonsberg, C., and Blohoff, R., Vitamin A is the key regulator for cell growth, cytokine production and differentiation in normal B cells, *J. Biological Chem.,* 267, 23788, 1992.

26. Zhao, Z. and Ross, A. C., Retinoic acid repletion restores the number of leukocytes and their subsets and stimulates natural cytotoxicity in Vitamin A-deficient rats, *J. Nutr.,* 125, 2064, 1995.

27. Lynch, S. R., Interaction of iron with other nutrients, *Nutr. Rev.,* 55, 102, 1997.

28. Carney, E. A. and Russell, R. M., Correlation of dark adaptation results with serum vitamin A levels in diseased adults, *J. Nutr.,* 110, 552, 1980.

29. Congdon, N., Sommer, A., Severns, M., Humphrey, J., Friedman, D., Clement, L., Shu-Fune, W. L., and Natadisastra, G., Pupillary and visual thresholds in young children as an index of population vitamin A status, *Am. J. Clinical Nutr.,* 61, 1076, 1995.

30. Sanchez, A. M., Congdon, N. G., Sommer, A., Rahmathullah, L., Venkataswamy, P. G., Chandravathi, P. S., and Clement, L., Pupillary threshold as an index of population vitamin A status among children in India, *Am. J. Clinical Nutr.,* 65, 61, 1997.

31. Hatchell, D. L. and Sommer, A., Detection of ocular surface abnormalities in experimental vitamin A deficiency, *Arch. Ophthalmol.,* 102, 1389, 1984.

32. Natadisatra, G., Wittpenn, J. R., Muhilal, West, K. P., Jr., Mele, L., and Sommer, A., Impression cytology for detection of vitamin A deficiency, *Arch. Ophthalmol.*, 105, 1224, 1987.

33. Olson, J. A., Recommended dietary intakes (RDI) of vitamin A in humans, *Am. J. Clinical Nutr.*, 45, 704, 1987.

34. Tanumihardjo, S. A., Furr, H. C., Erdman, J. W., Jr., and Olson, J. A., Use of the modified relative dose response (MRDR) assay in rats and its application to humans, *Eur. J. Clinical Nutr.*, 44, 219, 1990.

35. Tanumihardjo, S. A., Koellner, P. G, and Olson, J. A., The modified relative dose response (MRDR) assay as an indicator of vitamin A status in a population of well-nourished American children, *Am. J. Clinical Nutr.*, 53, 1064, 1990.

36. Habicht, J-P. and Stoltzfus, R. J., What do indicators indicate? *Am. J. Clinical Nutr.*, 66, 190, 1997.

37. Wickramasinghe, S. N., Morphology, biology and biochemistry of cobalamin- and folate-deficient bone marrow cells, *Bailliere's Clinical Haema.*, 8, 441, 1995.

38. Blount, B. C, Mack, M. M, Wehr, C. M., MacGregor, J. T., Hiatt, R. A., Wang, G., Wickramasinghe, S. N., Everson, R. B., and Ames, B. N., Folate deficiency causes uracil misincorporation into human DNA and chromosome breakage: implications for cancer and neuronal damage, *Proc. Nat. Acad. Sci. U.S.A.*, 94, 3290, 1997.

39. Green, R., Macrocytic and marrow failure anemias, *Lab. Med.*, 30, 595, 1999.

40. Green, R. and Miller, J. W., Folate deficiency beyond megaloblastic anemia: hyper-homocysteinemia and other manifestations of dysfunctional folate metabolism, *Semin. Hematol.*, 36, 47, 1999.

41. Carmel, R., Subtle and atypical cobalamin deficiency states, *Am. J. Hematol.*, 34, 108, 1990.

42. Boushey, C. J., Beresford, S. A., Omenn, G. S., and Motulsky, A. G., A quantitative assessment of plasma homocysteine as a risk factor for vascular disease: probable benefits of increasing folic acid intakes, *JAMA*, 274,1049, 1995.

43. Pancharuniti, N., Lewis, C. A., Sauberlich, H. E., et al., Plasma homocysteine, folate and vitamin B_{12} concentrations and risk for early onset coronary artery disease, *Am. J. Clinical Nutr.*, 59, 940, 1994.

44. Morrison, H. I., Schaubel, D., Desmules, M., and Wigle, D. T., Serum folate and risk of fatal coronary heart disease, *JAMA*, 275, 1893, 1996.

45. Rimm, E., B., Willett, W. C., Hu, F. B., Sampson, L., Colditz, G. A., Manson, J. E. Hennekens, C., and Stampfer, M. J., Folate and vitamin B_6 from diet and supplements in relation to risk of coronary heart disease among women, *JAMA*, 279, 359, 1998.

46. Christensen, B. and Rosenblatt, D. S., Effects of folate deficiency on embryonic development, *Bailliere's Clinical Haema.*, 8, 617, 1995.

47. Lindenbaum, J., Healton, E. B., Savage, D. G., Brust, J. C., Garrett, T.J., Podell, E. R., Marcell, P. D., Stabler, S. P., and Allen, R. H., Neuropsychiatric disorders caused by cobalamin deficiency in the absence of anemia or macrocytosis, *New Engl. J. Med.*, 318, 1720, 1988.

48. Healton, E. B., Savage, D. G., Brust, J. C. M., Garrett, T. J., and Lindenbaum, J., Neurologic aspects of cobalamin deficiency, *Medicine*, 70, 229,1991.

49. Metz, J., Cobalamin deficiency and the pathogenesis of nervous system disease, *Annu. Rev. Nutr.*, 12, 59,1992.

50. Chanarin, I., *The Megaloblastic Anaemias*, 2nd ed., Blackwell Scientific Publications, Oxford, 1979.

51. Selhub, J., Jacques, P. F., Wilson, P. W. F., Rush, D., and Rosenberg, I. H., Vitamin status and intake as primary determinants of homocysteinemia in an elderly population, *JAMA*, 270, 2693, 1993.

52. Clarke, R., Smith, A. D., Jobst, K. A., Refsum, H., Sutton, L., and Ueland, P. M., Folate, vitamin B_{12}, and serum total homocysteine levels in confirmed Alzheimer disease, *Arch. of Neurology,* 55, 1449, 1998.

53. Wickramasinghe, S. N., The wide spectrum and unresolved issues of megaloblastic anemia, *Semin. in Hematol.,* 36, 3, 1999.

54. Allen, L. H., Rosado, J. L., Casterline, J. E., Martinez, H., Lopez, P., Munoz, E., and Black, A. K., Vitamin B_{12} deficiency and malabsorption are highly prevalent in rural Mexican communities, *Am. J. Clinical Nutr.,* 62, 1013, 1995.

55. Allen, R. H., Stabler, S. P., Savage, D. G., and Lindenbaum, J., Metabolic abnormalities in cobalamin (vitamin B_{12}) and folate deficiency, *FASEB J.,* 7, 1344, 1993.

56. Green, R., Metabolite Assays in Cobalamin and Folate Deficiency, in Megaloblastic anemias, *Bailliere's Clinical Haema.,* 8, 533, 1995.

57. Herbert, V., Experimental nutritional folate deficiency in man, *Trans. of the Am. Assoc. Physicians,* 75, 307, 1962.

58. Herbert, V., The 1986 Herman award lecture. Nutrition science as a continually unfolding story: The folate and vitamin B12 paradigm, *Am. J. Clinical Nutr.,* 46, 387, 1987.

59. Lewis, C. A., Pancharuniti, M., and Sauberlich, H. E., Plasma folate adequacy as determined by homocysteine level, *Ann. N.Y. Acad. Sci.,* 669, 360, 1992.

60. Killmann, S.-A., Effect of deoxyuridine on incorporation of tritiated thymidine: difference between normoblasts and megaloblasts, *Acta Medica Scandinavica,* 175, 483, 1964.

61. Paulson, M. and Harvey, J. C., Hematological complications after total gastrectomy: evolutionary sequences over a decade, *JAMA,* 156, 1556, 1954.

62. Green R., Macrocytic anemias, in *Medicine for the Practicing Physician,* 4th ed., Hurst, J. W., Ed., Simon and Shuster, Stamford, CT, 1996, 814.

63. Hall, C. A. and Finkler, A. E., The dynamics of transcobalamin II. A vitamin B_{12} binding substance in plasma, *J. Lab. Clinical Med.,* 65, 459, 1965.

64. Lindenbaum, J. and Nath, B. J., Megaloblastic anaemia and neutrophilic hypersegmentation, *Br. J. Haema.,* 44, 511, 1980.

65. Carmel, R., Green, R., Jacobsen, D. W., and Qian, G. D., Neutrophil nuclear segmentation in mild cobalamin deficiency: relation to metabolic tests of cobalamin status and observations on ethnic differences in neutrophil segementation, *Am. J. Clinical Pathol.,* 106, 57, 1996.

66. Westerman, D. A., Evans, D., and Metz, J., Neutrophil hypersegmentation in iron deficiency anaemia: a case-control study, *Br. J. Haema.,* 107, 512, 1999.

67. Beard, M. E. and Weintraub, L. R., Hypersegmented neutrophilic granulocytes in iron deficiency anaemia, *Br. J. Haema.,* 16, 161, 1969.

68. Green, R. and Kinsella, L. J., Current concepts in the diagnosis of cobalamin deficiency (Editorial), *Neurology,* 45, 1435, 1995.

69. Gunter, E. W., Bowman, B. A., Caudill, S. P., Twite, D. B., Adams, M. J., and Sampson, E. J., Results of an international round robin for serum and whole-blood folate, *Clinical Chem.,* 42, 1689, 1996.

70. O'Broin, S. D. and Gunter, E. W., Screening of folate status with use of dried blood spots on filter paper, *Am. J. Clinical Nutr.,* 70, 359, 1999.

71. Stabler, S. P., Allen, R. H., Savage, D. G., and Lindenbaum, J., Clinical spectrum and diagnosis of cobalamin deficiency, *Blood,* 76, 871, 1990.

72. Fernandes-Costa, F. and Metz, J., Vitamin B12 binders (transcobalamins) in serum, *Crit. Rev. Clinical Lab. Science,* 18, 1, 1982.

73. Herzlich, B. and Herbert, V., Depletion of serum holotranscobalamin II: an early sign of negative vitamin B12 balance, *Lab. Investigation,* 58, 332, 1988.

74. Goh, Y. T., Jacobsen, D. W., and Green, R., Diagnosis of functional cobalamin deficiency: utility of transcobalamin-bound vitamin B12 determination in conjunction with total serum homocysteine and methylmalonic acid, *Blood,* 78(Suppl. 1), 100a, 1991.

75. Wickramasinghe, S. N. and Ratnayaka, I. D., Limited value of serum holo-transcobalamin II measurements in the differential diagnosis of macrocytosis, *J. Clinical Pathol.,* 49, 755, 1996.

76. Nygard, O., Vollset, S. E., Refsum, H., Brattstrom, L., and Ueland, P. M., Total homocysteine and cardiovascular disease, *J. Intern. Med.,* 246, 425, 1999.

77. Marangon, K., O'Byrne, D., Devaraj, S., and Jialal, I., Validation of an immunoassay for measurement of plasma total homocysteine, *Am. J. Clinical Pathol.,* 112, 757, 1999.

78. Cook, J. D., Finch, C. A., and Smith, N. J., Evaluation of the iron status of a population, *Blood*, 48, 449, 1976.

79. Expert Scientific Working Group, Summary of a report on the assessment of iron nutritional status of the United States, *Am. J. Clinical Nutr.,* 42, 1318, 1985.

80. Looker, A. C., Dallman, P. R., Caroll, M. D., Gunter, E. W., and Johnson, C. L., Prevalence of iron deficiency in the United States, *JAMA*, 277, 973, 1997.

81. Stoltzfus, R. J., Chwaya, H. M., Albonico, M., Schulze, K. J., Savioli., L., and Tielsch, J. M., Serum ferritin, erythrocyte protoporphyrin and hemoglobin are valid indicators of iron status of school children in a malaria-holoendemic population, *J. Nutr.,* 127, 293, 1997.

82. Skikne, B. S., Flowers, C. H., and Cook, J. D., Serum transferrin receptor: a quantitative measure of tissue iron deficiency, *Blood*, 75, 1870, 1990.

83. Cook, J. D., Skikne, B. S., Lynch, S. R., and Reusser, M. E., Estimates of iron sufficiency in the U. S. population, *Blood*, 58, 726, 1986.

84. Yip, R., Iron deficiency: contemporary scientific issues and international programmatic approaches, *J. Nutr.,* 124, 14795, 1994.

85. World Health Organization/United Nations Children's Fund/United Nations University, *Indicators for assessing iron deficiency and strategies for its prevention,* WHO, Geneva, 1997.

86. Dirren, H., Logman, M. H., Barclay, D. V., and Freire, W. B., Altitude correction for hemoglobin, *Eur. J. Clinical Nutr.*, 48, 625, 1994.

87. *Anemia Detection Methods in Low-Resource Settings: A Manual for Health Workers,* Program for Appropriate Technology in Health, Seattle, 1997.

4 Functional Consequences of Nutritional Anemia during Pregnancy and Early Childhood

Usha Ramakrishnan

CONTENTS

0-8493-8569-5/01/$0.00+$.50
© 2001 by CRC Press LLC

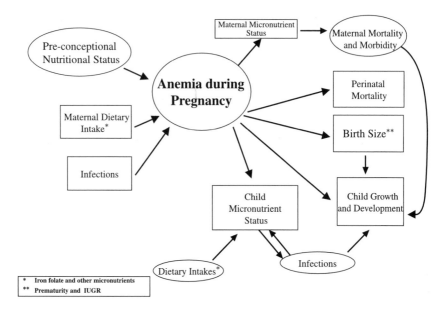

FIGURE 4.1 Functional consequences of anemia during pregnancy and early childhood.

4.1   INTRODUCTION

Pregnancy and early childhood are critical periods characterized by increased nutrient requirements due to high physiological needs and increased risk to the health and well being of both the mother and her infant. The prevalence of nutritional anemia is greatest during pregnancy and early childhood and has been associated with several adverse maternal and infant outcomes.[1,2] Nearly 600,000 women die each year in developing countries from complications of pregnancy, childbirth, and unsafe abortion, and many of these deaths are preventable.[3] Adverse infant related outcomes include increased mortality and morbidity, small birth size, and impaired growth and development during the early years.

This chapter will focus on functional consequences of nutritional anemia during pregnancy, lactation, and early childhood as shown in Figure 4.1. (Child development is addressed in Chapter 5.) A brief description of the physiology of nutritional anemia during these vulnerable periods is provided in the first section, followed by the evidence that relates nutritional anemia with specific functional consequences. Iron deficiency, the leading cause of nutritional anemia, the roles of nutrients such as folate and vitamins B_{12} and A, nutrient interactions, and multinutrient deficiencies are discussed.

4.2   PHYSIOLOGY OF NUTRITIONAL ANEMIA

4.2.1   PREGNANCY

Pregnancy is a period of rapid growth and development. Maternal requirements of several hemopoietic nutrients (iron, folate, vitamin B_{12}) are increased due to the increased burden of erythropoiesis. Iron needs increase substantially during pregnancy and so does the prevalence of iron deficiency and iron deficiency anemia (IDA).[4,5] It is important to recognize that even among iron sufficient women, hemoglobin levels fall during early pregnancy, reach a nadir in the second trimester of pregnancy, and rise again to prepregnant levels by term[6] as a result of normal changes in plasma volume during pregnancy.[7,8] Hallberg[9] estimated that the total iron requirement during a pregnancy is 1040 mg, of which 840 mg are permanently lost to the mother after delivery and 200 mg are retained to serve as a reservoir of iron when blood volume decreases after delivery. An additional 15 mg/day of iron averaged over the entire pregnancy was recommended by the U.S. Food and Nutrition Board Subcommittee on the tenth edition of the RDA (i.e., RDA of 30 mg/day). The subcommittee also recommended universal daily iron supplementation for all pregnant women irrespective of their iron stores based on the assertion that the additional iron requirements cannot be met by diet alone.[10] This has been challenged on the basis of limited evidence of benefits to the fetus and/or mother, which will be examined in the rest of this chapter.[11]

4.2.2 LACTATION

Iron requirements during lactation are not increased as they are during pregnancy. This is due to the low iron content of breast milk, the compensation by the absence of menstrual losses during lactation (at least part of it), and recuperation of iron reserves following delivery.[12] However, iron deficiency may continue during lactation among women who have small or no stores and/or have incurred substantial blood losses during pregnancy. Other nutrient deficiencies and parasitic infections such as malaria and helminthic infections may also contribute to anemia. Studies in Nepal and Indonesia reported that the prevalence of anemia among lactating women was 81% and 72%, respectively.[13] Most cases were mild to moderate; the prevalence of severe anemia (Hb <7 g/dl) was 14% and 3% respectively, raising the issue of the appropriateness of cutoff values.

4.2.3 EARLY CHILDHOOD

Infants and preschool age children are at increased risk of iron deficiency and anemia due to high physiological demands combined with low iron stores, inadequate dietary intake of bioavailable iron, and losses due to infections.[14] Healthy term infants are usually born with adequate reserves of iron stores that will last approximately 6 months, irrespective of the iron status of the mother. Iron stores of low birth weight (LBW) and premature infants may last only 2 to 3 months due to lower nascent stores and higher rates of postnatal growth in comparison to term infants.[15] Although breast milk is a poor source of iron, the bioavailability is high and is generally regarded adequate for the first 4 to 6 months. Recent studies suggest that exclusive breast feeding for 6 months may not protect a child from developing anemia especially if the infant has low birth weight (see Chapter 2). The appropriateness of the cutoff values to define anemia and iron deficiency during early infancy is debatable. In a recent review of complementary feeding practices, Gibson et al. concluded that diets in most developing countries cannot meet the daily iron requirements of young children and that additional iron in the form of supplements or fortified products is required.[16] Iron requirements can be further increased in the presence of infections that are common in many developing countries. For example, even a light intensity hookworm infection can double a preschooler's daily iron requirement.[17] In summary, low birth weight infants and children 6 months to 2 years of age are at the highest risk of iron deficiency anemia; current recommendations include the provision of daily iron supplements in areas where anemia is highly prevalent.[18]

4.3 FUNCTIONAL CONSEQUENCES DURING PREGNANCY

Although several studies have demonstrated the benefits of iron supplementation in reducing the prevalence of anemia and improving iron stores in pregnant women,[4,19] the data on the potential benefits for the fetus and other maternal outcomes are far from conclusive.[11,20-22] A brief review of existing data on the functional consequences of nutritional anemias, especially IDA, is presented in the following sections.

4.3.1 MATERNAL MORBIDITY AND MORTALITY

Anemia can contribute to maternal morbidity and mortality by increasing the chances of dying due to hemorrhage. Severe anemia (Hb <4 g/dl) is associated with an increased risk of dying.[23] The immediate cause of death in these cases is typically cardiorespiratory failure and shock as a result of excessive blood loss and impaired oxygen delivery. The relationship between moderate forms of anemia and maternal mortality is less clear and has been the focus of recent debates.[24,25] Rush challenged the notion that reducing nutritional anemia through the use of routine iron supplements provides benefits to the mother or fetus and suggests it may even be harmful.[24] While this view represents one extreme of the debate, it is true that the epidemiological evidence to support the role of nutritional anemia, especially IDA, as a causal factor of maternal deaths is limited due to the paucity of well designed trials. This is further complicated by the ethical dilemma in which we are placed, namely how can we justify randomized controlled trials (RCTs) that would examine the efficacy of interventions such as iron supplementation during pregnancy by comparing to a placebo group who will have to be denied a treatment that is known to reduce anemia?

The best evidence to date supporting the role of anemia in maternal mortality is provided in a meta-analyses by Ross and Thomas.[25] Based on a literature search of studies published since 1976, they included twelve hospital based studies from Africa (Table 4.1) and five studies from Asia (Table 4.2). It was estimated that direct anemia deaths accounted for 7.5 (±5.1)% and 10.8 (±5.1)% of all maternal deaths for Africa and Asia, respectively, and maternal deaths attributable to hemorrhage were 21.0 (±13.9)% and 19.2 (±10.2)%, respectively. The total number of maternal deaths attributable to anemia was then calculated as the sum of (1) direct anemia deaths, (2) 25% of hemorrhagic deaths, and (3) 10% of those due to other causes, and was estimated as 20% and 22.6% for Africa and Asia, respectively. Despite the shortcomings of this approach, these findings have made significant contributions

TABLE 4.1
Summary of Study Characteristics and Attributable Risks of Maternal Mortality Due to Anemia and Hemorrhage from 14 African Studies

Author	Country	Years of Study	Type of Study	Anemia Rate	% of Total Deaths Due to Anemia	% of Total Deaths Due to Hemorrhage	Maternal Mortality Ratio
Ampofo	Ghana	1963–67	Hospital based convenience sample	n/a	1.9%	16.7%	10.8 per 1000 deliveries
Armon	Tanzania	1974–77	Hospital based convenience sample	n/a	2.5%	7.5%	1.8/1000 births
Bullough	Malawi	1977	Hospital, other maternity wards, village, convenience sample	n/a	5.2%	24.1%	1.03/1000 births
Greenwood et al.	Gambia	1982–83	Community based convenience sample	n/a	6.7%	33.0%	22/1000 deliveries
Harrison	Nigeria	1976–79	Hospital based convenience sample	10% (survivors) 11% (deaths)	6.4% (unbooked patients)	21.0% (unbooked patients)	28.6/1000 deliveries (unbooked patients)
Hartfield	Nigeria	1958–70	Hospital based convenience sample	n/a	10.5%	19.4%	27.06/1000 live births (unbooked)
Kampikaho and Irwig	Uganda	1980–86	Hospital based convenience sample	38.00%	2.9%	11.6%	2.65/1000 deliveries (abortion excluded)
Kwast et al.	Ethiopia	1981–83	Community based, two stage probablity	n/a	2.2%	6.7%	4.8/1000 live births
Lawson	Nigeria	1957–60	Hospital based convenience sample	n/a	12.2%	5.3%	10.2/1000 deliveries
Malle et al.	Mali	1989–92	Hospitals, health centers, clinics, convenience sample	n/a	5.5%	58.8% (of deaths with known cause)	2.0/1000 live births
Mhango et al.	Zambia	1982	Hospital based convenience sample	n/a	3.3%	16.6%	1.2/1000 live births
Mtimavalye et al.	Tanzania	1974–77	Hospital based convenience sample	n/a	11.9%	25.0%	2.1/1000 deliveries
Oduntan and Odunlami	Nigeria	1972–73	Hospital based, random, and convenience	n/a	9.7%	30.1%	4.7/1000 births
Ojo and Savage	Nigeria	1962–71	Hospital based convenience sample	n/a	18.6%	15.8%	8.2/1000 deliveries

Source: From Ross, J. S. and Thomas, E. L., Profiles 3 Working Note Series No. 3: Iron Deficiency Anemia and Maternal Mortality, Academy for Educational Development, Washington, D.C., 1996. With permission.

TABLE 4.2
Summary of Study Characteristics and Attributable Risks of Maternal Mortality Due to Anemia and Hemorrhage from 7 Asian Studies

Author	Country	Years of Study	Type of Study	Anemia Rate	% of Total Deaths Due to Anemia	% of Total Deaths Due to Hemorrhage	Maternal Mortality Ratio
Alauddin	Bangladesh	1982–83	Community based convenience sample	n/a	4.2%	16.7%	5.7/1000 live births
Bhatia	India	1984–85	Hospital/community convenience/random	n/a	9.2%	6.9%	8.0/1000 live births; Rate = 14.25/10,000 women 15–49, rural areas
Chi et al.	Indonesia	1976–80	Hospital based convenience sample	47.7% (rural) 31.4% (urban)	n/a	38.0%	7.0/1000 maternal cases — anemic; 2.0/1000 maternal cases — non-anemic
Kumar et al.	India	1985–86	Community based convenience sample	n/a	16.4%	18.2%	2.3/1000 live births
Llewellyn-Jones	Malaysia	1953–62	Hospital based convenience sample	3.10%	n/a	n/a	15.5/1000 (anemic); 3.5/1000 (non-anemic) (denominator unknown)
Rao	India	1960–72	Hospital based convenience sample	n/a	8.7%	18.5%	16.7/1000 births
Seyal	Pakistan	1954–65	Hospital based convenience sample	80% (<10g %) 50% (<9g %)	15.7%	16.7%	19.1/1000 deliveries

Source: From Ross, J. S. and Thomas, E. L., Profiles 3 Working Note Series No. 3: Iron Deficiency Anemia and Maternal Mortality, Academy for Educational Development, Washington, D.C., 1996. With permission.

to policy decision making. The authors contend, since the studies are largely based on hospital studies, it is more likely that the magnitude has been underestimated as (1) emergency care and interventions to prevent deaths are more likely in hospital settings, and (2) anemia related emergencies may be underrepresented to the extent that the fatigue and lethargy associated with anemia prevent timely access to health care facilities. A key concern is that there is very little information on the causes of anemia (nutritional and non-nutritional) which may vary by setting, and the extent to which interventions such as the provision of iron-folate supplements will reduce maternal mortality remains unclear.

4.3.2   PERINATAL MORTALITY

Several large observational studies have found a U shaped relationship between maternal hemoglobin levels and perinatal mortality. Using data from the National Collaborative Perinatal Project that included nearly 60,000 births in the U.S., Garn et al.[26] found the lowest rates of fetal death among women with Hb values of 95 to 105 g/l in whites and 85 to 95 g/l in blacks. In England, the lowest death rate was seen at maternal Hb levels of 104 to 132 g/l in the Cardiff Births Survey (approximately 55,000 births).[27] Lister et al.[28] found a similar U shaped relationship between maternal hematocrit and perinatal mortality among singleton births (n = 18,000) in Nigeria. However, Onadeko et al. failed to detect an association between Hb levels and stillbirths in a study of over 4000 pregnancies in Nigeria.[29] Most recently, Mola et al.,[30] in a study of hospital based deliveries in Papua New Guinea, found that the lowest stillbirth rates (14 per 1000) were seen among women whose lowest Hb values during pregnancy were between 10 and 11 g/dl.[30] Women with severe anemia (<8 g/dl) remained at increased risk of stillbirth even after adjusting for other confounding variables such as age, parity, and hypertension (adjusted odds ratio = 1.6, 95% confidence interval: 1.3, 2.0). Malaria and hookworm infestation were endemic and the mean Hb value was 100 g/l in this population. Although these studies suggest that the effects of anemia on perinatal mortality are likely only if it is severe, the causes of anemia may be different in these varied settings; few intervention trials have examined this issue.[31,32] The trial in India reported significant reductions in neonatal deaths among the iron supplemented group, but the biases as a result of the high loss to followup (40%) cannot be overlooked. In contrast, an unexpected increase in perinatal mortality was detected among a group of Finnish women who received routine iron supplementation, compared to those who received only selective supplementation,[32] suggesting adverse consequences of providing too much iron to women who are not deficient. These findings need to be interpreted cautiously and more information is needed from settings where anemia is common. It is worth noting that perinatal mortality rates were much lower than the general population for the control groups who received routine iron-folate supplements in two large intervention trials conducted in the Gambia[33] and Tanzania.[34]

4.3.3   LOW BIRTH WEIGHT

Several studies have examined the association between anemia and low birth weight with varying results. Detailed reviews of the relationship between anemia especially

IDA and birth size have also been recently published.[20-22,35,36] The major limitations are that most of the studies are observational and suffer methodological flaws (lack of data on specific nutrient status, low sample size, failure to control for energy intake, etc.) that affect the interpretation of the results. Another serious weakness is that they did not account for normal physiologic changes in hematologic parameters that occur in response to plasma volume expansion during pregnancy. Some studies do not distinguish between preterm births and intra-uterine growth retardation (IUGR), and although both lead to smaller babies, the mechanisms involved may be quite different.

4.3.3.1 Iron Deficiency

Although the association between anemia and low birth weight has been examined in several observational studies, few have included other indicators of iron status such as serum ferritin and/or the use of iron supplements. Garn et al.[26] reported that when a hemoglobin concentration below 10 g/dl was reached during any stage of pregnancy, the likelihood of low birth weight, preterm birth, and perinatal mortality increased. Similar findings were noted by Murphy et al.[27] These studies have shown that high maternal hemoglobin or hematocrit during pregnancy have been associated with poor birth outcomes, although the measurements were often made later in pregnancy and may reflect inadequate plasma volume expansion and not iron status. Significant increases in the prevalence of LBW (65 vs. 27%) have been reported among primi-gravidae women detected with early pregnancy anemia* in a study in Papua New Guinea.[37] Findings from the CDC Pregnancy Nutrition Surveillance System (PNSS) suggest that anemia during the first trimester may be associated with a high risk for low birth weight.[38] Since the time of entry varied in these data, Scanlon et al.[39] defined anemia as hemoglobin values below −2 S.D. of mean values defined by weeks of gestation, and found that women who were anemic were 30% more likely to deliver infants prematurely as well as with IUGR. Most recently, Dreyfuss et al.,[40] in a large prospective study of pregnant women in Nepal, where both IDA and low birth weight are common, found a U-shaped relationship between maternal Hb measures at various stages of pregnancy and outcomes such as birth weight and preterm delivery.

Some studies suggest that iron supplementation may reduce the prevalence of low birth weight only for severe forms of iron deficiency anemia.[41,42] In one of the better designed prospective studies, Scholl et al.[43] found that the risk of low birth weight tripled and risk of preterm delivery more than doubled from iron deficiency based on serum ferritin values among 800 inner city gravidae in Camden, NJ. These risks remained even after adjusting for several confounding variables such as entry to prenatal care, age, etc. In contrast to the above findings, Goldenberg et al.[44] in a prospective follow up study of 580 African American women, found that those in the highest quartile of plasma ferritin levels at 26 weeks were at increased risk for preterm delivery and low birth weight compared to those with lower plasma ferritin levels. Tamura et al.[45] found that serum ferritin concentrations were negatively cor-related with gestational age at birth ($p = 0.034$) in a similar population. These

---

* Hemoglobin values below 8 g/dl.

findings suggest that increased serum ferritin levels act as a marker of subclinical infections and therefore pose a problem when used as a measure of iron status.

Although well designed, randomized, controlled trials (RCTs) provide clearer answers, few intervention trials have examined the impact of improving iron status on birth outcomes, especially in settings where the prevalence of nutritional anemia is high. This may be explained by the ethical difficulties of conducting studies in settings where routine prenatal care includes iron supplementation. A brief description of studies that examined the effects of iron supplements on birth outcomes is presented in Table 4.3.[31,32,46-55] The results of some of these trials are affected by inadequate sample size, poor predictive power, lack of blinding and random allocation of treatment. Two RCTs of iron supplementation done in Finland[32] and Denmark[54] failed to detect any significant differences in birth weight. The lack of blinding and suitability of the control group who received selective iron supplementation is a major concern in the study by Hemminki et al.[32] The study by Millman et al.[54] had a better design and included a placebo, but the small sample size (n = 120) may have limited their ability to detect significant differences. In the iron treated group (n = 63), maternal mean cell volume was negatively correlated to birth weight (r = –0.29, p <0.03), and in the placebo treated group (n = 66), maternal Hb and maternal serum erythropoietin were inversely correlated to birth length (r = –0.26, p <0.05). Finally, Achadi et al.[56] demonstrated in a prospective community based study in West Java, Indonesia, that the consumption of one or more iron tablets (200 mg ferrous sulphate and 0.25 mg folic acid) per week was associated with increased neonatal weight (172 g) and length (1 cm) even after controlling for several maternal and neonatal factors. Although of important policy significance, the absence of a control group and data on biochemical indicators makes it more difficult to interpret the findings.

Menendez et al.,[49] in a randomized placebo trial of pregnant women in The Gambia, reported that the mean birth weight of infants born to supplemented women increased by 56 g compared to the controls. Although this difference was not statistically significant, it represents an important effect (20% of a standard deviation) and was accompanied by significant reductions in the prevalence of anemia and iron deficiency; a positive dose response relationship was observed between birth weight and the degree of iron deficiency. Preziosi et al.[55] also found that infants born to women who began daily iron supplements (100 mg) beginning at 28 weeks of pregnancy were 30 g heavier and 0.7 cm longer at birth, compared to children of women who received placebos. Although the differences in birth weight were not statistically significant due to the small sample size and resulting lack of statistical power, these findings suggest the strong potential of iron supplementation in improving birth size in certain settings.

4.3.3.2 Folate and Vitamin B$_{12}$ Deficiency

The importance of preconceptual folate status in preventing neural tube defects has been well established.[57-59] Less is known, however, about the importance of folate and vitamin B$_{12}$ for outcomes such as fetal growth and length of gestation. Several prospective studies have reported a positive association between folate and birth weight.[35] For example, Scholl et al.[60] found that both low dietary intakes of folate

TABLE 4.3
Description of Experimental Trials of Iron Supplementation and Pregnancy Outcomes

Investigator (Year)	Study Site	Nature of Intervention[a]		Number of Subjects	Weeks Pregnant	Results		
		Experimental Group	Control Group			Birth Weight	Length of Gestation	Perinatal Mortality[b]
Paintin et al. 1966	Scotland	115 mg Fe	Placebo	173	20–36	—	n/a	n/a
Fleming et al. 1974	Australia	60 mg Fe + 5 mg FA	Placebo	146	20	—	n/a	n/a
Sood et al. 1975	India	30/60/120/240 mg Fe + 5 mg FA + 100 µg/2 wk B$_{12}$	Placebo	647	22	—	n/a	n/a
Whiteside et al. 1968	Australia	200 mg Fe	—	60	12	↑	—	n/a
Romslo et al. 1983	Finland	200 mg Fe	Placebo	45	???	—	n/a	n/a
Zittoun et al. 1983	France	105 mg Fe + 500 mg Vit C	Placebo	203	28	—	—	n/a
de Benaze et al. 1989	France	45 mg Fe	Placebo	191	22	n/a	—	n/a
Agarwal et al. 1991	India	60 mg Fe + 500 µg FA	Placebo	418	???	↑	→	→
Hemminki et al. 1991	Finland	100 mg Fe	50 mg Fe[c]	2694	10	—	→	→
Menendez et al. 1994	Gambia	60 mg Fe + 5 mg FA	5 mg FA	550	24	↑	—	n/a
Milman et al. 1994	Denmark	66 mg Fe	Placebo	120	14–16	—	—	n/a
Preizosi et al. 1997	Niger	100 mg Fe	Placebo	209	28	—	—	n/a

[a] Fe = elemental Fe; FA = folic acid; n/a = not available; Hb = hemoglobin; all are daily doses unless otherwise indicated.
[b] Perinatal mortality includes fetal deaths >28 weeks of gestation and neonatal deaths until the 7th day postpartum.
[c] Supplemented only if Hb < 100g

(<240 µg/day) and lower concentrations of serum folate measured at 28 weeks of pregnancy were associated with a twofold increased risk of preterm delivery and term LBW even after controlling for several maternal characteristics. Most of the experimental trials have compared iron-folate to iron alone and the findings are mixed (Table 4.4).[61-71] Two early studies, conducted in India reported increased birth weight using a design that compared iron to iron-folate supplementation. The dropout rates were large leaving in question the validity of the findings.[66,67] In an RCT conducted in Denmark, the infants in the folic acid group were 12.7% heavier than those in the control group (p <0.01).[70] In contrast, other studies conducted in developed countries showed no benefits of folic acid supplements on fetal growth. In summary, there is a need for well designed experimental trials in settings where folate deficiency and LBW are more common. There is even less information on the role of vitamin B_{12}.

4.3.3.3   Multinutrient Deficiencies

Based on our knowledge of the interrelationships between iron and other micronutrients, namely zinc, folate, and vitamin A metabolism, the potential benefits and disadvantages of these interactions on pregnancy outcomes are of interest. Zinc supplements can interfere with the absorption and availability of iron.[72] Zavaleta et al.[73] reported that the inclusion of 15 mg of zinc in the prenatal supplement containing iron did not adversely affect maternal and neonatal iron status; it improved zinc status and other infant outcomes in a large randomized controlled trial in Peru. There were no differences in birth weight. Cherry et al.,[74] in a randomized trial using a daily supplement of either zinc gluconate (30 mg zinc) or placebo that was combined with routine iron supplementation, found that women with lower ferritin values had infants who were longer compared to the infants of zinc treated women who entered prenatal care later and with adequate ferritin levels.* Head and chest circumferences were larger in infants born to zinc treated anemic women. Recent controlled trials have shown that improving vitamin A status during pregnancy improves hematological indices[75] and reduces maternal mortality by almost half,[76] but it is unlikely to reduce low birth weight.[34]

Anemia often results from the deficiency of several nutrients; it has been hypothesized that multiple micronutrient deficiencies rather than single nutrient deficiencies are more likely to cause adverse birth outcomes.[77] Several studies reported the benefits of multivitamin supplements, especially with folic acid, reducing the rate of neural tube and birth defects such as cleft palate and cleft lip, but few studies examined outcomes such as birth weight, maternal, and infant mortality, which are of greater public health significance. Kullander and Kallen, in a prospective study of drugs and pregnancy conducted in the 1960s in Sweden, found that the prevalence of LBW was significantly lower among women who reported the use of iron and/or multivitamin mineral supplements during pregnancy.[78] However, data on other potential confounding factors, such as the use of prenatal care, smoking, and other nutritional factors that may have been associated with supplement use were lacking. In the large RCT of periconceptual multivitamin supplementation in Hungary,[58]

---

* All women received iron supplementation upon entry into prenatal care.

TABLE 4.4
Description of Experimental Trials of Folic Acid Supplementation and Pregnancy Outcomes

Investigator (Year)	Study Site	Nature of Intervention[a]		Number of Subjects	Weeks Pregnant	Results		
		Experimental Group	Control Group			Birth Weight	Length of Gestation	Perinatal Mortality
Fleming et al. 1968	Nigeria	5 mg FA	Placebo	75	???	—	n/a	n/a
Baumslag et al. 1970	S. Africa	5 mg FA + 200 mg Fe	Placebo	183	24–28	↓c	↓c	n/a
Rae and Robb, 1970	Liverpool	5 mg FA + 200 mg Fe	200 mg Fe	698	13	↓c	n/a	n/a
Fletcher et al. 1971	England	5 mg FA + 200 mg Fe	200 mg Fe	643	???	—	n/a	n/a
Giles et al. 1971	Australia	5 mg FA+ 200 mg Fe	200 mg Fe	620	10–30	—	—	←
Iyengar et al. 1971	India	100 to 300 µg FA + 60 mg Fe	60 mg Fe	114	20–24	←	—	—
Iyengar et al. 1975	India	500 µg FA + 60 mg Fe	60 mg Fe	189	20–28	←	—	—
Trigg et al. 1976	England	0.05 mg FA + 50 mg Fe	50 mg Fe	158	???	—	n/a	n/a
Rolschau, 1979	Denmark	5 mg FA + MVM	MVM without FA	36	21–25	←	n/a	n/a
Tchernia et al. 1981	France	350 µg FA + 105 mg Fe	Fe	109	28	←	→	n/a
Fleming et al. 1986	Nigeria	1 mg FA + 60 mg Fe	60 mg Fe	200	<24	—	n/a	—
Cziezel et al. 1993	Hungary	MVM (incl 15 mg FA)	Trace elements	4704	<0b	→	—	—

[a] FA = folic acid; Fe = iron; MV = multivitamins; MVM = multivitamin mineral; all are daily doses

[b] Supplementation stopped at 12 weeks, whereas others were until delivery

[c] Significant effects

although the rates of LBW, prematurity, miscarriages, and stillbirths were similar for both study groups (Group I received multivitamins and trace elements whereas Group II received only trace elements preconceptually to 12 weeks gestation) suggesting a lack of any added benefit for periconceptual multivitamin supplementation. The most compelling evidence comes from a recent RCT of HIV+ pregnant women in Tanzania.[34] Significant reductions in low birth weight and mortality were found among those who received multivitamins compared to iron-folate supplements after 28 weeks of gestation. The generalizability of these findings needs to be confirmed and several trials are underway to address this question.

4.3.4   Iron Status of the Infant at Birth

Contrary to earlier findings, recent reviews point to evidence that (1) the maternofetal unit is dependent on exogenous iron, and (2) the level of iron stores in the newborn is related to maternal iron status during pregnancy.[19,21,79] Many of the studies that failed to detect an association were observational studies; they measured iron status late in pregnancy among women who were not iron deficient and used cord blood indicators of newborn iron status, which may not be reflective of iron stores. Studies from India and Nigeria have reported associations between maternal iron status at delivery and cord blood ferritin levels, in contrast to those conducted in settings where the prevalence of IDA is much lower.[31,41,80-82] As suggested by Allen,[21] the benefits of iron supplementation for infant outcomes may vary by the timing and duration of supplementation during pregnancy, compliance, and length of follow-up during infancy. Significant differences have been found in the iron status of older infants, i.e., after 2 months of age, when they are more susceptible to iron deficiency, if they do not receive additional iron from nonbreast milk sources, as a function of maternal iron status. De Benaze et al.[52] found that at 2 months postpartum, the serum ferritin values were double among infants whose mothers received 45 mg Fe (238 µg/dl) daily from early pregnancy (3 to 4.5 months after conception) to delivery compared to those who received placebos (111 µg/dl). A large epidemiologic investigation examined the relationship between maternal and infant iron deficiency. Infants of anemic mothers were almost 6 times more likely to become anemic by the first year of life even after adjusting for several confounding factors such as socioeconomic status, feeding practices, and morbidity.[83] Most importantly, the evidence from the few controlled trials of iron supplementation suggest that children born to iron treated mothers have higher serum ferritin levels compared to those who received a placebo.[50,54,55] Low birth weight infants are at greater risk of lowered iron stores at birth. They are more likely to develop anemia earlier and suffer the adverse consequences of impaired motor and mental development.

4.4   FUNCTIONAL CONSEQUENCES
DURING LACTATION

4.4.1   Breast Milk Volume and Composition

The mother's nutritional status during pregnancy and/or lactation should, in theory, affect the growth and development of the newborn during the early postnatal period by determining the level of nutrient reserves in the newborn and the breast milk quantity and quality, including micronutrient concentrations. Allen[84] identified iron as a priority II nutrient i.e., the iron content of breast milk is relatively protected and not influenced by maternal nutritional status, but depletion of maternal stores can result among poorly nourished women who are already anemic prior to lactation. Although few intervention trials have examined the effects of anemia on lactation performance, a randomized clinical trial of pregnant women in Niger[85] showed that iron supplementation during the last trimester of pregnancy did not alter the concentrations of iron, copper, selenium, and zinc in breast milk. In contrast, there is evidence that the breast milk level of other hemopoietic nutrients such as folic acid, vitamin A, and vitamin B_{12} are affected by maternal status.[84]

4.4.2 MATERNAL NUTRITIONAL STATUS

Studies have shown that anemia is common among lactating women,[13] which can have adverse consequences for the health, productivity, and ability to take care of the child. The consequences can be worse if she conceives again shortly after delivery. Scanlon et al.[86] reported a high prevalence of postpartum anemia among participants of the Womens Infants and Children (WIC) Program: the main predictor was anemia during pregnancy. The benefits of iron supplementation during pregnancy to reduce risk of anemia during pregnancy and improve iron stores beyond 6 months postpartum are well established.[21] It is important to note that these benefits have been seen even among women who received supplements later in pregnancy and women from industrialized nations who had adequate iron status.[54] Although providing supplements during lactation is not contraindicated, the efficiency of absorption is much higher during pregnancy. In contrast to iron, the requirements for folate and vitamin B_{12} are increased during lactation and megaloblastic anemia has been reported among lactating women.[87,88] Ensuring adequate intakes of all hemopoietic nutrients during pregnancy and lactation is critical. Studies which include lactating women are needed in settings where the prevalence of anemia is high.

4.5 FUNCTIONAL CONSEQUENCES DURING EARLY CHILDHOOD

4.5.1 CHILD MORBIDITY AND MORTALITY

Several micronutrients play essential roles in immune function, including vitamins A, B_1, B_2, B_6, B_{12}, C, E, folic acid, zinc, and iron. Deficiencies are likely to influence the rate of infection and/or duration and severity. Severe anemia, especially when encountered during times of physiological stress such as during an infection, is associated with increased morbidity and mortality rates in children. Anemia during pregnancy can indirectly increase infant mortality and poor growth and development from being born preterm and/or small for gestational age. Compared to newborns of normal weight, low birth weight infants are at higher risk of morbidity and mortality, growth retardation during the postnatal period, long term adverse effects on physical and mental performance, and perhaps an excess risk of adult chronic disease.[89] Less is known about the direct effects of maternal anemia on infant health outcomes. Higher Apgar scores were found at birth for infants born to mothers in the iron supplemented group compared to the placebo in the RCT conducted in Nigeria.[55] Van den Broeck et al. reported that among young children under 5 years of age in rural Zaire, severe anemia, primarily due to iron deficiency, was the second greatest cause of death.[90]

Iron deficiency anemia has been found to adversely affect immune function and to increase susceptibility to infection under laboratory conditions. Iron deficiency has been shown to both impair the responses of T cells to mitogens and decrease the bactericidal activity of neutrophils *in vitro*.[91] The relationship of iron status, immunity, and infections in young children remains controversial. Some studies have demonstrated impaired cell immunity as a result of iron deficiency,[92] whereas others did not show any effect.[93] Similarly, iron deficiency has been shown to have a protective effect on some infections such as malaria,[94] whereas intervention trials have shown that the incidence of morbidity is not affected[95,96] or even reduced by iron supplementation.[97] The reasons for these different findings may be due to confounding variables. For instance, acute infections are known to block erythropoiesis, thus reducing hemoglobin levels and complicating the causal relationship of iron deficiency and immune function. Evidence from the recent controlled trials in young children (see Table 4.5) indicates that short term iron supplementation does not increase the incidence of common childhood infections such as diarrhea or respiratory illness[98-102] or increase malaria susceptibility.[96,103]

4.5.2　CHILD GROWTH

Anemia, especially IDA is associated with poor physical growth. The evidence based on intervention trials is controversial and limited for preschool age children. The results of intervention trials using iron, vitamin B_{12}, folate, and multinutrient supplements to improve young child growth are described in the following sections.

4.5.2.1　Iron

Iron deficiency may impair growth through its effects on immunity and appetite as well as its metabolic role in thermogenesis and thyroid hormone metabolism.[104-106] Although many observational studies have examined the relationship between iron deficiency, especially anemia, and growth,[107-109] the results are difficult to interpret, primarily due to potential reverse causality and confounding. For example, rapid growth with marginal iron intakes can lead to iron depletion; children who grow slowly may appear iron replete. The common causes of iron deficiency, especially parasitic infections such as malaria and hookworm, may also have direct effects on child growth. Finally, poor iron intakes often coexist with a variety of other nutrient deficiencies, e.g., vitamin A, zinc, and protein, that may affect growth.

Well designed intervention trials, especially among preschool children, are surprisingly few in number.[110] The randomized placebo controlled intervention trials that have demonstrated the benefits of iron supplementation on child growth have

TABLE 4.5
Results of Intervention Trials of Iron Supplementation and Growth and Morbidity in Preschool Age Children

Investigators (Year)	Study Site	Ages of Subjects	Characteristics of Subjects	Sample Size	Intervention Dose/d	Intervention Duration	Results[a] Growth Weight Gain	Results[a] Growth Height Gain	Results[a] Morbidity
Judisch et al. (1966)	USA	<3 y	Anemic	156	6 mg/kg	8 wks[b]	+	n/a	n/a
Migasena et al. (1972)	Thailand	6 mo–5 y	Anemic	48	10 mg	16 wks	n.s.	n.s.	n/a
Auckett et al. (1986)	UK	1.5 y	Anemic	97	24 mg	8 wks	+	n/a.	n/a
Soewendo et al. (1989)	Indonesia	<3 y	All	127	50 mg	8 wks	n.s.	n.s.	n/a
Bhatia et al. (1993)	India	3–5 y	All	170	3 mg/kg	24 wks	+[d]	n/a	n/a
Angeles et al. (1993)	Indonesia	2–5 y	Anemic, low WAZ[c]	76	30 mg	8 wks	n.s.	+	+[e]
Idjradinata et al. (1994)	Indonesia	1–1.5 y	Fe-replete	47	3 mg/kg	16 wks	−	n.s.	n.s.
Rosado et al. (1997)	Mexico	18–36 mo	All	219	20 mg	16 wks	n.s.	n.s.	n.s.
Dewey et al. (2000)	Sweden Honduras	4 mo	Term, fully breastfed to 6 mo	232	1 mg/kg 1 mg/kg	4–9 mo 6–9 mo	n.s.	—	n/a
Hussein et al. (1988)	Egypt	2–6 y	All	319	25 mg	10 wks	n/a	n/a	+[e]
Mejia et al. (1988)	Guatemala	1–8 y	Anemic	99	3 mg/kg	2 mo	n/a	n/a	n.s.
Mitra et al. (1997)	Bangladesh	2–48 mo	All	349	12.5 mg	15 mo	n/a	n/a	n.s.

[a] = '+' — positive effects; '−' negative effects; n.s. = not significant; n/a = not available
[b] = no control group
[c] = WAZ = weight for age Z score
[d] = only in anemic children
[e] = differences found only in incidence not duration

been conducted, paradoxically, among older primary school age children.[111,112] A brief description of the intervention trials of iron supplementation on growth of young children is presented in Table 4.5. With respect to preschool age children, an early landmark study by Judisch et al.[113] found that oral iron supplements (6 mg/kg/day) given to severely anemic children (Hb <9 g/dl) improved weight gain and that the proportion of children below the third percentile for weight/age increased from 14.8 to 2.3%. The study had no control group for comparison and linear growth was not reported. Two other studies reported increased weight gains in nonanemic boys.[114,115] A relationship between iron nutriture and child growth is also suggested by an observational study from Bangladesh where children consuming tubewell water lower in iron content were shorter (HAZ = –2.45) than those drinking water with normal iron content (HAZ = –2.1)[116] though confounding by socioeconomic status is likely (HAZ = Height for age 'Z' score). In contrast, a study from Thailand failed to show any benefits of iron supplementation on the growth of preschool age children.[117] Since the hematologic response to treatment was mixed, other factors such as inadequate dosage, hookworm infection, and mixing of treatment with placebo (reported by others) may have affected these results. Rosado et al.[100] found that iron supplementation did not improve the growth of preschool Mexican children, despite a high prevalence of iron deficiency, a one year follow up period, and improvements in iron status based on serum ferritin values. Interestingly, both iron status and hemoglobin levels improved significantly in the placebo group for reasons unknown to the authors. Morbidity was similar in both groups.

To date, two randomized double blind intervention trials conducted in different populations (England, Indonesia) have shown that iron supplements improve the growth of anemic preschool age children.[118,119] Their results differ. In the British study,[118] anemic children aged 17 to 19 months received 24 mg iron/day with vitamin C for 8 weeks and had increased weight gain compared to the controls. Length was not reported. The study from Indonesia[119] reported the positive effect of iron supplementation only on linear growth (2.7 cm vs. 1.5 cm) among low-weight-for-age (<–2 weight for age Z score) anemic children following 8 weeks of supplementation. These effects were accompanied by reductions in morbidity and improved attention and performance.[120] Another controlled trial from India[121] also demonstrated increased weight gain among anemic preschool age children, but it is not clear whether the treatment was randomly assigned.

Although some have speculated that the duration of follow up may be inadequate in some of these studies, there are positive findings for similar follow up periods; the recent Mexican study failed to detect any improvements in growth even with a one year follow up period.[100] It appears more likely that there is a differential growth response to iron supplementation which depends on the degree of iron depletion, baseline nutritional status, and the underlying causes of iron deficiency. Few studies have included adequate measures of iron nutriture. The evidence to date suggests a nonlinear relationship between iron nutriture and child growth in that positive findings have been limited to anemic children who are severely iron deficient. Notably, evidence suggests potential adverse effects of iron supplementation on the growth of iron replete children.[122,123]

4.5.2.2   Vitamin B$_{12}$ and Folic Acid

Studies showing the importance of animal foods in promoting growth,[124] suggest a possible role of vitamin B$_{12}$ for optimal growth. These findings need to be interpreted cautiously since low intakes of animal foods are often associated with other potentially confounding factors such as socioeconomic status and poor diet diversity which contribute to inadequate intakes of other nutrients (protein, iron, zinc, and vitamin A) also related to growth. Neumann and Harrison[125] reported a positive association between maternal vitamin B$_{12}$ intake during lactation and linear growth of infants in Kenya even after controlling for maternal energy intake. Vitamin B$_{12}$ intake from complementary feeding also predicted length at 6 months. Unfortunately, no well designed intervention studies that examined the impact of vitamin B$_{12}$ on child growth could be identified in the literature.

In the only study of its kind, Foged et al.[126] found that daily folic acid supplementation did not affect postnatal growth in a randomized placebo controlled trial of small-for-gestational-age infants born at term. In contrast, Matoth et al.[127] reported that attained weight and length at 2 and 6 months were greater among infants whose folate levels were above the median in response to daily supplements of folic acid. The role of folic acid on child growth needs further examination.

4.5.2.3   Multinutrient Deficiencies

Few studies have examined the impact of multiple micronutrient supplementation on young child growth. One study in Thailand failed to detect any effect of multivitamin-mineral supplement on growth.[128] The extent of the deficiency and appropriateness of the dosage, whether treatment was randomly allocated, and whether the analysis accounted for the fact that the treatment was allocated at village level are unclear in this study. In China, a micronutrient fortified rusk containing extra zinc, iron, calcium, vitamins A, D and B$_{12}$, thiamin, riboflavin, niacin, and folic acid was used in a randomized double blind intervention trial of 236 children aged 6 to 13 months.[129] Although significant improvements in iron and vitamin A status were found, growth increments were similar in both groups. Unfortunately, data on breast feeding were not provided and it is plausible that benefits may not have been seen in this age group compared to older children, i.e., 12 to 24 months.

Two intervention trials using daily multiple micronutrient supplements found improved growth among subgroups of children namely those who were stunted at baseline[130] as well as among females and children under 12 months of age.[131] In contrast, two studies found no difference in growth among young children and school age children who received micronutrient fortified food supplements compared to unfortified food supplements.[129,132] No differences were seen at follow-up (1 to 2 years later) in the study from Mexico. A significant difference in height (0.6 cm) and HAZ (0.21) was originally observed among children who received multiple micronutrients when compared to those who received placebos.[131,133]

In conclusion, improvements in child growth following iron supplementation may be limited to anemic children who are severely iron deficient. These findings suggest that iron supplementation should be targeted and there is a need to better understand whether moderate to mild iron depletion impairs child growth. The role of other nutrients that cause anemia and multinutrient deficiencies need to be addressed as poor child growth seen in developing countries may be due to multiple nutrient deficiencies and poor dietary quality.

4.5.3 OTHER EFFECTS

Iron deficiency anemia has also been associated with an increased susceptibility to lead poisoning. Poor iron status has been shown to increase the gastrointestinal absorption and tissue concentrations of lead.[134] The adverse effects of lead toxicity appear to be more severe among iron deficient individuals.[134] Appetite can also be reduced as a result of nutritional anemia especially IDA, but this has not been examined in young children.

4.6 CONCLUSIONS

Nutritional anemias during the vulnerable periods of intrauterine life and early childhood have adverse consequences for both mother and child. The debate is related to the severity of the question. While there is clear evidence related to severe anemia, the relationships between moderate and mild forms of anemia are less clear especially for outcomes such as low birth weight and growth. It will be difficult to answer these questions by conducting placebo controlled trials in settings where the prevalence of anemia is high and has adverse consequences other than those related to reproductive health. The need is for well designed program evaluations that can provide useful answers for policy makers. The results of careful meta-analyses are also valuable. For example, Rasmussen[20] in a thorough review of the literature on IDA estimated the attributable risk for severe and moderate anemia ranged from 23 to 67% and 9 to 30%, respectively for a preterm baby. These estimates were 34 to 83% and 42 to 55%, respectively, for a low birth weight baby. Finally the interactions between other important infectious diseases such as malaria and HIV and nutrient deficiencies need to be examined.

REFERENCES

1. Koblinsky, M. A., Beyond maternal mortality: magnitude, interrelationship, and consequences of women's health, pregnancy-related complications and nutritional status on pregnancy outcomes, *Int. J. Gynecol. Obstet.,* 48, S21, 1995.
2. Fourth Report on the World Nutrition Situation, World Health Organization, Geneva, 2000.
3. Revised 1990 estimates of maternal mortality: a new approach, World Health Organization and United Nations Children's Fund, Geneva, April 1996, 20.
4. Institute of Medicine, *Nutrition during Pregnancy. Part II: Nutrient Supplements,* National Academy Press, Washington, D.C., 1990.
5. Bentley, D. P., Iron metabolism and anaemia during pregnancy, *Clinical Haema.,* 14(3), 613, 1985.
6. Centers for Disease Control, CDC Criteria for anaemia in children and child bearing-aged women, *MMWR,* 38, 400, 1989.

7. Klebanoff, M. A., Shiono, P. H., Berendes, H. W., Rhoads, G. G., Facts and artifacts about anemia and preterm delivery, *J. Am. Med. Assoc.,* 262, 511, 1990.

8. Scholl, T. O. and Hediger, M. L., Anemia and iron deficiency anemia: compilation of data on pregnancy outcome, *Am. J. Clinical Nutr.,* 59 (2 Suppl.), 492S, 1994.

9. Hallberg, L., Iron balance in pregnancy, in *Vitamins and Minerals in Pregnancy and Lactation,* Berger, H., Ed., Raven Press, New York, 115, 1988.

10. National Research Council, Recommended Dietary Allowances, 10th ed., National Academy Press, Washington, D.C., 1989.

11. United States Preventive Services Task Force, Routine iron supplementation during pregnancy, policy statement. *J. Am. Med. Assoc.,* 23(270), 2846, 1993.

12. Institute of Medicine, Meeting maternal nutrient needs during lactation, in *Nutrition during Lactation,* National Academy Press, Washington, D.C., 213, 1990.

13. Stoltzfus, R. J., Rethinking anaemia surveillance, *Lancet,* 349, 1764, 1997.

14. Yip, R. and Dallmann, P., Iron, in *Present Knowledge in Nutrition,* Ziegler, E. and Filer, L., Eds., ILSI Press, Washington, D.C., 277, 1995.

15. Dallman, P. R., Siimes, M.A., et al., Iron deficiency in infancy and childhood, *Am. J. Clinical Nutr.,* 33(1), 86, 1980.

16. Gibson, R. S., Ferguson, E L., et al., Complementary foods for infant feeding in developing countries: their nutrient adequacy and improvement, *Eur. J. Clinical Nutr.,* 52(10), 764, 1998.

17. Stoltzfus, R. J., Dreyfuss, M. L., Chwaaya, H. M., and Albinoco, M., Hookworm control as a strategy to prevent iron deficiency, *Nutr. Rev.,* 55(6), 223, 1997.

18. Stolzfus, R. J. and Dreyfuss, M. L., Guidelines for the use of iron supplements to prevent and treat iron deficiency anemia, International Anemia Consultative Group, World Health Organization, and United Nations Children's Fund, Washington, D.C., 1998.

19. Milman, N., Bergholt, T., Byg, K.E., Eriksen, L., and Graudal, N., Iron status and iron balance during pregnancy. A critical reappraisal of iron supplementation, *Acta Obstet. Gynecol. Scan.,* 78, 749, 1999.

20. Rasmussen, K.M., Is there a causal relationship between iron deficiency or iron deficiency anemia or anemia and weight at birth, length of gestation and perinatal mortality? Cornell University, February, 2000 (in preparation).

21. Allen, L H., Anemia and iron deficiency: effects on pregnancy outcome, *Amer. J. Clinical Nutr.,* 71(5S), 1280S, 2000.

22. Mahomed, K., Routine iron supplementation in pregnancy, in *Pregnancy and Childbirth Module, Cochrane Database of Systematic Reviews,* 2nd ed., Enkin, M. W., Keirse, M. J. N. C., Renfrew, M. J., and Neilson, J. P., Eds., Oxford, U.K., 1993.

23. The Prevalence of Anemia in Women: A Tabulation of available information, 2nd ed., World Health Organization, Geneva, 1992, 1.

24. Rush, D., Nutrition and maternal mortality in the developing world, paper prepared for OMNI and INACG, 1998.

25. Ross, J. S. and Thomas, E. L., PROFILES 3 Working Notes Series No. 3: Iron Deficiency Anemia and Maternal Mortality, Academy for Educational Development, Washington, D.C., 1996.

26. Garn, S. M., Ridella, S. A., Petzold, A. S., and Falkner, F., Maternal hematologic levels and pregnancy outcomes, *Semin. Perinatol.,* 5, 155, 1981.

27. Murphy, J. F., O'Riordan, J., Newcombe, R. G., Coles, E. C., and Pearson, J. F., Relation of hemoglobin levels in first and second trimesters to outcome of pregnancy, *Lancet,* 1, 992, 1986.

28. Lister, U. G., Rossiter, C. E., and Chong, H., Perinatal mortality, *Br. J. Obstet. Gynaecol. Suppl.,* 5, 86, 1985.

29. Onadeko, M. O., Avokey, F., Lawoyin, T. O., Observations on stillbirths, birthweight and maternal haemoglobin in teenage pregnancy in Ibadan, Nigeria, *Afr. J. Med. Sci.,* 25, 81, 1996.

30. Mola, G., Permezel, M., Amoa, A. B., and Klufio, C. A., Anaemia and perinatal outcome in Port Moresby, *Aust. N.Z. J. Obstet. Gynaecol.,* 39(1), 31, 1999.

31. Agarwal, K. N., Agarwal, D. K., and Mishra, K. P., Impact of anaemia prophylaxis in pregnancy on maternal haemoglobin, serum ferritin and birth weight, *Indian J. Med. Res.,* 94, 277, 1991.

32. Hemminki, E. and Rimpela, U., A randomized comparison of routine versus selective iron supplementation during pregnancy, *J. Am. Coll. Nutr.,* 10(1), 3, 1991.

33. Ceesay, S. N., Prentice, A. M., Cole, T. J., Foord, F., Weaver, L. T., Poskitt, E. M. E., and Whitehead, R. G., Effects on birth weight and perinatal mortality of maternal dietary supplements in rural Gambia: 5 year randomized controlled trial, *Br. Med. J.,* 315, 786, 1997.

34. Fawzi, W. W., Msamanga, G. I., Spiegelman, D., et al., Randomized trial of effects of vitamin supplements on pregnancy outcomes and T cell counts in HIV-1-infected women in Tanzania, *Lancet,* 351, 1477, 1998.

35. Steer, P. J., Maternal hemoglobin concentration and birth weight, *Amer. J. Clinical Nutr.,* 71(5S), 1285S, 2000.

36. Ramakrishnan, U., Manjrekar, R., Rivera, J., Gonzales-Cossio, T., and Martorell, R., Micronutrients and Pregnancy Outcome: A Review of the Literature, *Nutr. Res.*, 19(1), 103, 1999.

37. Brabin, B. J., Ginny, M., Sapau, J., Galme, K., and Paino, J., Consequences of maternal anaemia on outcome of pregnancy in a malaria endemic area in Papua New Guinea, *Ann. Trop. Med. Parasitol.,* 84(1), 11, 1990.

38. Kim, I., Hungerford, D. W., Yip, R., Kuester, S. A., Zyrkowski, C., and Trowbridge, F. L., Pregnancy nutrition surveillance system, United States, 1979-1990, *MMWR CDC Surveillance Summaries,* 41(7), 25, 1992.

39. Scanlon K. S., personal communication 1997.

40. Dreyfuss, M. L., Stolzfus, R. J., Shrestha, J. B., Khatry, S. K., Shrethsa, S. R., Pradhan, E. K., and West, K. P., Jr., Pregnancy anemia and neonatal weight in rural Nepal, International Congress of Nutrition, Montreal, July 27–August 1, 1997.

41. Bhargava, M., Kumar, R., Iyer, P. U., Ramji, S., Kapani, V., and Bhargava, S. K., Effect of maternal anemia and iron depletion on foetal iron stores, birthweight and gestation, *Acta Ped. Scand.,* 78, 321, 1989.

42. Swain, S., Singh, S., Bhatia, B.D., Pandey, S., and Krishna, M., Maternal hemoglobin and serum albumin and fetal growth, *Indian Pediatr.,* 31(7), 777, 1994.

43. Scholl, T. O., Hediger, M. L., Fischer, R. L., and Shearer, J. W., Anemia vs. iron deficiency: increased risk of preterm delivery in a prospective study, *Am. J. Clinical Nutr.,* 55(5), 985, 1992.

44. Goldenberg, R. L., Tamura, T., Dubard, M., Johnston, K. E., Copper, R. L., and Neggers, Y., Plasma ferritin and pregnancy outcome, *Am. J. Obstet. Gynecol.,* 175, 1356, 1996.

45. Tamura, T., Goldenburg, R. L., Johnston, K. E., Cliver, S. P., and Hickey, C., Serum Ferritin: a predictor of early spontaneous preterm delivery, *Obstet. Gynecol.,* 87, 360, 1996.

46. Paintin, D. B., Thomson, A. M., and Hytten, F. E., Iron and the hemoglobin level in pregnancy, *J. Obstet. Gynaecol. Br. Commonw.,* 73, 181, 1966.

47. Whiteside, M. G., Ungar, B., and Cowling, D. C., Iron, folic acid and vitamin B_{12} levels in normal pregnancy, and their influence on birth weight and the duration of pregnancy, *Med. J. Aust.,* 338, 1968.

48. Fleming, A. F., Martin, J. D., and Stenhouse, N. S., Obstetric outcome in pregnancies complicated by recurrent anaemia, with observations on iron and folate metabolism, bacteriuria and pre-eclampsia, *Aust. N.Z. J. Obstet. Gynaecol.,* 14, 204, 1974.

49. Sood, S. K., Ramachandran, K., and Mathur, M., WHO sponsored collaborative studies on nutritional anaemia in India. 1. The effect of supplemental oral iron administration to pregnant women, *Q. J. Med.,* 174, 251, 1975.

50. Romslo, I., Haram, K., Sagen, N., and Augensen, K., Iron requirement in normal pregnancy as assessed by serum ferritin, serum transferrin saturation and erythrocyte protoporphyrin determinations, *Br. J. Obstet. Gynaecol.,* 90(2), 101, 1983.

51. Zittoun, J., Blot, I., Hill, C., Papiernik, E., and Tchernia, G., Iron supplements versus placebo during pregnancy: its effects on iron and folate status on mothers and new-borns, *Annu. Nutr. Metab.,* 27, 320, 1983.

52. De Benaze, C., Galan, P., Wainer, R., and Hercberg, S., Prevention de l'anemie ferriprive au course de la grossesse par une supplémentation martiale précoce: un essai controlé. (Prevention of iron deficiency anemia in pregnancy by using early iron supplementation: a controlled trial), *Rev. Epidémiol. Santé Publique.,* 37, 109, 1989.

53. Menendez, C., Todd, J., Alonso, P. L., Francis, N., Lulat, S., Ceesay, S., M'Boge, B., and Greenwood, B. M., The effects of iron supplementation during pregnancy, given by traditional birth attendants, on the prevalence of anaemia and malaria, *Trans. R. Soc. Trop. Med. Hyg.,* 88(5), 590, 1994.

54. Milman, N., Agger, A. O., Nielsen, O. J., Iron status markers and serum erythropoietin in 120 mothers and newborn infants: effect of iron supplementation in normal pregnancy, *Acta Obstet. Gyn. Scan.,* 73, 200, 1994.

55. Preziosi, P., Prual, A., Galan, P., Daouda, H., Boureima, H., and Hercberg, S., Effect of iron supplementation on the iron status of pregnant women: consequences for newborns, *Am. J. Clinical Nutr.,* 66, 1178, 1997.

56. Achadi, E. L., Hansell, M. J., Sloan, N. L., and Anderson, M. A., Women's nutritional status, iron consumption and weight gain during pregnancy in relation to neonatal weight and length in West Java, Indonesia, *Int. J. Gyn. Obs.,* 48 (Suppl S103), 1995.

57. MRC Vitamin Study Research Group, Prevention of neural tube defects, *Lancet,* 338, 131, 1991.

58. Czeizel, A. E., Controlled studies of multivitamin supplementation on pregnancy outcomes, *Annu. N.Y. Acad. Sci.,* 678, 266, 1993.

59. Oakley, G. P., Jr., Adams, M. J., and Dickinson, C. M., Folic acid for everyone, now, *J. Nutr.,* 126, 751S, 1996.

60. Scholl, T. O., Hediger, M. L., Scholl, J. I., Khoo, C. S., and Rischer, R. L., Dietary and serum folate: their influence on the outcome of pregnancy, *Am. J. Clinical Nutr.,* 63, 520, 1996.

61. Fleming, A. F., Henrickse, J. V., and Allan, N. C., The prevention of megaloblastic anaemia in pregnancy in Nigeria, *J. Obstet. Gynaecol. Br. Commonw.,* 75, 425, 1968.

62. Rae, P. G. and Robb, P. M., Megaloblastic anemia of pregnancy: a clinical and laboratory study with particular reference to the total and labile serum folate levels, *J. Clinical Path.,* 23, 379, 1970.

63. Baumslag, N., Edelstein, T., and Metz, J., Reduction of incidence of prematurity by folic acid supplementation in pregnancy, *Br. Med. J.,* 1, 16, 1970.

64. Fletcher, J., Gull, A., Fellingham, F. R., Pranherd, T. A. J., Brant, H. A., and Menzies, D. N., The value of folic acid supplements in pregnancy, *J. Obstet. Gynaecol. Br. Commonw.,* 78, 781, 1971.

65. Giles, P. F. H., Harcourt, A. G., and Whiteside, M. G., The effect of prescribing folic acid during pregnancy on birth weight and duration of pregnancy: a double-blind trial, *Med. J. Aust.,* 2, 17, 1971.

66. Iyengar, L., Folic acid requirements of Indian pregnant women, *Am. J. Obstet. Gynecol.*, 111, 13, 1971.

67. Iyengar, L. and Rajalakshmi, K., Effect of folic acid supplementation on birth weights of infants, *Am. J. Obstet. Gynecol.*, 122(3), 332, 1975.

68. Tchernia, G., Blot, I., Rey, A., and Papiernik, E., Carences maternelles en fer et folates: répercussion sur le nouveau-né, *Sem Hôptiaux Paris*, 59, 416, 1983.

69. Trigg, K. H., Rendall, E. J. C., Johnson, A., Fellingham, F. R., and Prankerd, T. A. J., Folate supplements during pregnancy, *J. R. Coll. Gen. Pract.*, 26, 228, 1976.

70. Rolschau, J., Date, J., and Kristoffersen, K., Folic acid supplement and intrauterine growth, *Acta Obstet. Gynecol. Scand.*, 58, 343, 1979.

71. Fleming, A. F., Chatoura, G. B. S., Harrison, K. A., Briggs, N. D., and Dunn, D. T., The prevention of anaemia in pregnancy in primigravidae in the guinea savanna of Nigeria, *Annu. Trop. Med. Parasitol.*, 80, 211, 1986.

72. Caballero, B., Nutritional implications of dietary interactions: a review, *Food Nutr. Bull.*, 10(2), 9, 1988.

73. Zavaleta, N., Caulfield, L. E., and Garcia, T., Changes in iron status during pregnancy in Peruvian women receiving prenatal iron and folic acid supplements with or without zinc, *Am. J. Clinical Nutr.*, 71(4), 956, 2000.

74. Cherry, F. F., Sandstead, H. H., and Wickremasinghe, A. R., Adolescent pregnancy. Zinc supplementation and iron effects, *Annu. N.Y. Acad. Sci.*, 678, 330, 1993.

75. Suharno, D., West, C. E., Muhilal, Karyadi, D., and Hautvast, J. G., Supplementation with Vitamin A and iron for nutritional anaemia in pregnant women in West Java, Indonesia, *Lancet*, 342(8883), 1325, 1993.

76. West, K. P., Jr., Katz, J., Khatry, S. K., LeClerq, S. C., Pradhan, E. K., and Shrestha, S. R. et al., Double blind, cluster randomized trial of low dose supplementation with vitamin A or beta carotene on mortality related to pregnancy in Nepal, *Br. Med. J.*, 27, 318(7183), 570, 1999.

77. Keen, C. L. and Zidenberg, Cherr, S., Should vitamin mineral supplements be recommended for all women with childbearing potential? *Am. J. Clinical Nutr.*, 59(2)(Suppl. 532S), 1994.

78. Kullander, S. and Kallen, B., A prospective study of drugs and pregnancy. 4. Miscellaneous drugs, *Acta Obstet. Gynecol. Scand.*, 55(4), 287, 1976.

79. Blot, I., Diallo, D., and Tchernia, G., Iron deficiency in pregnancy: effects on the newborn, *Curr. Opinions Hematol.*, 6(2), 65, 1999.

80. Milman, N., Ibsen, K. K., and Christiansen, J. J., Serum ferritin and iron status in mothers and new born infants, *Acta Obstet. Gynecol. Scand.*, 66, 205, 1987.

81. Ajayi, O. A., Iron stores in pregnant Nigerians and their infants at term, *Eur. J. Clinical Nutr.*, 42, 23, 1988.

82. Okuyama, T., Tawada, T., Furuya, H., and Villee, C. A., The role of transferrin and ferritin in the fetal-maternal-placental unit, *Am. J. Obstet. Gynecol.*, 152(3), 344, 1985.

83. Colomer, J., Colomer, C., Gutierrez, D., Jubert, A., Nolasco, A., Donat, J., et al., Anaemia during pregnancy as a risk factor for infant iron deficiency: report from the Valencia Infant Anaemia Cohort (VIAC) study, *Paediat. Perinatal. Epidemiol.*, 4(2), 196, 1990.

84. Allen, L. H., Maternal micronutrient malnutrition: effects on breast feeding, infant nutrition, and priorities for intervention, in Maternal and Child Nutrition, *SCN News*, 11,21, 1994.

85. Arnaud, J., Prual, A., Preziosi, P., Cherouvrier, F., Favier, A., Galan, P., and Hercberg, S., Effect of iron supplementation during,pregnancy on trace element (Cu, Se, Zn) concentrations in serum and breast milk from Nigerian women, *Annu. Nutr. Metab.*, 37(5), 262, 1993.

86. Bodnar, L. M., Scanlon, K. S., Cogswell, M. E., Freedman, A. M., and Siega-Riz, A. M., High prevalence of postpartum anemia in U.S. Low income women, *FASEB J.,* 14(4), A754, 2000.

87. Casterline, J. E., Allen, L. H., and Ruel, M. T., Vitamin B_{12} deficiency is very prevalent in lactating Guatemalan women and their infants at three months postpartum, *J. Nutr.,* 127(10), 1966, 1997.

88. Ingram, C. F., Fleming, A. F., Patel, M., and Galpin, J. S., Pregnancy and lactation-related folate deficiency in South Africa — a case for folate food fortification, *S. Afr. Med. J.,* 89(12), 127, 1999.

89. Martorell, R., Undernutrition during pregnancy and early childhood: consequences for cognitive and behavioral development, in *Early Childhood Development: Investing in our Children's Future,* Young, M. E., Ed., Elsevier, New York, 1997, 39.

90. Van Den Broeck, J. and Eeckels, R. et al., Influence of nutritional status on child mortality in rural Zaire, *Lancet,* 341(8859), 1491, 1993.

91. Walter, T., Olivares, M., Pizarro, F., and Munoz, C., Iron, anemia and infection, *Nutr. Rev.,* 55(4), 111, 1997.

92. Chandra, R. K. and Saraya, A. K., Impaired immunocompetence associated with iron deficiency, *J. Pediatr.,* 86, 899, 1975.

93. Thibault, H., Galan, P., Selz, F., Preziosi, P., Olivier, C., Badoual, J., and Hercberg, S., The immune response in iron-deficient young children: effect of iron supplementation on cell-mediated immunity, *Eur. J. Pediatr.,* 152, 120, 1993.

94. Oppenheimer, S. J., Iron and infection in the tropics : paediatric clinical correlates, *Annu. Trop. Paed.,* 18 (Suppl. S81), 1998.

95. Berger, J., Dyck, J. L., Galan, P., Aplogan, A., Schneider, D., Traissac, P., and Hercberg, S., Effect of daily iron supplementation on iron status, cell-mediated immunity, and incidence of infections in 6-36 month old Togolese children, *Eur. J. Clinical Nutr.,* 54(1), 29, 2000.

96. Harvey, P. W. J., Heywood, P. F., Nesheim, M. C., Galme, K., Zegans, M., and Habicht, J. P. et al., The effect of iron therapy on malarial infection in Papua New Guinean school children, *Am. J. Trop. Med. Hyg.,* 40, 12, 1989.

97. Beisel, W. R., Single nutrients and immunity, *Am. J. Clinical Nutr.,* 35, 417, 1982.

98. Mitra, A. K., Akramuzzaman, S. M., Fuchs, G. J., Rahman, M. M., and Mahalanabis, D., Long-term oral supplementation with iron is not harmful for young children in a poor community of Bangladesh, *J. Nutr.,* 127(8), 1451, 1997.

99. Heresi, G., Pizarro, F., Olivares, E., Cayazzo, M., Hertrampf, E., Walter, T., Murphy, J. R., and Steckel, A., Effect of supplementation with an iron-fortified milk on incidence of diarrhea and respiratory infection in urban-resident infants, *Scand. J. Infect. Dis.,* 27(4), 385, 1995.

100. Rosado, J. L., Lopez, P., Munoz, E., and Allen, L. H., Lack of an effect of iron and zinc supplementation on the growth of Mexican children, *Am. J. Clinical Nutr.,* 8, 5, 4743, 1997.

101. Mejia, L. A. and Arroyave, G., The effect of vitamin A fortification of sugar on iron metabolism in Central American children, *Am. J. Clinical Nutr.,* 36, 87, 1982.

102. Hussein, M. A., Hassan, H. A., Abdel-Ghaffar, A. A., and Salem, S., Effect of iron supplements on the occurrence of diarrhoea among children in Egypt, *Food Nutr. Bull.,* 10(2), 35, 1988.

103. Menendez, C., Kahigwa, E., Hirt, R., Vounatsou, P., Aponte, J. J., Font, F., et al., Randomised placebo-controlled trial of iron supplementation and malaria chemoprophylaxis for prevention of severe anaemia and malaria in Tanzanian infants, *Lancet,* 350(9081), 844, 1997S.

104. Lawless, J. W., Latham, M. C., Stephenson, L. S., Kinoti, S. N., and Pertet, A. M., Iron supplementation improves appetite and growth in anemic Kenyan primary school children, *J. Nutr.,* 124, 5, 645, 1994.

105. Bhaskaram, P., Immunology of iron-deficient subjects, in *Nutrition and Immunology,* Chandra, R. K., Ed., A.R. Liss, New York, 149, 1988.

106. Beard, J. L., Haas, J. D., and Hurtado G. L., The relationship of nutritional status to oxygen transport and growth in highland Bolivian children, *Hum. Biol.,* 55, 151, 1983.

107. Lozoff, B., Brittenham, G. M., Viteri, F. E., Wolf, A. W., and Urrutia, J. J., Developmental deficits in iron-deficient anemic infants: effects of age and severity of iron lack, *J. Pediatr.,* 101, 948, 1982.

108. Owen, G. M., Lubin, A. H., and Garry, P. J., Preschool children in the United States: who has iron deficiency? *J. Pediatr.,* 79, 563, 1971.

109. Rao, K. V., Radhaiah, G., and Raju, S. V., Association of growth status and the prevalence of anaemia in preschool children, *Indian J. Med. Res.,* 71, 237, 1980.

110. Pollitt, E., Effects of a diet deficient in iron on the growth and development of preschool and school-age children, *Food Nutr. Bull.,* 13, 2, 110, 1991.

111. Chwang, L. C., Soemantri, A. G., and Pollit, E., Iron supplementation and physical growth of rural Indonesian children, *Am. J. Clinical Nutr.,* 47, 496, 1988.

112. Latham, M. C., Stephenson, L. S., Kinoti, S. N., Zaman, M. S., and Kurz, K. M., Improvements in growth following iron supplementation in young Kenyan school children, *Nutrition,* 6, 159, 1990.

113. Judisch, J. M., Naiman, J. L., and Oski, F. A., The fallacy of the fat iron-deficient child, *Pediatrics,* 37, 987, 1966.

114. Burman, D., Haemoglobin levels in normal infants aged 3 to 24 months, *Arch. Dis. Child.,* 47, 261, 1972.

115. Lammi, A. T. and Lovric, V. A., Assessment of iron deficiency in children without anaemia, *Med. J. Aust.,* 2, 540, 1973.

116. Briend, A., Hoque, B. A., and Aziz, K. M., Iron in tubewell water and linear growth in rural Bangladesh, *Arch. Dis. Child.,* 65, 224, 1990.

117. Migasena, P., Thurnham, D. I., Jintaknon, K., and Pongpaew, P., Anemia in Thai children: the effect of iron supplement on hemoglobin and growth, *SE Asian J. Trop. Med. and Public Health,* 3, 255, 1972.

118. Auckett, M. A., Parks, Y. A., Scott, P. H., and Wharton, B. A., Treatment with iron increases weight gain and psychomotor development, *Arch. Dis. Child.,* 61, 849, 1986.

119. Angeles, I. T., Schultink, W. J., Matulessi, P., Gross, R., and Sastroamidjojo, S., Decreased rate of stunting among anemic Indonesian preschool children through iron supplementation, *Am. J. Clinical Nutr.,* 58, 339, 1993.

120. Soewondo, S., Husaini, M., and Pollitt, E., Effects of iron deficiency on attention and learning processes in preschool children: Bandung, Indonesia, *Am. J. Clinical Nutr.,* 50, (3 Suppl.), 667, 1989.

121. Bhatia, D. and Sheshadri, S., Growth performance in anaemia following iron supplementation, *Indian Paediatrics,* 30, 195, 1993.

122. Idjradinata, P., Watkins, W. E., and Pollitt, E., Adverse effect of iron supplementation on weight gain of iron-replete young children, *Lancet,* 343, 1252, 1994.

123. Dewey, K. G., Domellof, M., Cohen, R. J., Landa Rivera, L., Hernell, O., and Lonnerdal, B. L., Effects of iron supplementation on growth and morbidity of breast-fed infants: a randomized trial in Sweden and Honduras, *FASEB J.,* 14(4), 9, 2000.

124. Allen, L. H., Backstrand, J. R., Pelto, G. H., Mata, M. P., and Chavez, A., The interactive effects of dietary quality on the growth and attained size of young Mexican children, *Am. J. Clinical Nutr.,* 56, 353, 1992.

125. Neumann, C. G. and Harrison, G. G., Onset and evolution of stunting in infants and children. Examples from the Human Nutrition Collaborative Research Support Program. Kenya and Egypt studies, *Eur. J. Clinical Nutr.,* 48 (Suppl. 1), S90, 1994.

126. Foged, N., Lillquist, K., Rolschau, J., and Blaabjerg, O., Effect of folic acid supplementation on small-for-gestational-age infants born at term, *Eur. J. Pediatr.,* 149, 1, 65, 1989.

127. Matoth, Y., Zehavi, I., Topper, E., and Klein, T., Folate nutrition and growth in infancy, *Arch. Dis. Child.,* 54, 9, 699, 1979.

128. Gershoff, S. N., McGandy, R. B., Nondasuta, A., and Tantiwongse, P., Nutrition studies in Thailand: effects of calories, nutrient supplements, and health interventions on growth of preschool Thai village children, *Am. J. Clinical Nutr.,* 48, 1214, 1988.

129. Liu, D-S., Bates, C. J., Yin, T-A., Wang, X-B., and Lu, C-Q., Nutritional efficacy of a fortified weaning rusk in a rural area near Beijing, *Am. J. Clinical Nutr.,* 57, 506, 1993.

130. Thu, D. B., Schultink, W., Dillon, Drupadi, Gross, R., Leswara, N. D., and Khoi, H. H., Effect of daily and weekly micronutrient supplementation on micronutrient deficiencies in young Vietnamese children, *Am. J. Clinical Nutr.,* 69, 80, 1999.

131. Rivera, J., Romero, M., Flores, M., Rivera, M., Gonzalez-Cossio, T., Tellez, M., and Rosado, J., Multiple Micronutrient Supplementation improves the growth of Mexican girls and children under 12 months of age, *FASEB J.,* 13(4), A207, abs. 190.7, 1999.

132. Van Stuijvenberg, M. E., Kvalsvig, J. D., Faber, M., Kruger, M., Kenoyer, D. G., and Benade, A. J., Effect of iron-, iodine-, and B-carotene fortified biscuits on the micronutrient status of primary school children: a randomized controlled trial, *Am. J. Clinical Nutr.,* 69, 497, 1999.

133. Noel, J., Ramakrishnan, U., Rivera, J., Romero, M., Flores, M., Rivera, M., and Gonzales-Cossio, T., Long-term Effects of Multiple Micronutrient Supplements on Growth of Young Mexican Children, *FASEB J.,* 13(4), A207, abs. 190.8, 1999.

134. Mahaffey, K. R., Nutrition and lead: strategies for public health, *Environ. Health Perspect.,* 103 (S6), 191, 1995.

5 Functional Correlates of Nutritional Anemias in Infancy and Early Childhood — Child Development and Behavior

Betsy Lozoff and Theodore D. Wachs

CONTENTS

This chapter describes alterations in normal cognitive, social-emotional, and motor development as functional correlates of nutritional anemia in infants and young children. The primary focus will be on iron deficiency anemia, given its high prevalence. Evidence on short and long term outcomes from therapeutic and preventive trials and possible underlying mechanisms will be described. Nutritional anemias caused by deficiencies in vitamins and trace minerals other than iron will also be discussed in a separate section.

5.1   IRON DEFICIENCY ANEMIA IN INFANCY

Anemia was once thought to be the main reason to be concerned about iron deficiency in infants and toddlers. Even then, anemia was considered of little consequence unless it was severe enough to compromise cardiovascular function (that is, when hemoglobin levels fall below 50 to 60 g/l). The situation changed dramatically in the 1970s, beginning with the work of Frank Oski and colleagues. Oski wanted to pursue earlier anecdotal observations that infants with iron deficiency anemia showed behavioral improvements within days of iron treatment (e.g., less irritability, more activity, improved appetite). To do so, Oski and Honig[1] used a strong experimental design in which a standard test of infant development was given to 9 to 26 month old infants with iron deficiency anemia before and one week after randomly assigned intramuscular iron or a placebo injection. One week after treatment, the anemic infants who received intramuscular iron showed statistically significant increases in mental test scores. The increases among placebo treated anemic infants were not significant.

Oski and Honig interpreted these results as evidence that iron deficiency produces developmental alterations in infants that are rapidly reversible with iron therapy. They suggested that iron's activity in various neurotransmitters and cytochromes was responsible and that such biochemical processes might respond to iron therapy before the anemia was corrected. However, the findings of the study were actually equivocal. As Oski and Honig pointed out, the difference between the iron and placebo treated groups in improved mental test scores (+14 vs. +6 points) was not statistically significant. Thus, the study did not demonstrate a clear effect of iron treatment over and above the effect of repeating the same test within a short period of time. Nonetheless, these results were intriguing and stimulated a number of other investigators to undertake related research.

Several subsequent studies have examined developmental and behavioral aspects of iron deficiency in infancy. Collectively, the studies address the following specific issues: (1) differences in developmental tests scores and other behavioral measures prior to treatment; (2) the degree of iron deficiency at which differences are observed; (3) effects of short term iron therapy; (4) effects of a full course of treatment; and (5) differences years after the period of deficiency. Summaries of the studies, including specifics of research design and results, can be found in recent reviews.[2,3] It should be noted that making direct comparisons among studies is still limited by differences in the ages of the infants and differences in the timing, duration, or severity of iron deficiency.

A longitudinal study by Lozoff and associates in Costa Rica[4] is described in some detail, because it addresses all the above issues. Regarding each of the key questions, we will note how the results of this study relate to those of other studies. Only those findings that are statistically significant with a probability of 0.05 or less are reported here as positive results. A subsequent section will consider mechanisms that could explain the findings.

The original study in Costa Rica involved 191 infants from an urban community near San Jose. The study included all 12- to 23-month-old infants in the community who had been born with birth weights ≥2.5 kg, of singleton uncomplicated births, who were free of acute or chronic medical problems, and had normal physical examinations. These healthy infants had relatively low lead levels, no evidence of growth failure or other nutrient deficiencies, and were generally free of parasites. Iron status in infancy varied from sufficiency to moderate iron deficiency anemia. Comprehensive information was collected about the child and family, including demography, birth history, nutrition, socioeconomic status, stimulation in the home, and parental IQ. Developmental tests were administered before and one week and three months after intramuscular or closely supervised oral administration of iron with appropriate placebo controls.[4]

5.1.1   DIFFERENCES PRIOR TO TREATMENT

5.1.1.1   Development Test Scores (Motor and Mental)

Infants with moderate iron deficiency anemia (Hb ≤100 g/l and 2 of 3 abnormal iron measures) were found to have lower mental and motor test scores. Infants with mild anemia (Hb = 101 to 105 g/l) scored lower on motor scores but not on mental scores. Differences in mental and motor test scores remained statistically significant after controlling for factors related to birth, nutrition, family background, lead, parental IQ, and home environment. These findings are consistent with seven other studies of iron deficient anemic infants distinguished by the use of careful definitions of iron status and the inclusion of comparison groups.[5-11] All showed that mental test scores of iron deficient anemic infants were lower than the scores of comparison group infants before treatment (averaging 6 to 16 points lower). Four of the six other studies reporting motor test scores found them to be lower as well (averaging 9 to 17 points lower).

Infants with lesser degrees of iron deficiency did not have impairments in developmental test performance. This result is consistent with the other studies that examined differing degrees of iron deficiency.[6,10] It appears that iron deficiency must be severe and chronic enough to cause anemia before differences on a global measure such as a test of overall development will be observed. It is possible that more sensitive measures would detect differences at lesser degrees of iron deficiency.

5.1.1.2   Behavioral Differences Other Than Developmental
Test Scores

A variety of other behavioral differences were noted among the infants with iron deficiency anemia in the Costa Rica study.[12] Anemic infants maintained closer contact with caregivers during play and motor testing. They showed less pleasure/delight during the mental test, and some were wary or hesitant throughout the motor test. More iron deficient anemic than comparison group infants received behavior ratings indicating little endurance and excess fatigability, and there were other indications that they were less active. During play, they were more likely to be low in vocalization and initiating changes in proximity to their mothers, thus creating fewer opportunities for interaction. Observations at home showed that iron deficient anemic infants were more likely to be carried by their mothers and to be asleep, irritable, alone in a playpen, or doing activities that did not involve interaction with caregivers.

These findings seem to fit with other research, even though there is nothing directly comparable to the study's quantitative analyses during developmental testing and observations in the home. The results are consistent with previous behavioral ratings suggesting affective changes among iron-deficient infants during developmental testing[8-10,13,14] and with an earlier pilot study indicating closer proximity to caregivers during play.[15]

The Costa Rica study also found that both the tester and primary caregivers (generally mothers) related differently to infants with iron deficiency anemia. In play, the caregivers of iron deficient anemic infants showed less obvious pleasure in the children, even though the caregivers initiated interaction more often. Caregivers showed less affection during both mental and motor testing. During motor testing, both the caregiver and the tester tried less frequently to get the iron deficient anemic infants to perform the tasks, and the motor test sessions were shorter for them.

5.1.2 THERAPEUTIC TRIALS

5.1.2.1 Short-Term Treatment

The Costa Rica study compared the short term effects of placebo, oral, and intramuscular iron. After one week of treatment, no differences in developmental test scores and hematologic parameters between iron deficient infants who received intramuscular iron and those who received oral iron were observed. Intramuscular and oral iron were therefore combined for comparison with placebo treatment. After one week, researchers noted a significant increase in mental test scores regardless of whether the infants were anemic and treated with iron or placebo or nonanemic and treated with iron or placebo. Similarly, iron treatment had no short term effects on motor test scores. The lack of short term treatment effects, whether with oral or intramuscular iron, was confirmed in most studies.[4,7,10,16] There is no explanation for the improvements in developmental test scores with 7 to 10 days of therapy reported in earlier studies by Oski and associates[7,13] and Walter et al.[9] However, those studies did not include both nonanemic comparison groups and placebo conditions.

5.1.2.2 Full Course Treatment

The initial search for rapid behavioral changes with iron therapy was motivated by a desire to attribute improvements in behavior and test scores to improved function of iron dependent central nervous system enzymes rather than to the correction of iron deficiency anemia. However, the failure to replicate improvements after short term therapy led researchers to assess behavior and development after a full course of iron therapy. This is the more pertinent question from a clinical perspective. Although trying to detect rapid change is interesting, the important issue is whether iron therapy corrects the behavioral abnormalities, regardless of how soon changes might be detectable.

The study in Costa Rica[4] was specifically designed to examine the effects of the course of treatment commonly used in practice (3 months of oral iron therapy). After the short term treatment part of the study, all iron deficient and iron depleted children were treated with iron for 3 months; the iron sufficient group was randomly assigned to oral iron or placebo treatment. After treatment, all iron deficient anemic infants corrected their anemia, but the majority (64%) still had biochemical evidence of iron deficiency, suggesting greater severity or chronicity. As a group, formerly anemic infants still had lower developmental test scores after treatment. However, the minority who became iron sufficient showed improvement in motor scores and did not show the declines in mental scores observed in the rest of the sample.[4] (A decline in mental test scores is frequently observed in the second year of life in disadvantaged groups.)

Despite this encouraging response for a subset of infants, it was worrisome that lower mental and motor test scores persisted among the majority of initially anemic infants. Similar results, indicating that the majority of anemic infants do not show improvement after iron therapy, have been obtained in several other studies. In one other study, improvements were seen in a minority of infants who showed the best hematologic response but the majority still had lower scores.[4,17] Two other studies, which included iron therapy for up to 6 months, found no overall improvement.[8,10] Only one study reported an overall increase in mental and motor scores after 4 months of iron therapy.[6] The explanation of this result, which conflicts with the other four studies, is unknown.

To summarize, all eight studies that included careful definitions of iron status and appropriate comparison groups reported that iron deficient anemic infants had lower mental test scores than infants with better iron status.[4-11] Five studies showed lower motor scores as well.[4-7,10] A variety of behavioral differences, especially in emotional responses and mood, have been reported.[8-10,12-14] No association between lower pretreatment test scores or behavioral ratings and lesser degrees of iron deficiency has been documented.[4,6,10,17] After one week of treatment, the effects on scores for the intramuscular and oral iron group did not differ from the placebo group.[4,7,10,16,19] After a full course of iron, one study reported an overall improvement in mental and motor test scores,[6] while differences in developmental test scores and behavior remained for the majority of formerly anemic infants in the other studies.[4,8,10,12,18] Thus, the ability of iron therapy to correct the lower test scores and behavioral differences, or the conditions under which iron therapy can effect improvements remain open questions. In this context, it is also important to emphasize that global measures of infant development might not detect effects of mild iron deficiency and/or iron therapy.

5.1.3 PREVENTIVE TRIALS

Given the uncertainty about the reversibility of test score differences with iron therapy, an important related question is whether preventing iron deficiency will prevent poorer developmental test performance. Several preventive trials have been published. The first, conducted in Papua New Guinea,[20] compared 1-year-old infants, half of whom received intramuscular iron (3 ml iron dextran and 150 mg elemental iron) at 2 months; half received placebo injections. Although the design of the study was strong, the results were difficult to interpret, because malaria was endemic, all groups were anemic at 12 months, and iron status measures did not clearly indicate iron deficiency. However, it seemed that iron treated infants who were negative for malaria showed better attentional abilities.

Another preventive trial[21] included a relatively large sample of Native American infants in Canada, half of whom received iron fortified formula and half received unfortified formula from birth, with follow-up until 15 months. The groups were comparable in iron status, development, and family background at 6 months but diverged in hemoglobin, iron status, and psychomotor test scores at 9 and 12 months, with poorer outcomes in the unfortified group. Because of its design, this study provides convincing evidence that iron deficiency caused lower test scores in infancy. Two findings qualify this conclusion: (1) no differences in mental scores were noted, even though they have been consistently found in case-control studies, and (2) the differences in motor scores resolved spontaneously by 15 months. These observations raise the possibility that some other factor explains the differences in mental and motor development in iron deficient anemic infants.

A third preventive trial was recently conducted in England.[22] Infants were randomly assigned to receive unmodified cow's milk or iron supplemented formula between approximately 8 and 18 months of age. Developmental test scores were similar at the time of enrollment and declined in both groups during the study. There were no differences between groups at 18 months, but by 2 years of age, the decrease in developmental test quotient was more marked in the group receiving unmodified cow's milk (decline of 14.7 points vs. 9.3 points in the supplemented group), and differences in personal and social scores were most pronounced. This study also suggests a causal link between iron deficiency and poor development, but the lack of differences at 18 months is puzzling.

Another well-designed, relatively large preventive trial in the UK randomly assigned 9-month-old infants to cow milk, unfortified formula, or iron-fortified follow-on formula.[23] The groups were comparable at study entry. At 18 months, there were no differences in mental or motor development and thus no evidence for a beneficial effect of supplemental iron in late infancy and early toddlerhood.

A small, but intensive study at West Java compared behavior and development in infants at risk for growth faltering who were randomly assigned to receive a high energy and micronutrient supplement, micronutrients only, or control between 6 and 18 months of age.[24,25] The greatest developmental benefits were observed in those who received the combined energy-micronutrient supplement. However, the micronutrient condition by itself was also associated with increased vocalization, more playing, less carrying of the infant[24] and, among infants with iron-deficiency anemia, increased activity and improved motor development.[25]

By far, the largest preventive trial to date has been conducted in Chile (Lozoff et al., unpublished). Over 1600 healthy 6-month-old infants were randomly assigned to receive supplemental iron or no added iron until 12 months of age. Analysis of this study has recently been completed, and results should be forthcoming soon.

The reasons for differing results in the various preventive trials is unclear. Clues to explanation are likely to lie in differences in sample characteristics, outcome measures other than global tests, timing of iron supplementation, and/or duration and severity of iron deficiency.

5.1.4 LONG-TERM CORRELATES OF IRON DEFICIENCY IN INFANCY

The studies described above cannot determine whether ill effects associated with iron deficiency persist into childhood, because traditional infant developmental tests, such as the Bayley Scales, are not good predictors of later intellectual functioning.[26] To identify long term effects, the children in the Costa Rica study were reevaluated when they were 5 years old[27] and again at 11 to 14 years.[28,29] At each assessment, 85 to 87% of the original cohort participated. All the children had excellent hematologic status and growth. At 5 years of age, children who had moderate iron deficiency anemia as infants (Hb ≤100 g/L) still tested lower than the rest of the sample in mental and motor functioning. In general, the magnitude of test score differences were greater for tasks requiring nonverbal skills, visual-motor integration, and motor coordination than for purely verbal tasks. An unexpected finding was that children with initial Hb >100 g/L, for whom 3 months of iron therapy did not fully correct iron deficiency, also had poorer outcomes at 5 years. They showed no statistically significant differences on mental and motor tests in comparison with formerly moderately anemic children, and both groups tested lower than the other children in a variety of areas.[27]

The results were similar at 11 to 14 years.[28,29] Children who had severe chronic iron deficiency in infancy scored lower on measures of overall mental and motor functioning. More of them repeated a grade and/or were referred for special services or tutoring. They showed a delay or disruption of shifts in cognitive processing expected in early adolescence. The iron deficient group had more difficulty on a motor test and on tasks involving visual-spatial memory and selective recall for visual stimuli. Parents and teachers had more concerns about the behavior of formerly iron deficient children in several areas. Both parents and teachers reported that the iron deficient group showed more anxiety/depression, social problems, and attention problems, with a corresponding increase in summary measures of internalizing problems and total problems.

A handful of other studies reassessed cognitive functioning and school achievement among children who were anemic as infants. In Israel, Chile, and France, follow-up studies at 4 to 8 years found that children who were anemic as infants or toddlers tested lower than peers several years after iron treatment.[30-35] Two studies reassessed children at older ages, close to those in the most recent Costa Rica follow-up. Walter and associates in Chile reevaluated a subset of their original infant cohort at 10 years of age. Preliminary analyses show that the formerly anemic group had poorer school functioning and lower achievement test scores.[36] In a population based study of Women, Infants, and Children (WIC) participants in Florida, Hurtado and associates reported an inverse relationship between hemoglobin level in infancy and the risk of mild to moderate mental retardation at age 10 years.[37] The consistency of the results from five countries is striking. The findings show that anemia, presumably due to iron deficiency or severe, chronic iron deficiency in infancy, identifies children with poorer overall cognitive functioning and lower school achievement test scores years later.

5.1.5 Mechanisms for Long Lasting Ill Effects of Early Iron Deficiency

Figure 5.1 provides a conceptual model of mechanisms for poorer behavior and developmental outcomes associated with iron deficiency in early childhood. Both biological and environmental influences are shown to combine to produce poorer outcomes. There is little doubt that iron deficiency affects disadvantaged infants disproportionately.[38,39] For instance, in the Costa Rica study, infants with iron deficiency anemia had mothers with lower IQ scores and more depressive symptoms, received less stimulation in the home, were less likely to be breastfed, and were weaned earlier.[4] Statistical control for differences in these factors did not eliminate the significant effect of chronic and severe iron deficiency on behavior and development in infancy or at 5 or 12 years. However, such disadvantageous conditions are known to have adverse effects on child development, and environmental disadvantage

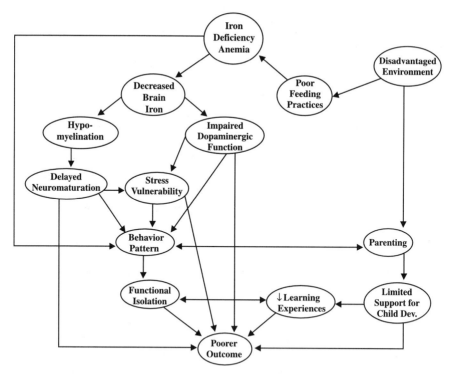

FIGURE 5.1 Conceptual model of mechanisms for poorer development in iron deficient anemic infants. The left side of the figure focuses on the child, beginning with more biological mechanisms. The right side focuses on the environment, indicating factors that might limit support for child development. Both biological and environmental influences are shown to combine to produce poorer outcome. From Lozoff, B. et al., Behavior of infants with iron deficiency anemia, *Child Dev.*, 69, 24, 1998. With permission.

has been shown to adversely affect parenting behavior.[40] In a transactional fashion, parental behavior might combine with biologically based changes in infant behavior to produce poorer developmental outcome.

The link between iron deficiency and environmental risk is strong, but the evidence for biologically based changes in infant behavior is also compelling. Information on iron's role in the developing brain has steadily accumulated, inviting cautious interpretation of some findings in studies of iron deficiency in infancy. In animal models of iron deficiency, dietary iron deficiency during maximal brain growth has consistently led to a deficit in brain iron that is not reversed with treatment.[41-45] New studies indicate that this decrease in brain iron is distributed heterogeneously. Iron-deficient weanling rats showed lower amounts of iron in cortex and hippocampus compared to controls, while other regions were quite unaffected.[46] Similarly, in rats with perinatal iron deficiency, cytochrome oxidase activity (an iron containing enzyme involved in oxidative phosphorylation, whose activity reflects neuronal metabolism) was reduced most markedly in the brain regions involved in higher cognitive functions.[47] Older research, extended by recent studies, shows that function of the dopamine neurotransmitter system, perhaps especially involving the D_2 receptor, is altered in early iron deficiency.[48-50] In parallel to the recent basic science research on iron deficiency, other investigators have been defining the role of dopamine in higher cognitive function and characterizing related neural networks.[51,52] One neural system where dopamine plays a particularly prominent role is the prefrontal-striatal system.[53] There are many dopamine D_2 receptors in the prefrontal cortex, dopamine levels are higher in the striatum (caudate/putamen) than anywhere else in the brain, and the basal ganglia are rich in iron.[54,55] The results of the Costa Rica follow-up study showing differences in certain specific cognitive functions may fit with new understanding of iron's role in the prefrontal-striatal and hippocampal systems.

Persisting lower motor scores may also relate to central nervous system effects of iron deficiency earlier in development. Although it has been known for some time that high iron concentrations are found in brain regions involved with motor function and coordination (basal ganglia, cerebellum, etc.),[54] iron's essential role in myelin formation and maintenance has been described only recently.[56-60] Perhaps the most direct evidence for an effect in human infants that could be due to impaired myelination comes from a recent study showing that young infants with iron deficiency anemia had slower nerve conduction through the auditory pathway, even after effective iron therapy.[61]

In contrast to plausible central nervous system mechanisms that account for motor and cognitive differences, there is less basis for hypothesizing the neural underpinnings of behavior problems reported in formerly iron deficient children. While there is insufficient literature linking nutritional deficiencies to variability in infant temperament,[62] recent basic work on iron and the brain has not focused on issues directly relevant to socioemotional development and therefore does not support any speculation. Behavioral differences that begin in infancy could contribute to poorer developmental outcome in the future. This line of reasoning is based on a transactional model of development.[63] Attributes of the infant affect the caregiver, whose behavior in turn influences the infant. The behavioral pattern of wariness, unhappiness, and hesitance in an unfamiliar setting[8-10,12-15] suggests that infants with chronic and severe iron deficiency might be functionally isolated. They seek and/or receive less stimulation from the physical and social environment, resulting in adverse effects on development.[12] This behavior pattern could combine with limitations in parental behavior and other environmental disadvantages to produce poorer outcomes. In addition, infant characteristics such as passive, withdrawn behavior might also increase risk for subsequent nutritional deficiencies, further compounding the impact of the original nutritional insult.[62] Behavior problems after the period of deficiency, like those observed in the Costa Rica follow-up, have the potential to continue to interfere with ability to learn. Thus, behavioral differences could contribute to lower achievement test scores and other outcomes that depend on formal and informal learning.

5.1.6 SUMMARY AND IMPLICATIONS

The explanations for long lasting ill effects of iron deficiency in infancy considered above are not mutually exclusive. Different mechanisms may be involved, perhaps depending on the domain in question. For instance, a deficit in visual-spatial/working memory, with adverse effects on learning math, might be a direct result of lower iron levels in certain brain regions, and long lasting motor differences might result from delayed myelination. Indirect effects, which might still begin with central nervous system changes, could also be postulated. Lowered brain iron levels, altered neurotransmitter function, or impaired myelination during infancy could disrupt the process of laying down the neural bases for some cognitive, socioemotional, and motor fundamentals. This disruption could place iron deficient children on developmental trajectories that differ from those of peers who have better iron status. Behavioral changes in infancy might produce long lasting effects through their impact on caregivers in a transactional fashion. In contrast, poorer school achievement and grade repetition might be influenced heavily by family disadvantages and limitations. It seems likely that several of the above mechanisms combine to produce poorer outcomes in the various domains.[12]

5.2 IRON DEFICIENCY ANEMIA IN THE PRESCHOOL PERIOD

While our review documents ample evidence on the functional-behavioral consequences of iron deficiency anemia during infancy and a similar literature also covers the school age period,[64] curiously, less evidence is available for the intervening preschool period between 2 and 5 years. While some cognitive differences have been reported favoring more iron replete preschool children,[65] studies generally report no differences between anemic and nonanemic preschoolers[66,67] or significant differences in some behavioral outcomes such as emotional tone but not in other outcomes such as responsivity.[68]

Similarly, while gains in cognitive performance following iron treatment of anemic preschoolers have been reported,[65-67] not all studies have reported significant gains.[68] Further, even among those studies reporting improvements, gains do not occur uniformly across the cognitive or behavioral spectrum. Improvements after iron therapy are more likely to appear for more demanding cognitive tasks that require shifting previously successful problem solving strategies[67] or for aspects of behavior that involve reactivity to a structured testing situation.[77,79]

The potential developmental implications of links between iron deficiency and deficits in specific cognitive functions can also be understood in light of the evidence of preschool consequences of concurrent iron deficiency anemia. As discussed earlier, gains following iron treatment in the preschool years are restricted to relatively specific cognitive or behavioral outcomes. Such specificity could explain both the conclusions drawn from our review as well as related reviews,[83] all of which indicate that the majority of treated anemic infants show poorer cognitive and academic performance in the school years even when their anemia has been corrected. The preschool results suggest that it will be important in long term follow-up studies to look for specific treatment gains in certain areas, even though global measures may remain lowered.

5.3   THE NON-IRON DEFICIENCY ANEMIAS

While iron deficiency anemia (IDA) is perhaps the most common type of nutritionally related anemia, it is not the only type. Other nutritional anemias, namely macrocytic/megaloblastic anemias associated with folate or vitamin B_{12} deficiencies[70,71] or even copper, zinc or thiamine,[72-75] have also been associated with a variety of developmental behavioral abnormalities. At least 150 years of history link pernicious anemia to a variety of psychiatric symptoms[76] and this linkage has been confirmed in the modern scientific literature.[77,78] Similarly, a body of evidence shows how anemias related to folate deficiency are associated with increased risk of affective disorders such as depression.[77,78]

The links between non-IDA anemias and behavioral developmental deviations will be the major focus of this final section. Before discussing such linkages, it is important to note what will not be considered in this section. Given that our focus is on nutritional anemias, the behavioral developmental consequences of anemias related to inborn errors of metabolism are not addressed. Detailed reviews of the nature and consequences of anemias related to inborn metabolic errors can be found in a number of recent sources.[80,81] Our focus is on the developmental period between conception and the first few years of life with the exception of research involving pregnant and lactating women. Reviews of the nature and consequences of anemia in older age populations are available in the literature.[71,82] Anemias that occur as a result of disease process (e.g., sickle cell disease) have not been included.[81]

5.3.1   PREGNANCY

The combination of growing fetal demands for folate plus the relatively moderate level of stored maternal folate means that maternal folate depletion can occur in unsupplemented pregnant women within 4 months, with a consequent increased risk of megaloblastic anemia.[70,84] It has been assumed that because of the efficiency of folate transfer between mother and fetus, the fetus is adequately buffered even in cases where maternal folate deficiency has progressed to the level of severe anemia.[70] However, the well documented relation of maternal folate deficiency to an increased risk of offspring neural tube defect,[85] as well as an increasing amount of evidence linking maternal folate deficiency to an increased risk of preterm birth or low birth weight, suggests that fetal buffering is not total.[81,85] Under such conditions, maternal folate deficiency that progresses to the stage of megaloblastic anemia may act as an indirect developmental risk, given the adverse behavioral developmental consequences associated with low birth weight and preterm birth.[86]

Maternal megaloblastic anemia associated with vitamin B_{12} deficiency appears to be less of a prenatal developmental risk factor. The maternal and fetal requirement for this vitamin is relatively low, and vitamin B_{12} is relatively available from a high level of stored B_{12}.[70,85] Metabolic interactions between vitamin B_{12} and folate can result in a deficit of folate at the erythrocyte level as a result of poor vitamin B_{12} status,[70] which may partially account for the presence of neural tube defects in offspring of women with low B_{12} status.[81]

5.3.2 INFANCY AND EARLY CHILDHOOD

In discussing the consequences of non-iron deficiency anemia in the early years of life, we have organized our review based on the presumed nutritional deficit underlying the anemias. The reader must be cautioned that such separation may be artifactual, for example, in the case of prolonged breast feeding by a nutritionally deficient mother living under poverty conditions. In such cases, resulting anemias may be associated with coexisting deficits of a variety of micronutrients including iron, vitamin B_{12}, and folate.[87] The distinctions we have made must be regarded as an organizational tool rather than as a reflection of existing realities.

5.3.2.1 Vitamin B_{12} Deficiency

While it is assumed that vitamin B_{12} driven anemia is seen only in adulthood, this assumption is not correct. The most common exceptions are breast fed infants of mothers who are vegan or strict vegetarians. Such infants are at elevated risk for megaloblastic anemia.[81] High levels of maternal folate intake may mask B_{12} deficiencies in strict vegetarians, so it is not surprising to find anemic infants whose vegetarian mothers show few signs of vitamin B_{12} deficiency.[88] Vitamin B_{12} related megaloblastic anemia has also been found in breast fed infants whose mothers have undergone gastric or intestinal bypass procedures.[89] Common to both exceptions is the combination of low infant B_{12} storage at birth plus breast feeding by a mother who has compromised vitamin B_{12} status. The developmental-behavioral consequences associated with B_{12} linked anemia in infancy are shown in Table 5.1.

These data indicate that perhaps the most common symptom pattern involves an increase in lethargy and irritability. Infants with B_{12} linked anemia appear to become increasingly less responsive to outside stimulation. When they react, the reaction tends to be primarily negative — increased irritability. Another symptom is slowing of normally developing psychomotor performance and cognitive functioning. The loss of cognitive and psychomotor function seen in infants with B_{12} megaloblastic anemia may be the result of progressive retardation of myelination, especially in the temporal and frontal lobe areas.[90]

TABLE 5.1
Behavioral Developmental Consequences Associated with Vitamin B$_{12}$ Linked Anemia in Infancy

Consequences	References
Increased irritability	Higgenbottom et al., 1978[88]
	Saraya et al., 1970[87]
	Sklar, 1986[92]
Increased lethargy: e.g., decreased activity level, lack of reactivity to stimulation, loss of emotional responsiveness, apathy	Lampkin, Shore, and Chadwick, 1996[91]
	Higgenbottom et al., 1978[88]
	Sklar, 1986[92]
Loss of normally developing psychomotor function or cognitive delay	Higgenbottom et al., 1978[88]
	Sklar, 1986[92]

Treatment of such infants with increased dosages of vitamin B$_{12}$ appears to greatly reduce both apathy and irritability.[88,91,92] Evidence is still equivocal on whether there can be complete recovery of psychomotor or cognitive losses following such treatment.[88,92,93]

5.3.2.2 Folate Deficiency

In contrast to vitamin B$_{12}$ linked anemia in infancy, which is mostly associated with strict maternal vegetarian diets, folate deficiency linked anemias are much more likely to occur in the context of overall child malnutrition.[87,94] The covariation of malnutrition and folate deficiency anemia makes it difficult to isolate the unique functional consequences of folate deficiency anemia. Given the role folate deficiencies play in fetal malformations[85] and adult affective disorders[95] and the impact of folate deficiency upon serotonin metabolism,[96] we would expect to see behavioral or developmental consequences associated with early folate deficiency anemia. Congenital errors of folate metabolism resulting in severe megaloblastic anemia have been associated with mental retardation.[97,98] A greater risk of attention deficit hyperactive disorder has been reported in older children born to severely folate deficient mothers.[99]

Unfortunately, evidence on the functional consequences of anemia associated with early deficiencies in dietary intake of folate is extremely difficult to find and results tend not to be statistically significant. In nonanemic populations variability in folate levels was unrelated to neonatal habituation, 6-month motor performance, or level of symbolic play in the second year of life.[62,100] Whether significant results would have occurred if folate deficiencies were severe enough to produce anemia remains an unanswered question. However, neither perinatal nor postnatal biomedical complications were found in infants whose mothers had severe folate driven megaloblastic anemia.[101] Whether deficiencies in dietary folate intake severe enough to cause anemia have functional behavioral and developmental consequences in the early years of life is an area that clearly requires further investigation.

5.3.2.3   Other Nutritional Anemias

Although relatively rare, some case studies have reported vitamin E responsive hemolytic anemia in low birth weight preterm infants[102] and macrocytic anemia in infants with protein energy malnutrition.[103] Both types of anemias appear to be responsive to vitamin E therapy. At present, the functional consequences of these types of anemias are unknown.

Low birth weight infants fed cow's milk or formula that was not copper supplemented are also at increased risk of copper deficiency anemia.[72,102] Copper deficiency anemia has also been reported in an exclusively breast fed infant given high levels of zinc supplement.[104] At present, no evidence links neurological or developmental abnormalities with copper deficiency anemia,[72] although apathy and failure to thrive may be early manifestations of this condition.[104]

5.3.3   CONCLUSIONS

Despite the small data base on behavioral developmental consequences associated with non-iron deficiency anemia occurring prenatally or in early childhood, sufficient data are available to indicate that consequences occur. A critical question is whether such consequences are the result of the anemia or whether both the consequences and the anemia are the result of a third factor, namely the nutritional deficiencies that led to the anemia. Even less data are available on this question, but the currently available information that is available allows us to reach some tentative conclusions.

Of particular relevance are a number of studies showing that folate or vitamin B_{12} deficiencies can result in neuropsychiatric or developmental problems such as depression, cognitive deficit, or a failure to thrive even before the onset of anemia.[76,78,85,105-107] While the majority of studies in this area involved individuals with inherited metabolic vitamin disorders, a similar pattern of findings has also been reported for dietary related vitamin deficiency anemias.[81] Failure to thrive and cognitive delay are seen in nonanemic infants who have low levels of vitamin B_{12} as a result of low maternal B_{12} levels.[80] This pattern suggests the possibility of a progressive process, wherein vitamin deficiencies initially lead to behavioral developmental consequences and then, in a later stage, to anemia.[84] Within this process, observed linkages between anemia and adverse behavioral developmental consequences are due to the impact of a third factor — vitamin deficiency — rather than anemia. This conclusion is supported by evidence showing how vitamin treatment can reverse anemia but still have no effect on neuropsychiatric symptoms,[79,81] as in the case when folate treatment masks vitamin B_{12} deficiency anemia but has little effect on associated neuropsychiatric symptoms.[85] Further supportive evidence is seen in studies showing no relation between severity of neuropsychiatric symptoms and severity of anemia[76,77,108] or a lack of neurological symptomatology even in the presence of severe anemia.[109]

The majority of the above studies deal with hereditary anemias or older populations. The consistency of evidence suggests that the functional consequences associated with non-iron deficiency anemias in early childhood are more likely due to dietary deficiencies and that anemia is a covariate rather than a causal influence.

An alternative line of support for this conclusion is seen in evidence on the covariance between dietary non-iron deficiency anemias in the prenatal or early perinatal period and other developmental risk factors. Nutritionally driven non-iron deficiency anemia has been shown to covary with low socioeconomic status, multiple offspring in the family,[70] general malnutrition[81] or specific eating disorders,[110] and a lack of or inadequate prenatal care.[82] Given the covariance of nutritional anemias with other developmental risk factors, it is difficult to determine whether adverse outcomes are a result of the anemia or whether the anemia is simply a marker for an individual who is at high risk for adverse outcomes due to the operation of nonanemia based developmental risks.

REFERENCES

1. Hofstadter, M. and Reznick, J. S., Response modality affects human infants' delayed-response performance., *Child. Dev.*, 67, 646, 1996.
2. Lozoff, B., Explanatory mechanisms for poorer development in iron-deficient anemic infants, in *Recent Advances in Research on the Effects of Health and Nutrition on Children's Development and School Achievement in the Third World*, Grantham, McGregor, S., Ed., Pan American Health Organization, 162, Washington, D.C., 1998.
3. Nokes, C., van den Bosch, C., and Bundy, D., *The Effects of Iron Deficiency and Anemia on Mental and Motor Performance, Educational Achievement, and Behavior in Children*, International Nutritional Anemia Consultative Group, Washington, D.C., 1998.
4. Lozoff, B., Brittenham, G. M., Wolf, A. W., et al., Iron deficiency anemia and iron therapy: effects on infant developmental test performance, *Pediatrics*, 79, 981, 1987.
5. Grindulis, H., Scott, P. H., Belton, N. R., et al., Combined deficiency of iron and vitamin D in Asian toddlers, *Arch. Dis. Child.*, 61, 843, 1986.
6. Idjradinata, P. and Pollitt, E., Reversal of developmental delays in iron-deficient anaemic infants treated with iron, *Lancet*, 341, 1, 1993.
7. Lozoff, B., Brittenham, G. M., Viteri, F. E., et al., The effects of short-term oral iron therapy on developmental deficits in iron deficient anemic infants, *J. Pediatr.*, 100, 351, 1982.
8. Lozoff, B., Wolf, A. W., and Jimenez, E., Effects of extended oral-iron therapy on infant developmental test scores, *J. Pediatr*, 129, 382, 1996.
9. Walter, T., Kovalskys, J., and Stekel, A., Effect of mild iron deficiency on infant mental development scores, *J. Pediatr*, 102, 519, 1983.
10. Walter, T., de Andraca, I., Chadud, P., et al., Iron deficiency anemia: adverse effects on infant psychomotor development, *Pediatrics*, 84, 7, 1989.
11. Wasserman, G., Graziano, J. H., Factor-Litvak, P., et al., Independent effects of lead exposure and iron deficiency anemia on developmental outcome at age 2 years, *J. Pediatr.*, 121, 695, 1992.
12. Lozoff, B., Klein, N. K., Nelson, E. C., et al., Behavior of infants with iron deficiency anemia, *Child. Dev*, 69, 24, 1998.
13. Honig, A. S. and Oski, F. A., Solemnity: A clinical risk index for iron deficient infants, *Early Child Develop. Care*, 16, 69, 1984.
14. Lozoff, B., Wolf, A. W., Urrutia, J. J., et al., Abnormal behavior and low developmental test scores in iron-deficient anemic infants, *J. Dev. Behav. Pediatr.*, 6, 69, 1985.
15. Lozoff, B., Klein, N. K., and Prabucki, K. M., Iron-deficient anemic infants at play, *J. Dev. Behav. Pediatr.*, 7, 152, 1986.

16. Moffatt, M. E. K., personal communication, 1987.

17. Aukett, M. A., Parks, Y. A., Scott, P. H., et al., Treatment with iron increases weight gain and psychomotor development, *Arch. Dis. Child.,* 61, 849, 1986.

18. Oski, F. A., Honig, A. S., Helu, B., et al., Effect of iron therapy on behavior performance in nonanemic, iron-deficient infants, *Pediatrics,* 71, 877, 1983.

19. Oski, F. A. and Honig, A. S., The effects of therapy on the developmental scores of iron-deficient infants, *J. Pediatr.,* 92, 21, 1978.

20. Heywood, A., Oppenheimer, S., Heywood, P., et al., Behavioral effects of iron supplementation in infants in Madang, Papua New Guinea, *Am. J. Clinical Nutr.,* 50, 630, 1989.

21. Moffatt, M. E. K., Longstaffe, S., Besant, J., et al., Prevention of iron deficiency and psychomotor decline in high risk infants through iron fortified infant formula: a randomized clinical trial, *J. Pediatr.,* 125, 527, 1994.

22. Williams, J., Wolff, A., Daly, A., et al., Iron supplemented formula milk related to reduction in psychomotor decline in infants for inner city areas: randomized study, *Br. Med. J.,* 318, 693, 1999.

23. Morley, R., Abbot, R., and Fairweather-Tait, S., Iron fortified follow on formula from 9-18 months improves iron status but not development or growth: a randomised trial, *Arch. Dis. Child.,* 81, 247, 1999.

24. Pollitt, E., Saco-Pollitt, C., Jahari, A. B., and Huang, J., Effects of an energy and micronutrient supplement on mental development and behavior under natural conditions in undernourished children in Indonesia, *Eur. J. Clinical Nutr.,* 54:S80-S90, 2000.

25. Harahap, H., Jahari, A. B., Husaini, M., Saco-Pollitt, C., and Pollitt, E., Effects of an energy and micronutrient supplement on iron deficiency anemia, physical activity, and motor and mental development in undernourished children in Indonesia, *Eur. J. Clinical Nutr.,* 54:S114-S119, 2000.

26. Bornstein, M. H. and Sigman, M. D., Continuity in mental development from infancy, *Child Dev.,* 57, 251, 1986.

27. Lozoff, B., Jimenez, E., and Wolf, A. W., Long-term developmental outcome of infants with iron deficiency, *New Eng. J. Med.,* 325, 687, 1991.

28. Lozoff, B., Wolf, A., Mollen, E., et al., Functional significance of early iron deficiency, *Pediatr. Res., Abstr.,* 41, 15A, 1997

29. Lozoff, B., Jimenez, E., Hagen, J., et al., Poorer behavioral and developmental outcome more than 10 years after treatment for iron deficiency in infancy, *Pediatrics,* e51:1, 2000.

30. Palti, H., Pevsner, B., and Adler, B., Does anemia in infancy affect achievement on developmental and intelligence tests? *Hum. Biol.,* 55, 189, 1983.

31. Palti, H., Meijer, A., and Adler, B., Learning achievement and behavior at school of anemic and non-anemic infants, *Early Hum. Dev,* 10, 217, 1985.

32. Dommergues, M. P., Archambeaud, B., Ducot, Y., et al., Iron deficiency and psychomotor development scores: a longitudinal study between ages 10 months and 4 years, *Arch. Fr. Pediatr.,* 46, 487, 1989.

33. Walter, T., de Andraca, I., Castillo, M., et al., Cognitive effect at 5 years of age in infants who were anemic at 12 months: a longitudinal study, *Pediatr. Res., Abstr.,* 295, 1990.

34. DeAndraca, I., Walter, T., Castillo, M., et al., Iron deficiency anemia and its effects upon psychological development at preschool age: a longitudinal study, in *Nestle Foundation Nutrition Annual Report 1990,* Nestec Ltd., Vevey, Switzerland, 53, 1991.

35. Walter, T., Impact of iron deficiency on cognition in infancy and childhood, *Eur. J. Clinical Nutr.,* 47, 307, 1993.

36. Rivera, F. and Walter, T., Effects on school performance at age ten years of former iron deficiency anemia in infancy, *Rev. Child. Pediatr.,* 67, 141, 1996.

37. Hurtado, E. K., Claussen, A. H., and Scott, K. G., Early childhood anemia and mild/moderate mental retardation, *Am. J. Clinical Nutr.,* 69, 115, 1999.

38. Lozoff, B., Has iron deficiency been shown to cause altered behavior in infants? in *Brain, Behaviour, and Iron in Infant Diet,* Dobbing, J., Ed., Springer-Verlag, New York, 107, 1990.

39. McLoyd, V. and Lozoff, B., Racial and ethnic trends in children's behavior and development, in *America Becoming: Racial trends and their Consequences,* Smelser, N., Wilson, W. J., Mitchell, F., Eds., National Academy Press, Washington, D.C., 2000.

40. Brody, G., Flor, D., and Neubaum, E., Coparenting processes and child competence among rural African-American families, in *Families, Risk and Competence,* Lewis, M. and Feiring, C., Eds., Lawrence Erlbaum, Mahwah, NJ, 227, 1998.

41. Dallman, P. R., Siimes, M., and Manies, E. C., Brain iron: persistent deficiency following short-term iron deprivation in the young rat, *Br. J. Haema.,* 31, 209, 1975.

42. Findlay, E., Reid, R. L., Ng, K. T., et al., The effect of iron deficiency during development on passive avoidance learning in the adult rat, *Physiol. Behav.,* 27, 1089, 1981.

43. Weinberg, J., Levine, S., and Dallman, P. R., Long-term consequences of early iron deficiency in the rat, *Pharmacol. Biochem. Behav.,* 11, 631, 1979.

44. Felt, B. T. and Lozoff, B., Brain iron and behavior of rats are not normalized by treatment of iron deficiency anemia during early development, *J. Nutr.,* 126, 693, 1996.

45. Chen, Q., Connor, J. R., and Beard, J. L., Brain iron, transferrin and ferritin concentrations are altered in developing iron-deficient rats, *J. Nutr.,* 125, 1529, 1995.

46. Erikson, K. M., Pinero, D. J., Connor, J. R., et al., Regional brain iron, ferritin and transferrin concentrations during iron deficiency and iron repletion in developing rats, *J. Nutr.,* 127, 2030, 1997.

47. Deungria, M., Rao, R., Wobken, J. D., Luciana, M., Nelson, C. A., and Georgieff, M. K., Perinatal iron deficiency decreases cytochrome oxidase (CYTOX) activity in selected regions of neonatal rat brain, *Pediatr. Res.,* 48, 169, 2000.

48. Youdim, M. B. H., Neuropharmacological and neurobiochemical aspects of iron deficiency, in *Brain, Behaviour, and Iron in the Infant Diet,* Dobbing, J., Ed., Springer-Verlag, New York, 83, 1990.

49. Beard, J. L., Connor, J. R., and Jones, B. C., Iron in the brain, *Nutr. Rev.,* 51, 157, 1993.

50. Lozoff, B., Behavioral alterations in iron deficiency, *Adv. Pediatr,* 35, 331, 1988.

51. Alexander, G. E., DeLong, M. R., and Strick, P. L., Parallel organization of functionally segregated circuits linking basal ganglia and cortex, *Annu. Rev. Neuroscience,* 9, 357, 1986.

52. Middleton, F. A. and Strick, P. L., Anatomical evidence for cerebellar and basal ganglia involvement in higher cognitive function, *Science,* 266, 458, 1994.

53. Selemon, L. D. and Goldman-Rakic, P. S., Longitudinal topography and interdigitation of corticostriatal projections in the rhesus monkey, *J. Neurosci.,* 5, 776, 1985.

54. Hill, J. M., The distribution of iron in the brain, in *Brain Iron: Neurochemical and Behavioural Aspects,* Youdim, M. B. H., Ed., Taylor and Francis, London, 1988.

55. Hallgren, B. and Sourander, P., The effect of age on the non-haemin iron in the human brain, *J. Neurochem.,* 3, 41, 1958.

56. Connor, J. R. and Benkovic, S. A., Iron regulation in the brain: histochemical, biochemical, and molecular considerations, *Annu. Neurol.,* 32 (Suppl. S51), 1992.

57. Connor, J. R. and Menzies, S. L., Altered cellular distribution of iron in the central nervous system of myelin deficient rats, *Neuroscience,* 34, 265, 1990.

58. Larkin, E. C. and Rao, G. A., Importance of fetal and neonatal iron: adequacy for normal development of central nervous system, in *Brain, Behaviour, and Iron in the Infant Diet,* Dobbing, J., Ed., Springer-Verlag, New York, 43, 1990.

59. Yu, G. S., Steinkirchner, T. M., Rao, G. A., et al., Effect of prenatal iron deficiency on myelination in rat pups, *Am. J. Path.,* 125, 620, 1986.

60. Connor, J. R. and Menzies, S. L., Relationship of iron to oligodendrocytes and myelination, *GLIA,* 17, 83, 1996.

61. Roncagliolo, M., Garrido, M., Walter, T., et al., Evidence of altered central nervous system development in infants with iron deficiency anemia at 6 mo: Delayed maturation of auditory brain stem responses, *Am. J. Clinical Nutr.,* 68, 683, 1998.

62. Wachs, T. D., Linking nutrition and temperament, in *Temperament and Personality Development across the Life Span,* Molfese, D. and Molfese, V., Eds., Lawrence Erlbaum, Mahwah, NJ, 2000, in press.

63. Sameroff, A. J. and Chandler, M. J., Reproductive risk and the continuum of caretaking casualty, in *Review of Child Development Research,* Horowitz, F. D., Ed., University of Chicago Press, Chicago, 1975, 187.

64. Watkins, W. E. and Pollitt, E., Iron deficiency and cognition among school-age children, in *Recent Advances in Research on the Effects of Health and Nutrition on Children's Development and School Achievement in the Third World,* Grantham McGregor, S., Ed., Pan American Health Organization, Washington, D.C., 1998, 179.

65. Pollitt, E., Leibel, R. L., and Greenfield, D. B., Iron deficiency and cognitive test performance in preschool children, *Nutr. Behav.,* 1, 137, 1983.

66. Seshadri, S. and Gopaldas, T., Impact of iron supplementation on cognitive functions in preschool and school-aged children: the Indian experience, *Am. J. Clinical Nutr.,* 50, 675, 1989.

67. Soewondo, S., Husaini, M., and Pollitt, E., Effects of iron deficiency on attention and learning processes in preschool children: Bandung, Indonesia, *Am. J. Clinical Nutr.,* 50, 667, 1989.

68. Deinard, A. S., List, A., Lindgren, B., et al., Cognitive deficits in iron-deficient and iron-deficient anemic children, *J. Pediatr.,* 108, 681, 1986.

69. Grantham-McGregor, S., Fernald, L., and Sethuraman, K., Effects of health and nutrition on cognitive and behavioral development in the first 3 years of life. Part 2. Infections and micronutrient deficiencies: iodine, iron and zinc, *Food Nutr. Bull.,* 20, 76, 1999.

70. Campbell, B. A., Megaloblastic anemia, *Clinical Obstr. Gynecol.,* 38, 455, 1995.

71. Colon-Otero, G., Menke, D., and Hook, C. C., A practical approach to the differential diagnosis and evaluation of the adult patient with macrocytic anemia, *Med. Clinical North Am.,* 76, 581, 1992.

72. Uauy, R., Olivares, M., and Gonzales, M., Essentiality of copper in humans, *Am. J. Clinical Nutr.,* 67, 952S, 1998.

73. Fiske, D. N., McCoy, H. E., and Kitchens, C. S., Zinc-induced sideroblastic anemia: report of a case, review of the literature, and description of the hematologic syndrome, *Am. J. Hematol.,* 46, 147, 1994.

74. Anonymous. Thiamine-responsive megaloblastic anemia, *Nutr. Rev.,* 38, 374, 1980.

75. Schuh, S., Rosenblatt, D. S., Cooper, B. A., et al., Homocystinuria and megaloblastic anemia, *New Engl. J. Med.,* 310, 686, 1984.

76. Zucker, D. K., Livingston, R. L., Nakra, R., et al., B$_{12}$ deficiency and psychiatric disorders: Case report and literature review, *Biol. Psychiatry,* 16, 197, 1981.

77. Bender, D. A., Review: B vitamins in the nervous system, *Neurochem. Int.,* 6, 297, 1984.

78. Saracaceanu, E., Tramoni, A. V., and Henry, J. M., An association between subcortical dementia and pernicious anemia — a psychiatric mask, *Compr. Psychiatry,* 38, 349, 1997.

79. Hutto, B. R., Folate and cobalamine in psychiatric illness, *Compr. Psychiatry,* 38, 305, 1997.

80. Kapadia, C. R., Vitamin B$_{12}$ in health and disease. Part I: inherited disorders of function, absorption, and transport, *Gastroenterologist,* 3, 329, 1995.

81. Rosenblatt, D. S. and Whitehead, V. M., Cobalamine and folate deficiency: acquired and hereditary disorders in children, *Sem. Hematol.,* 36, 19, 1999.

82. Williams, M. D. and Wheby, M. S., Anemia in pregnancy, *Med. Clinical North Am.,* 76, 631, 1992.

83. Stabler, S. P., Screening the older population for cobalamin vitamin B$_{12}$ deficiency, *J. Am. Geriatr. Soc.,* 43, 1290, 1995.

84. Wickramasinghe, S. N., The wide spectrum and unresolved issues of megaloblastic anemia, *Sem. Hematol.,* 36, 3, 1999.

85. Green, R. and Miller, J. W., Folate deficiency beyond megaloblastic anemia: hyperhomocysteinemia and other manifestations of dysfunctional folate status, *Sem. Hematol.,* 36, 47, 1999.

86. Friedman, S. and Sigman, M., *The Psychological Development of Low Birth Weight Children,* Albex, Norwood, MA., 1992.

87. Saraya, A. K., Singla, P. N., Ramachandran, K., et al., Nutritional macrocytic anemia of infancy, *Am. J. Clinical Nutr.,* 23, 1378, 1970.

88. Higginbottom, M. C., Sweetman, L., and Nyhan, W. L., A syndrome of methylmalonic aciduria, homocystinuria, megaloblastic anemia and neurologic abnormalities in a vitamin B$_{12}$-deficiency breast-fed infant of a strict vegetarian, *New Engl. J. Med.,* 299, 317, 1978.

89. Grange, D. K. and Finlay, J. L., Nutritional vitamin B$_{12}$ deficiency in a breastfed infant following maternal gastric bypass, *Pediatr. Hem. Oncol.,* 11, 311, 1994.

90. Lovblad, K., Ramelli, G., Remonda, L., et al., Retardation of myelination due to dietary vitamin B$_{12}$ deficiency: cranial MRI findings, *Pediatr. Radiol.,* 27, 155, 1997.

91. Lampkin, B. C., Shore, N. A., and Chadwick, D., Megaloblastic anemia in infancy secondary to maternal pernicious anemia, *New Engl. J. Med.,* 274, 1168, 1996.

92. Sklar, R., Nutritional vitamin B$_{12}$ deficiency in a breast-fed infant of a vegan-diet mother, *Clinical Pediatr.,* 25, 219, 1986.

93. Monfort-Gouraud, M., Bongiorno, A., Le Gall, M. A., et al., Severe megaloblastic anemia in child breast fed by a vegetarian mother, *Ann. Pediatr.,* 40, 28, 1993.

94. Taha, S. A., The pattern of severe protein-calorie malnutrition in Sudanese children attending a large hospital in the Sudan, *Am. J. Clinical Nutr.,* 32, 446, 1979.

95. Alpert, J. and Fava, M., Nutrition and depression: the role of folate, *Nutr. Rev.,* 55, 129, 1997.

96. Bottiglieri, T., Folate, Vitamin B$_{12}$, and neuropsychiatric disorders, *Nutr. Rev.,* 54, 382, 1996.

97. Lubani, M. M., al-Saleh, Q. A., Teebi, A. S., et al., Cystic fibrosis and *Helicobacter pylori* gastritis, megaloblastic anaemia, subnormal mentality and minor anomalies in two siblings: a new syndrome? *Eur. J. Pediatr.,* 150, 253, 1991.

98. Zittoun, J., Congenital errors of folate metabolism, *BailliERES Clinical Haematol.,* 8, 603, 1995.

99. Greenblatt, J. M., Huffman, L. C., Reiss, A. L., Folic acid in neurodevelopment and child psychiatry, *Prog. Neuro-Psychopharmacol Biol. Psychiatr.,* 18, 647, 1994.

100. Kirksey, A., Wachs, T. D., Srinath, U., et al., Relation of maternal zinc nutrition to pregnancy outcome and early infant development in an Egyptian village, *Am. J. Clinical Nutr.,* 60, 782, 1994.

101. Pritchard, J. A., Scott, D. E., Whalley, P. J., et al., Infants of mothers with megaloblastic anemia due to folate deficiency, *JAMA,* 211, 1982, 1970.

102. Freycon, F. and Pouyau, G., Rare nutritional deficiency anemia: deficiency of copper and vitamin E, *Semaine des Hopitaux,* 59, 488, 1983.

103. Majaj, A. S., Vitamin E-responsive macrocytic anemia in protein-calorie malnutrition. Measurements of vitamin E, folic acid, vitamin C, Vitamin B_{12} and iron, *Am. J. Clinical Nutr.,* 18, 362, 1966.

104. Botash, A. S., Nasca, J., Dubowy, R., et al., Zinc-induced copper deficiency in an infant, *Am. J. Dis. Child.,* 146, 709, 1992.

105. Lindenbaum, J., Healton, E. B., Savage, D. G., et al., Neuropsychiatric disorders caused by cobalamin deficiency in the absence of anemia or macrocytosis, *New Engl. J. Med.,* 318, 1720, 1988.

106. Verbanck, P. and LeBon, O., Changing psychiatric symptoms in a patient with vitamin B_{12} deficiency, *J. Clinical Psychiatr.,* 52, 182, 1991.

107. Wulffraat, N. M., De Schryver, J., Bruin, M., et al., Failure to thrive is an early symptom of the Imerslund Grasbeck syndrome, *Am. J. Pediatr. Hematol. Oncol.,* 16, 177, 1994.

108. Shorvon, S. D., Carney, M. W., Chanarin, I., et al., The neuropsychiatry of megaloblastic anaemia, *Br. Med. J.,* 281, 1036, 1980.

109. Al Essa, M., Sakati, N. A., Dabbagh, O., et al., Inborn error of vitamin B_{12} metabolism: a treatable cause of childhood dementia/paralysis, *J. Child. Neurol.,* 13, 239, 1998.

110. Kam, T., Birmingham, C. L., and Goldner, E. M., Polyglandular autoimmune syndrome and anorexia nervosa, *Int. J. Eating Dis.,* 16, 101, 1994.

6 Functional Consequences of Nutritional Anemia in School Age Children

Santosh Jain Passi and Sheila C. Vir

CONTENTS

6.1 INTRODUCTION

Nutritional anemia, particularly iron deficiency anemia (IDA), is perhaps clinically the most widespread nutritional deficiency disorder in the world today.[1] Anemia is a public health problem, not only among pregnant mothers, infants, and young children but also among school age children including adolescents. Growing children require large amounts of iron for continuous increase in body mass and are therefore vulnerable to iron deficiency and its consequences. At a meeting of the International

Nutritional Anemia Consultative Group (INACG, 1999), it was stated that school children aged 5 to 14 years must be recognized as a high risk group because the percentage of anemic children is as high as that of the pregnant women.[2]

6.2   PREVALENCE

Recent estimates suggest that over one-third of the school population is anemic; the problem is most pronounced in sub-Saharan Africa and Southeast Asia where anemia is linked to poverty.[1] Most studies have focussed on pregnant women and preschool age children; data for preadolescent school aged children are limited. More data are becoming available for older school age children because of the increasing concern for this target group. Studies from developing countries indicate that the incidence of anemia varies widely. Prevalence data from a multicountry study on the nutritional status of adolescents report anemia prevalence ranging from 32 to 55%.[3] While anemia and vitamin A deficiency are common nutritional disorders in school children (aged 5 to 15 years) in India,[4] the prevalence of anemia (Hb <12 g/dL) in Sri Lanka was only 3.7% among adolescent females; however the prevalence of depleted iron stores (serum ferritin <12 µg/L) was 59%.[5] Three of the 4 studies from the multi-country study supported by International Center for Research on Women (ICRW) did not find any gender differences except in Ecuador where the prevalence was higher among boys (20%) compared to girls (15%). In contrast, studies from Asia indicate that the prevalence of iron deficiency anemia (IDA) is higher in females than in males, especially teenage girls.[6-9] The prevalence of IDA in China was 61.8% and 46.8% among girls and boys, respectively, and the associated morbidity was 15.8 and 32.6%, respectively. The study from Taiwan[6] identified teenaged females at risk of IDA, with the prevalence ranging from 9.38 to 26.4%. Although the prevalence of anemia was similar for both sexes (17% in boys and 18% in girls) among Pakistani school children (13 to 20 years), the prevalence of iron deficiency (based on serum ferritin) was higher in girls (54%) compared to boys (30%). Limited availability of dietary iron for children belonging to a lower socioeconomic group was proposed to be the major contributory cause.[9] In the study conducted by the Nutrition Foundation of India (1999), including 520 urban and 185 rural adolescent girls (aged 11 to 19 years), nearly 17% of the rural and 9.6% of the urban adolescent girls had Hb levels <10g/dl.[4] In another study from India, the prevalence of anemia was 25% among school age girls and increased with the attainment of menarche.[7] Although the iron density in the diets of boys and girls is similar, the lower food intake by the adolescent girls compared to boys, combined with menstrual losses, cause adolescent girls to be at greater risk of iron deficiency and anemia.

Studies have also shown that adolescent girls of high and low socioeconomic groups have alarmingly high incidence of iron deficiency anemia.[7,10] A nutrition survey report from Tanzania[11] found that the hemoglobin status was lower in school children (aged 5 to 14 years) and adolescents. The main causes were low dietary intakes of iron and parasitic infections. The prevalence of anemia in female teenagers from Brazil was reported to be 17.6% and was higher in the group that had not reached menarche. Other predictors of anemia included socioeconomic status,

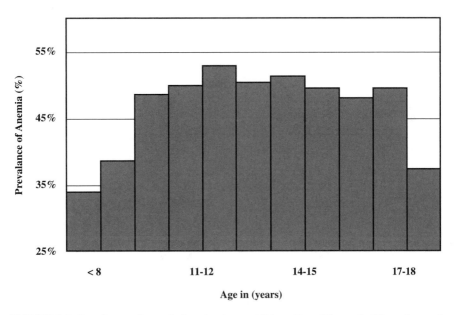

FIGURE 6.1 Prevalence of anemia in school age children (8 to 18 years). (From Agarwal, D.K., Upadhyay, S.K., Tripathi, A.M., and Agarwal, K.N., Nutrition Foundation of India, Scientific Report 6, 1987, 40. With permission.)

schooling of parents, and specific home characteristics. Surprisingly, the occurrence of anemia was not associated with the interval between menstrual cycles.[12]

Many studies suggest that the incidence of anemia in school age children tends to increase with age and is highest during periods of growth and adolescence. In India, the prevalence of anemia amongst adolescent girls increased from 10 years old upward and remained high until 18 years of age (Figure 6.1).[7,13] The highest prevalence was between the ages of 12 to 15 years with over 50% children being anemic. A study of 2224 children and adolescents (12 to 18 years) in Madrid found that the prevalence of iron deficiency was the highest in the age group of 13 to 15 years old, although the magnitude of the problem was smaller. The actual prevalence of iron deficiency and iron deficiency anemia (IDA), was only 4.94% and 0.94%, respectively.[14] The increase in the prevalence of IDA with age may be explained by the steady increase in body mass, which can be correlated to variation in the growth of adolescents.[15,16]

Data from developed countries in America and Europe indicate a much lower prevalence of anemia among adolescent populations. However, studies in Japan, Sweden, Australia, and the U.S. indicate a greater frequency of iron deficiency in affluent societies.[17] A study from England indicates that while the overall prevalence of anemia (Hb <120 g/L) was 20%, it was 11% for Caucasian girls compared to 22 to 25% for Asian girls.[18] The prevalence of anemia was higher (25%) among girls who tried to lose weight in the previous year and among those who belonged to a lower social class. Data from a survey in the U.S. indicate that the prevalence

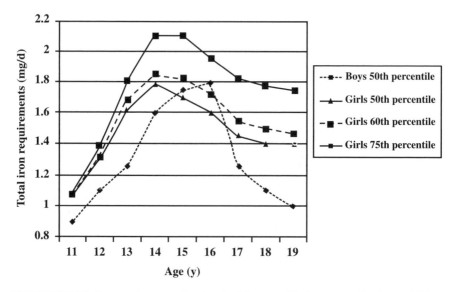

FIGURE 6.2 Median requirements for absorbed iron (mg/day) among school age children. (From Beard, J.L., *J. Nutr.*, 130(25), 4405, 2000. With permission.)

of iron deficiency was between 8 to 10% among adolescent girls aged 12 to 19 years, whereas it was <1% in boys of the same age group.[19]

6.3 CAUSES OF NUTRITIONAL ANEMIA

Iron deficiency is the major cause of anemia. It is apparent from Figure 6.2 in which the median requirement for absorbed iron (mg/day) is shown, that the risk of iron deficiency is proportional to growth velocity and increases during the adolescent growth spurt — the risk is high for both boys and girls.[15,20] Following the growth spurt, the risk continues to remain high for girls because of menstrual blood loss, but subsides for boys. Losses of iron due to frequent parasitic infections, dietary factors, and menstrual loss contribute to IDA. It is important to recognize that in many settings, the etiology of nutritional anemias is multicausal. Low dietary intakes of iron and/or other nutrients such as folate and vitamins A, and B$_{12}$, coupled with poor absorption and exacerbated by malaria and hookworm infestation result in nutritional anemias. The role of other underlying factors such as gender discrimination in intra-household food allocation and early marriage leading to early pregnancy also needs to be considered in certain settings (Figure 6.3).

6.3.1 DIETARY CAUSES

Low intake and poor bio-availability of iron are the most important causes of IDA (Allen et al., Chapter 2). Cereal based diets in many developing countries have high concentrations of inhibitors and low concentrations of enhancers. Szarfarc and De-Souza[21] found that the typical Brazilian diet is poor in bio-available iron. The amount of meat and beans, the two main food items that contribute to total iron intake in

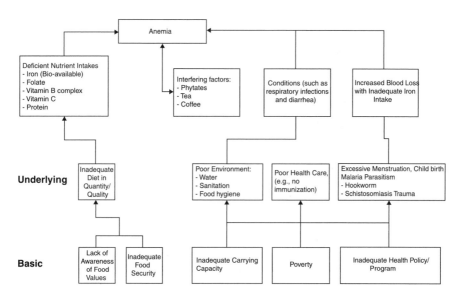

FIGURE 6.3 Causes of anemia. (*Source:* UNICEF-WHO Joint Committee on Health Policy, 1994.)

the habitual Brazilian diet, has been decreasing during the last two decades. Pooled data from the National Nutrition Monitoring Bureau (NNMB) indicate that the diets of Indian girls aged between 13 and 18 years provide much lower levels of iron than diets of the boys in the same age groups.[22] The prevalence of anemia is reported[23] to be significantly higher in Indian adolescents consuming a vegetarian diet (45.8%) as compared to those consuming a mixed diet, which includes animal foods (30.0%). Moreover, habitual consumption of tea/coffee immediately after meals by adolescent girls was associated with a higher prevalence of anemia (50%) compared to those who did not consume tea/coffee after meals (34%).

In developed urban areas of developing countries, symptoms of iron deficiency have been on the increase and have been linked to changing dietary intakes.[7] Dietary intakes of iron and vitamin C are often inadequate even in industrialized countries. Diets of school age children tend to include fewer vegetables, fruits, and unrefined cereals which are often replaced by the widely available snack foods such as carbonated colas, chips, candies, etc., which are of low protein and micronutrient density.[24] High iron requirements, combined with lower food intakes due to the desire to lose weight often lead to insufficient dietary iron and produce high incidence of iron deficiency in affluent societies.[25]

6.3.2 INFECTIONS

Hookworm infestation results in chronic blood loss and is an important cause of anemia in some settings. It affects nearly one billion people worldwide, and the prevalence increases with age, reaching a plateau in late adolescence. Urbani et al.[26] found a significant correlation between anemia and intestinal parasitic infection (*Schistosoma haematobium*) in an epidemiological survey of 1297 school children aged 5 to 12 years in Mauritania. The overall prevalence of intestinal parasitic infections and anemia (Hb <11 g/dl) was 38.1% and 50.4%, respectively. Stoltzfus et al.[27] reported that in school age children with more than 2000 hookworm eggs per gram of feces, the incidence of high protoporphyrin levels and moderate to severe anemia (Hb <9 g/dl) was significantly higher in Zanzibar. In a study in India, one-third of adolescent girls had a history of passing worms. The prevalence of anemia was double in these girls (53.6%) compared to those who were not infected (25%).[23]

Malaria increases the risk of anemia. It adversely affects its severity by causing hemolytic anemia that leads to less iron in the hemoglobin and more iron sequestered in stores.[28,29] Malaria is associated with some impairment in the release of iron from reticulo-endothelial stores. The victims of HIV infections are also reported to suffer from anemia.[24]

6.4 CONSEQUENCES OF NUTRITIONAL ANEMIA

Anemia during childhood and adolescence has serious implications for a wide range of outcomes: impaired physical growth and mental development; weakened behavioral and cognitive development; reduced physical fitness and work performance/capacity, and diminished concentration in work and school performance. A detailed review of the effect of iron deficiency on children's growth and mental, cognitive, and behavioral development has been documented by many.[30,31] The role of anemia in adolescent girls posing a major threat to safe motherhood also has to be recognized.[32]

6.4.1 GROWTH RETARDATION

The body weights of children suffering from IDA are often lower than those of normal children, which can partly be attributed to anorexia and the altered intestinal functions associated with this deficiency disorder. Young school age children (6 to 8 years) with low iron stores were significantly more stunted than iron replete children in a study in South Africa.[33] Several controlled studies have shown that iron supplementation improved growth of school age children in different settings.[34-38] A study conducted in Indonesia[34] reported significant increases in weight, height, and mid upper arm circumference (MUAC) only among anemic children following 12 weeks of daily iron supplementation. Latham et al.[35] found a significant increase only in weight gain (2.1 kg compared to 1.2 kg after 15 weeks) in their study of Kenyan school children with low Hb levels. However, subsequent studies by the same group[36,39] have reported improvements in linear growth as well. The more recent studies in India[37,38] failed to detect an effect on linear growth, which may be due to limited sample size, limited response only to those who are anemic, and short duration of intervention. It is also important to note that the age ranges of subjects varied in these studies and included both pre- and post-pubertal children who may respond differently. For example, the studies from Indonesia and Kenya included primary school children, whereas those from India also included postmenarcheal girls. Of note, are the findings by Kanani and Poojara[53] in which the greatest response in weight gain and body mass index (BMI) was seen among younger children (10 to

14 years), although older girls (15 to 18 years) benefited as well.[37] Some of these studies suggest that iron supplementation possibly affects growth by improving appetite and total food intake.[36,37] The effects of iron fortified soup consumption and deworming have also demonstrated that combined interventions had a greater impact on improving iron status and the growth of South African 6 to 8 year old children.[33] Similarly, Ash et al. demonstrated the benefits of a multinutrient approach.[39] Walker[40] has reported that iron deficiency adversely affects the growth rate in children and causes impaired cognitive function.

In light of the recent interest in intermittent iron supplementation as a strategy to prevent and control anemia, the results of two recent studies from India are described in detail.[38] Fifty adolescent girls aged 14 to 16 years and 40 elementary school girls aged 6 to 7 years received Fe-B_{12} tablets twice a week for 8 weeks from their school teachers for *on the spot* consumption. Proper records were maintained.[38] The experimental group registered a significant improvement in the Hb levels in both age groups; the mean increase was 1.42 g/dl in adolescent girls who received tablets containing 100 mg elemental iron and 500 µg vitamin B_{12}, and 1.19 g/dl in elementary school girls who received 20 mg elemental iron and 100 µg vitamin B_{12}. In contrast, the changes in mean Hb levels were negligible in the control groups (0.1 g/dl and 0.16 g/dl). These changes were accompanied by significant increases in weight gain for both the supplemented groups; 1.34 kg and 1.51 kg for adolescents and elementary school girls, compared to 0.34 kg and 0.8 kg in the respective control groups. There was no effect on linear growth. The younger girls were more enthusiastic about receiving the Fe-B_{12} supplements and attached a lot of importance to the fact that anything received from their teacher had to be in their benefit. In another group of primary school children which included both boys and girls aged 8 to 9 years, belonging to lower socioeconomic strata, tablets containing 20 mg elemental iron and 100 µg vitamin B_{12} were distributed by the schoolteachers twice a week for on the spot consumption along with the mid-day meal food supplement. The study was carried out for a period of 2 months and the results indicated that the experimental group (n = 57) registered a significant increase in mean Hb levels (0.71 g/dl) compared to the control group (n = 54) who received only the food supplements (0.09 g/dl). Significant increases in mean body weight (1.07 kg) and MUAC (0.21 cm) were seen for the supplemented group compared to the control group who gained only 0.36 kg in body weight and 0.10 cm in MUAC. There were no differences in height increments between the groups.[38] This study demonstrates how school feeding programs can be used as effective channels for the distribution of micronutrient supplements at a nominal cost.

6.4.2   POOR PHYSICAL PERFORMANCE

Work capacity, work output, and endurance are impaired due to iron deficiency. Moderate and severe forms of anemia result in reduced endurance, i.e., individuals take a longer time to complete tasks.[41] Mild anemia can have an adverse effect on productivity, there is evidence of lowered work capacity and reduced immunocompetence in mild iron deficiency without anemia.[42] It has been estimated that each 1% decrease in hemoglobin results in a 1.5% decrease in work capacity and a 1 to 2% decrease in work output which can result in serious economic consequences.[43]

Although few studies have examined work performance among adolescents, this age group is often involved in productive activities. A close correlation between the degree of growth retardation and the degree of physical and functional impairment was observed in a study of 1336 children between the ages of 6 to 8 years studying in rural schools of Uttar Pradesh, India. The prevalence of anemia and growth retardation (85%) was extremely high in this population.[43] Similarly, a reduction in endurance capacity was noted among those who were moderately or severely anemic in another study of school age girls (6 to 14 yrs of age) in India.[44] Anemia has been correlated with physical functional handicaps as well.

6.4.3 IMPAIRED MENTAL AND PSYCHOMOTOR FUNCTIONS

Anemic children are reported to exhibit poor attentiveness, poor memory, and poor academic performance. They are often disruptive, irritable, and restless and show behavioral abnormalities like lack of attention, fatigue, insecurity, and reduced learning ability. Poor attention span, memory, and concentration, as well as concept acquisition leading to poor school performance have been attributed to anemia during this phase of critical learning. Recent studies have established the fact that anemia in school age children is related to poor mental capabilities, lower IQ, lowered scholastic performance, and behavioral modifications resulting in poor social interactions and other related problems.

In a study carried out by Nutrition Foundation of India (n = 469), there were a significantly higher proportion of children with IQs above 110 and a significantly lower proportion with IQs below 90 in the nonanemic group when compared to the severely anemic children. Both the verbal and performance IQ scores of the children decreased progressively with falls in Hb levels. These findings suggest that all functions are not affected in anemia; and that among those affected, different functions are compromised at different levels of severity of anemia. The results of analysis of variance (ANOVA) highlighted that the observed influence of anemia could be attributed to the associated undernutrition rather than anemia per se. The children's mean arithmetic test scores were found to decrease with the severity of anemia. The authors conclude that while anemia impairs attention and concentration, its effect on intellectual ability could be attributed to associated malnutrition.[13] Webb and Oski[45] and Soemantri et al.[46] reported that anemia results in poor attention, concentration and scholastic performance.

In a study conducted in Egypt (n = 68; mean age = 9.5 years), the efficiency in problem solving was found to be positively associated with iron status.[47] The responses of children who were not anemic were significantly faster and more accurate compared to those with IDA. In a large study of 8000 randomly selected children aged 9 to 13 years in Jamaica, ascaris infection and anemia predicted poorer school attendance; even mild undernutrition and geohelminthic infections were associated with poorer school achievement levels on the wide range achievement test.[48] The prevalence of anemia (Hb <10 g/dl) was 14.7%, and helminthic infections were common in this population. Similarly, Hurtado et al.[49] found in a study of 5411 children, aged 10, that anemia was associated with increased likelihood of mild/moderate mental retardation even after controlling for confounding factors such as birth weight, gender, race, maternal age/education. In a study conducted in Philadelphia with 193 economically deprived children aged 12 to 14 years, anemic students obtained significantly lower achievement scores in the Iowa Test of Basic Skills compared to the nonanemic children.[45] Anemic students took significantly longer time in reporting a visual after image task than the nonanemics, which could perhaps be attributed to altered cerebral metabolism. These findings suggest that anemia is associated with disturbances in attention and perception resulting in poor academic achievements.

The only exception is a study from China[8] which showed no significant effects of IDA on intelligence, IQ, and school performance. However, speed and endurance capabilities of students of both sexes were correlated directly with hemoglobin levels. Anemic female students in Australia demonstrated higher psychological distress based on the General Health Questionnaire (GHQ) than nonanemic subjects.[50] Iron deficiency, however, was not associated with nonspecific symptoms of psychological distress. Among iron deficient subjects, those using oral contraceptive pills reported significantly more symptoms than non-users.

Most of the consequences of anemia related to cognitive outcomes in school age children are based on the role of iron deficiency, which has been associated with longterm impairments in brain maturation, attention span, intelligence scores, and school performance.[51] The role of iron deficiency on developmental effects is not well defined but the requirement of iron for myelination of developing neurons within the central nervous system and being an essential component of several neurotransmitters provide some possible explanations (see Chapters 5 and 7). Lozoff[30] has reported that iron deficiency adversely affects behavior by impairing cognitive development disturbances and by limiting activity and work capacity. It has been proposed that iron deficiency causes alterations in attention processes. Iron therapy may bring about improvement in some cognitive functions but lower developmental IQ and achievement test scores continue even after iron is taken. The behavioral effects of IDA have been associated with changes in neurotransmission. Pollitt[52] contends that learning disabilities and mental retardation can be due to general developmental lag or to specific cognitive dysfunctions that, when combined, interfere with school performance in most or all of the areas of learning. He reported that the existing data do not suggest that IDA interferes with several of the cognitive functions; in fact, the particular functions at the highest risk remain unknown.

Earlier work by Hill[53] has shown that iron is not equally distributed in all regions of the brain and therefore it is unlikely that all of the neural substrates of cognitive function are going to be affected equally due to IDA. It has been reported that the associations between IDA and long term intellectual deficits are mediated by either anatomic or neurochemical changes. Although most of the evidence to date is based on treatment of IDA, some studies have shown that iron deficiency even in the absence of anemia may adversely affect mental performance. Improved verbal learning and memory were found in a study among nonanemic iron deficient American children treated with oral ferrous sulfate.[54] In contrast, results of earlier intervention trials found that only IDA, but not the less severe forms of iron deficiency, cause impairments in mental development.[52] Iron therapy in school age children suffering from IDA results in improvement in certain behavioral tests and school performance. Significant improvements in the school test performance were seen among iron deficient anemic children (9 to 12 years) who received iron supplements in a controlled trial in Indo-nesia.[46] Although this study did not examine the effect of iron deficiency on the specific cognitive processes which interfere with learning, the authors suggest that attention maintenance, selective attention, concentration, perceptual organization, short-term memory, and conceptual learning are some of the cognitive processes that are likely to be affected. Similarly, in the study from Egypt, significant improvements were seen among anemic children following 4 months of daily iron supplementation (50 mg of iron as ferrous sulfate) when compared to those who received the placebo. Nonanemic children did not benefit from iron supplementation. It is not clear whether iron repletion will compensate for the accrued deficits in learning.

In summary, the impact of anemia on mental development and cognitive per-formance can be equal to the impact of mild childhood lead poisoning, i.e., 0.5 to 1.0 standard deviations (SD) lower. Improvement in cognitive scores of 1 SD has been associated with a 17% to 23% increase in hourly earnings of primary/secondary school children in Kenya.[55] The World Bank has estimated that a 1 SD rise in cognitive achievement can be equated with a 7 to 12% increase in earnings.[56] The economic consequences of anemia can thus be grave. However, many of the ill effects of IDA may not be corrected by iron therapy alone, and therefore the prevention of anemia and iron deficiency among school age children should be treated as an absolute priority.

6.4.4 MATERNAL MORTALITY AND LOW BIRTH WEIGHT

Scholl et al. demonstrated the increased risk of preterm delivery in adolescents with anemia, but there are very few intervention trials in this population.[57] The deleterious effects of IDA on reproductive health and later pregnancy outcome are more likely if girls are anemic through adolescence and enter pregnancy with depleted stores. Poor iron stores before conception constitute one of the main causes of IDA during pregnancy.[58] Iron stores are depleted during adolescence due to increased needs for iron for rapid growth and loss of iron with the onset of menarche. A vicious cycle of nutritional anemia thus sets in (Figure 6.4).

The high prevalence of anemia and growth retardation among girls who conceive during adolescence might partly account for lowered mean birth weight and higher perinatal and neonatal mortality.[59] This is of significant public health concern in developing countries where one-third of adolescent girls are reported to be anemic[60] and the average age at marriage ranges between 15 to 17 years.[61] The role of adequate iron status in promoting birth weight, gestational age, and adolescent growth in developing countries is of special significance. There is however, limited evidence from developing countries on the adverse consequences of IDA on pregnancy out-comes in adolescent girls and whether improving iron status during adolescence will improve pregnancy outcomes.

6.4.5 OTHER CONSEQUENCES

Other clinical symptoms due to iron deficiency anemia include anorexia, nausea, flatulence, dimness of vision, and headache, all of which may ultimately affect a school age child's performance. Anemia also causes listlessness, fatigue, and reduced work

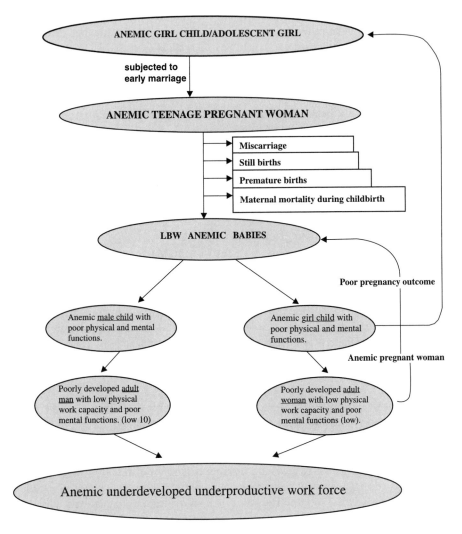

FIGURE 6.4 Vicious cycle of nutritional anemia in children.

capacity; even mild anemia results in impaired work capacity and reduced physical activity. Beaton and Patwardhan[62] reported that as anemia becomes severe, the individuals may experience headache, dizziness, nausea, flatulence, and irregularity in menstruation as well as disturbances in gastrointestinal, renal, and neuromuscular functions. Regularization of menstrual cycle has been reported following iron supplementation.[63] Other effects of anemia include reduced immunity, increased morbidity,[64] and recently it has been reported that the response to iodine intervention can also be hampered by iron deficiency, since thyroperoxidase is a heme containing enzyme.[65]

In summary, nutritional anemias contribute toward the morbidity, mortality, and dropout rates among school children. Poor attendance in school and poor school performance/achievements suggest that efforts need to be directed toward reducing the incidence of anemia and improving not only the nutritional and health status of these children, but improving their retention at school and achieving the goal of universal primary education.

6.5 INTERVENTION MEASURES

Several food based (dietary improvement, fortification of foods with iron) and non-food based (iron supplementation and helminth control) strategies can be used effectively to prevent and control nutritional anemias in school age children. Recent experiences and future directions in relation to this important target group are summarized in this final section.

6.5.1 FOOD BASED STRATEGIES

6.5.1.1 Dietary Diversification

Dietary diversification has been recognized as the most effective long term sustainable strategy for overcoming the multiple nutrient deficiencies that may play a role in the etiology of nutritional anemia. To achieve this, nutrition education coupled with horticultural programs to increase production and consumption of micronutrient (including iron) rich food groups, especially vegetables and fruits, is of utmost importance.[66,67] Promoting appropriate dietary habits through effective nutrition education has been reported to have a positive impact on reducing IDA in Indonesia and in improving Hb levels in India.[68] Studies undertaken in Baroda[69] demonstrated that children who consume green leafy vegetables frequently (once a week or more) tend to have higher Hb levels than those who are infrequent or nonconsumers (10.2% vs. 9.5%). Daily supplementation of guava fruit with the two major meals resulted in significant increases in Hb of 2.2 g/dl in young anemic women while the unsupplemented subjects showed nonsignificant increases of 0.3 g/dl. No change in serum ferritin was noted. Similar positive impacts of nutrition education have been reported in urban poor schoolgirls (8 to 13 years) who were encouraged to improve their dietary practices using inexpensive local foods.[70] The nutrition communication strategy with a focus on qualitative and quantitative improvement of the diets resulted in highly significant increases in energy, protein, iron, and vitamin C intakes, increased awareness of the importance of preventing iron deficiency, and increased Hb levels. The mean Hb increment was 0.8 g/dl in the experimental group. These findings clearly indicate that the promotion of iron rich food items should form a part of a comprehensive nutrition communication strategy with a focus on (1) regular consumption of iron and vitamin C rich foods/enhancers; (2) reduced intake of inhibitors of iron absorption such as tea/coffee immediately following meals; (3) promoting household food processing methods such as fermentation, germination, and malting which increase iron absorption by lowering phytic acid or tannin or both (see Chapter 10 for details).[71]

6.5.1.2 Fortification

At the population level, food fortification is the best option if a suitable food vehicle can be identified. The successful experience in Latin America is described by Walter et al. (see Chapter 9). Iron fortification of wheat flour is under study in other parts of the world. As part of the anemia prevention policy, Zambia has a program of food fortification; in many other countries, some foods are being fortified; although, as yet, they have no policies on food fortification. Still others, like Ethiopia and Madagascar, are considering food fortification (INACG). India has no such program yet except fortification of a few food items by some food companies.

School feeding programs providing energy protein rich food supplements fortified with micronutrients (including iron) have been quite successful in reducing the prevalence of anemia in different settings.[72] Gopaldas et al.[73] have demonstrated the significant impact of iron-folate, vitamin A, and deworming in reducing anemia and improving iron status and growth of midday meal program beneficiaries in western India. Most recently, in a placebo controlled trial conducted in South Africa, micronutrient fortified biscuits and cold drinks were given to 6- to 11-year-old school children (N = 252) for 12 months; significant improvements in serum ferritin, serum iron, transferrin saturation, hemoglobin, and hematocrit levels were seen in the experimental groups. The greatest benefits were for children with poorer iron status.[74] The intervention also resulted in a significant improvement in performing certain cognitive tasks, particularly those related to intellectual skills.[75] This study indicated that biscuits and cold drinks can easily be used as suitable vehicles for fortification in school feeding, particularly in view of their high energy content, relatively low cost, and ease of consumption, storage, distribution, and monitoring. Ash et al. have demonstrated the efficacy of a commercially prepared multinutrient fortified beverage in reducing anemia among school age children in Kenya.[39] These findings show how a feasible, cost effective, and practical strategy, along with nutrition education can help in addressing the problem of micronutrient malnutrition in school age children.

6.5.2 SUPPLEMENTATION

Most iron supplementation programs typically do not include school age children. However, this has been suggested as a promising strategy in the prevention and control of anemia, especially in settings where diets have poor iron bioavailability and the overall prevalence of anemia is high as seen in South Asia. Viteri[76] proposed that weekly iron supplementation for school age children (36 to 50 doses of 60 mg of iron per year) could serve as a cost effective, community based strategy, aimed at the primary prevention of iron deficiency as well as increasing iron reserves among adolescents and adult women. In addition to the benefits of improved growth and school performance in young children, the needs of adolescent girls warrant special attention.[77] Weekly pharmaceutical supplements have been suggested as a cost effective method of addressing the problem of anemia in adolescent girls since the requirement for iron tablets will be reduced to 52 per year, and weekly doses may ensure more effective absorption of iron with reduced side effects and possibly higher compliance. In a technical workshop of UNICEF/UNU/WHO/MI,[78] it was proposed that in countries where anemia prevalence exceeds 40% of pregnant women, universal supplementation of adolescent girls (at a minimum those aged 12 to 16 years) and women of childbearing age is warranted. Based on the preliminary findings of the ongoing multicentric study in three regions of India (Table 6.1), the expert working group at

TABLE 6.1
Multicentric Study on School Age Girls (10–18 years) in India (1996–1997)

Study Parameter	Gujarat Seshadri et al. (1998)[80]	Mumbai Mehta et al. (1998)[63]	Delhi Agarwal et al. (1998)[79]
Sample size	1513	1748	2170
Iron intake (mg)	8.1–9.3	8.11–12.3	—
Energy intake (kcal)	908–945	960–1062	—
Anemia (%)	57–65	62–65	48–50
Reduction in anemia with daily iron supplements (%)	63–45	61.6–26.2	—
Reduction in infections (%)	57–66	65–33.9	

the National Consultation recommended that adolescent girls upon reaching menarche should consume weekly dosages of one IFA tablet containing 100 mg elemental iron and 500 μg folic acid — accompanied by appropriate dietary counselling.[65,79,80]

A recent meta-analysis of controlled trials (Table 6.2) examined the efficacy of intermittent iron supplementation compared to daily iron supplementation to reduce the prevalence of IDA in developing countries. Beaton et al.[81] concluded that while weekly iron supplementation was efficacious in reducing the prevalence of anemia in adolescents compared to controls (RR = 0.76 to 1.10), the evidence demonstrates that a daily regimen is better than a weekly one with a summary relative risk value of 1.44 (95% CI = 1.33, 1.56) based on nine studies. More importantly, the authors highlighted that in situations other than pregnancy when daily supplementation is recommended, weekly iron supplementation should be introduced only in situations where compliance will be higher, i.e., under supervised administration. The implications of these recommendations raise questions as to the effectiveness of weekly supplementation in field based programs in supervised settings such as schools that do not cover all adolescents, especially girls. More work is needed in this area.

A "girl-to-girl" approach has been recommended for reaching adolescent girls, i.e., linking one schoolgirl with 4 to 5 girls in the community who are not at school. The school network offers an excellent opportunity to reach "captive" adolescent girls. A group of girls could be trained (supplying, counselling, and monitoring of IFA tablets) to take on the responsibility for nonstudent girls. A group of 42 adolescent girls (aged 12 to 18 years) participating in the girl-to-girl approach of the Integrated Child Development Program (ICDS) was recruited for a study; they received 25 iron folate tablets containing 100 mg of elemental iron and 500 μg of folate and were advised to consume one tablet per day. After 8 weeks, unlike the schoolgirls, the ICDS beneficiaries showed little improvement in Hb, weight, or height status. The poor impact could be attributed to noncompliance, irregularity of consumption, or lack of motivation and monitoring. In the case of the school children, the teachers performed the monitoring function very well.[38] This strategy needs to be further tested in different settings through linkages with schools and other development programs.

TABLE 6.2
Comparison of Weekly versus Daily Iron Supplementation in Reducing the Prevalence of Anemia[a] among School Age Children (10–18 years)

Study	Treatment	N	Baseline (%)	Final (%)
Baroda, India	Weekly	438	53.8	66.2
	Daily	441	63.5	44.4
	Control	311	62.7	60.1
East Jakarta	Weekly	134	17.9	6.7
	Daily	64	15.6	7.8
	Control	75	17.3	21.3
Bombay, India	Weekly	680	65.0	33.9
	Daily	558	61.6	26.2
	Control	510	64.8	58.4
Delhi, India	Weekly Supervision	506	49.0	48.2
	Daily	480	49.6	43.0
	Daily Supervision	617	47.0	30.9
	Control	401	44.6	57.8
Mali	Weekly	115	29.6	38.0
	Daily	116	37.1	30.9
	Control	114	28.9	39.0
Peru	Weekly	98	18.4	17.3
	Daily	116	19.8	10.9
	Control	97	15.5	22.7

[a] Hb <120g/l.

Source: From Beaton, G.H. and McCabe, G.P., Efficacy of intermittent iron supplementation in the control of iron deficiency anaemia in developing countries: an analysis of experience, Third final report of the Micronutrient Initiative, Toronto, 1999.

Other alternatives such as the social marketing of tablets, currently being pilot tested by Parivar Seva Sanasthan — a non-governmental organization and the Delhi government with UNICEF support, also need to be reviewed and promoted especially in urban schools.[82] A successful weekly supplementation program has been reported from northern Thailand where families have been encouraged to purchase iron tablets.[78] In a Nutrition Foundation of India study conducted in Delhi and Rajasthan, the increases in Hb levels of adolescent girls were greater among those who received vitamin C along with iron and folic acid supplements compared to those who received only iron-folate supplements alone; these benefits were seen only among iron deficient anemic children.[83] No change was observed in nonanemic children given iron supplementation or anemic children who received placebos. These findings support the need to examine multinutrient strategies and appropriate targeting of supplementation.

Finally, although iron deficiency promotes infection by lowering the body's resistance to infectious diseases, the administration of iron supplements, especially to iron replete individuals, may have adverse effects such as increased morbidity. Pathogenic bacteria may compete effectively for iron in circulation and thereby exacerbate existing infections. Wright[84] has cautioned against the indiscriminate use of iron supplements, particularly in view of the relationship between iron deficiency and lead poisoning, which are the causes of neurocognitive toxicity. In light of these concerns, it is recommended that iron supplements should be distributed with caution and preferably targeted only to those who are iron deficient or those who continue to live in lead exposed environments.

6.5.3 CONTROL OF PARASITIC INFECTIONS

Control of infections, particularly those producing chronic blood loss is another important strategy. Routine deworming has been recommended as a cost effective strategy to control anemia, especially in areas where hookworm infestation is heavily endemic. It has been shown to improve iron status, appetite, and even growth (weight) of school age children in several controlled trials (Hall et al., see Chapter 10). Studies that failed to detect any benefit may have been conducted in areas where the load of parasitic infections is relatively low.[38,85] It is necessary to determine the extent to which iron deficiency, factors such as other nutrient deficiencies, and malaria, helminth, and other chronic or acute infections play a role in the etiology of anemia in different settings in order to better implement strategies to reduce the prevalence of nutritional anemia.

In conclusion, the functional consequences of nutritional anemias, especially IDA in school age children indicate the urgency for addressing this public health problem in many developing countries. Public health services and school health policy need to assign a high priority to this preventable micronutrient deficiency disorder. It has significant adverse effects not only on school performance but also on future work productivity, health, and the wellbeing of the next generation by influencing birth outcomes and child growth and development. A concerted advocacy effort is required to appreciate the linkages of IDA with the World Summit goals for universal primary education, reduction of incidence of low birth weight, and reduction of maternal mortality.

REFERENCES

1. Indicators for assessing iron deficiency and strategies for its prevention. Draft based on WHO/UNICEF/UNU Consultation 6–10 December 1993, New York.
2. Internatinoal Nutritional Anaemia Consultative Group Symposium, Durban, March 12, 1999.
3. Kurz, K. M. and Johnson-Welch, C., The nutrition and lives of adolescents in developing countries: findings from the nutrition of adolescent girls research programmes, International Center for Research on Women, Washington, D.C., 1994.
4. Awate, R. V., Ketkar, Y. A. and Somaiya, P. A., Prevalence of nutritional deficiency disorders among rural primary school children (5–15 years), *J. Indian Med. Assoc.*, 95(7), 410, 1997.

5. Atukorala, T. M. and de Silva, L. D., Iron status of adolescent females in three schools in an urban area of Sri Lanka, *J. Trop. Pediatr.,* 36(6), 316, 1990.

6. Shaw, N. S., Iron deficiency anemia in school children and adolescents, *J. Formosa Med. Assoc.,* 95(9), 692, 1996.

7. Vasanthi, G., Pawashe, A. B., Susie, H., Sujatha, T., and Raman, L., Iron nutritional status of adolescent girls from rural area and urban slum, *Indian Pediatr.,* 31(2), 127, 1994.

8. Cai, M. Q. and Yan, W. Y., Study of iron nutritional status in adolescence, *Bio. Med. Environ. Sci.,* 3(1), 113, 1990.

9. Agha, F., Saddrudin, A., Khan, R. A., and Ghafoor, A., Iron deficiency in adolescence, *J. Pak. Med. Assoc.,* 42(1), 3, 1992.

10. Verma, M., Chhatwal, J., and Kaur, G., Prevalence of anemia among urban school children of Punjab, *Indian Pediatr.,* 35, 1181, 1998.

11. Tatala, S., Svanberg, U., et al., Low dietary iron availability is a major cause of anemia: a nutrition survey in the Lindi District of Tanzania, *Am. J. Clinical Nutr.,* 68(1), 171, 1998.

12. Fujimari, E., Szarfara, S., and de Oliverira, I. M., Prevalence of iron deficiency anaemia in female adolescents in Taboaoa da Serro, Brazil, *Rev. Lat. Am. Enferma-gem.,* 4, 49, 1996.

13. Agarwal, D. K., Upadhyay, S. K., Tripathi, A. M., and Agarwal, K. N., Nutritional status, physical work capacity and mental function in school children, Nutrition Foundation of India, New Delhi, Scientific Report 6, 1987, 40.

14. Caballo, Roig N., Garcia, P., Valdemera, M., Del Castello, M. L., Santos Tapia, M., Gonzales Vargaz, A., Arias Alvarez, M. A., Serna Saugan, C., Merino, J. M., and Teresa, M. A., The prevalence of anaemia in children and adolescents of Madrid, *Annu. Espana Pediatr.,* 39(3), 219, 1993.

15. Beard, J. L., Iron requirements in adolescent females, *J. Nutr.,* 130(2S), 440S, 2000.

16. Vir, S., Adolescent growth in girls — the Indian perspective, *Indian Pediatr.,* 27(12), 1249, 1991.

17. Hallberg, L., Hulten, L., Lindstedt, G., Lundberg, P. A., Mark, A., Purens, J., Svan-berg, B., and Swolin, B., Prevalence of iron deficiency in Swedish adolescents, *Pediatr. Res.,* 34(5), 680, 1993.

18. Nelson, M., Bakalion, F., and Trivedi, A., Iron deficiency anaemia and physical performance in adolescent girls from different ethnic backgrounds, *Br. J. Nutr.,* 72(3), 427, 1994.

19. Dallman P., Looker A.C., Johnson, S.L., and Carroll, M., Influence of age on laboratory criteria for the diagnosis on iron deficiency anemia and iron deficiency in infants and children, in *Nutrition in Health and Disease,* Hallberg, L. and Asp, N-G., Eds., John Libbey & Co., London, 165–182, 1996.

20. Dallman, P.R., Simes, M.A., and Stekel, A., Iron deficiency in infancy and childhood, *Amer. J. Clinical Nutr.,* 33, 86, 1980.

21. Szarfarc, S.C. and De Souza, S.B., Prevalence and risk factors in iron deficiency and anemia, *Arch. Latinoam. Nutr.,* 47(2 Suppl. 1), 35, June 1997.

22. National Institute of Nutrition, National Nutrition Monitoring Bureau Report, Hyderabad, India, 1998.

23. Rawat, C.M.S., An epidemiological study of anaemia in adolescent girls in the rural areas of Meerut, M.D. thesis, Chaudhary Charan Singh University, Meerut, India, 2000.

24. Gillespie, S., *Major Issues in the Control of Iron Deficiency,* Micronutrient Initiative, Ottawa, 1998.

25. Maede, M., Yamamoto, M., and Yamuchi, K., Prevalence of anaemia in Japanese adolescence: 30 years experience in screening of anaemia, *Int. J. Hematol.,* 69(2), 75, 1999.

26. Urbani, C., Toure, A., Hamed, A. O., Albonico, M., Kane, I., Cheikna, D., Hamed, N. O., Montresor, A., and Savioli, L., Intestinal parasitic infections and schistosomiasis in the valley of the Senegal River in the Islamic Republic of Mauritania, *Med. Trop.,* 57(2), 157, 1997.

27. Stoltzfus, R. J., Albonico, M., Chwaya, H. M., Tielsch, J. M., Schulze, K. Z., and Savioli, L., Effects of the Zanzibar school-based deworming program on iron status of children, *Am. J. Clinical Nutr.,* 68(1), 179, 1998.

28. Brabin, B. J., The role of malaria in nutritional awareness, in Fomon, S.J. and Zloktin, S., Eds., *Nutritional Awareness,* Nutrition Nestle Workshop, Series 30, Raven Press, New York, 1992.

29. Kaviks, J., Iron Deficiency: a widespread cause of anaemia in coastal area of New Guinea, *Med. J. Aust.,* 2, 1289, 1969.

30. Lozoff, B., Iron and learning potential in childhood, *Bull. N.Y. Acad. Med.,* 65(10), 1050, 1989.

31. Grantham-McGregor, S., Fernald, L. C., and Sethuraman, K., Effects of health and nutrition on cognitive and behavioural development in children in the first three years of life, *Food Nutr. Bull.,* 20(1), 76, 1999.

32. Vir, S., Control of iron deficiency anaemia — A public health programme priority, *Proceedings of XXXI Nutrition Society of India Meeting* 26-27 November 1998.

33. Kruger, M., Badenhorst, C. J., Manswelt, E. P. G., Laubscher, J. A., and Spinnler Benada, A. J., Effects of iron fortification in school feeding scheme and anthelminthic therapy on the iron status and growth of six to eight years' old school children, *Food Nutr. Bull.,* 17, 11, 1996.

34. Chwang, L. C., Soemantri, A. C., and Pollit, E., Iron supplementation and physical growth of rural Indonesian children, *Am. J. Clinical Nutr.,* 47, 496, 1988.

35. Latham, M. C., Stephenson, L. S., Kinote, S. N., Zaman, M. S., and Kurz, K. M., Improvements in growth following iron supplementation in young age children, *Nutrition,* 6, 159, 1990.

36. Lawless, J. W., Latham, M. C., Stephenson, L. S, Kinoti, S. N., and Pertet, A., Iron supplementation improves the appetite and growth in anaemic Kenyan primary school children, *J. Nutr.,* 124, 645–654, 1994.

37. Kanani, S. and Poojara, R. H., Supplementation with iron and folic acid enhances growth in adolescent Indian girls, *J. Nutr.,* 130(2S), 452S, 2000.

38. Passi, S. J., Tamber, B., Murgai, T., and Anand, M., Impact of iron-folate supplementation among school age children and adolescents, 2000, in preparation.

39. Ash, D. M., Latham, M. C., Tatala, S. R., Mehansho, H., Ndossi, G. D., and Frongillo, E. A., Jr., Effect of a multiple micronutrient fortified beverage on anemia, vitamin A status and growth in Tanzanian school children, INACG Symposium, Durban, March 12, 1999.

40. Walker, S. P., Powell, C. A., and Grantham-McGregor, S., Early childhood supplementation and cognitive development, during and after intervention, in *Nutrition, Health, and Child Development,* Pan American Health Organization, Scientific Publication No. 566, 69, 1998.

41. Gledhill, N., Warburton, D., and Jamnik, V., Haemoglobin, blood volume, cardiac function, and aerobic power, *Can. J. Appl. Physiol.,* 24(1), 54, 1999.

42. Buzina, R., Bates, C. G., Van der Beek, J., Brubacher, G., Chandra, R. K., Hallberg, L., Heseker, J., Mertz, W., Pietrzik, K., Pollitt, E., Pradilla, A., Suboticanec, K., Sandstead, H. H., Schalch, W., Spurr, G. B., and Westenhofer, J., Workshop on functional significance of mild to moderate malnutrition, *Am. J. Clinical Nutr.,* 50, 172, 1989.

43. Levin, H. M., A benefit-cost analysis of nutritional programs for anaemia reduction, *Res. Observer*, 1, 219, 1986.

44. Murthy, N. K., Srinivasan, S., and Ravi, P., Anaemia and endurance capacity among children and women aged 6–26 years, *Indian J. Nutr. Diet.*, 26, 319, 1989.

45. Webb, T. E. and Oski, F. A., Behavioural status of young adolescents with iron deficiency anemia, *J. Spec. Educ.*, 8, 153–6, 1974.

46. Soemantri, A. G., Pollitt, E., and Kim, I., Iron deficiency anemia and educational achievement, *Am. J. Clinical Nutr.*, 42, 1221, 1985.

47. Pollitt, E., Effects of iron deficiency with or without anemia on cognitive development, in Johnston, F. (ed), *Nutrition in Anthropology*, Alan Liss Press, New York, 1985.

48. Hutchinson, S. E., Powell, C. A., Walker, S. P., Chang, S. M., and Grantham-McGregor, S. M., Nutrition, anemia, geohelminth infection and school achievement in rural Jamaican primary school children, *Eur. J. Clinical Nutr.*, 51(11), 729, 1997.

49. Hurtado, E. K., Claussen, A. H., and Scott, K. G., Early childhood anemia and mild or moderate mental retardation, *Am. J. Clinical Nutr.*, 69(1), 115, 1999.

50. Ranjan, A. M., Blight, C. D., and Binnus, C.W. Iron status and non-specific symptoms of female students, *J. Am. Coll. Nutr.*, 17(4), 1351, 1998.

51. Pollitt, E., Iron deficiency and cognitive function, *Ann. Rev. Nutr.*, 13, 521, 1993.

52. Pollitt, E., Early iron deficiency anemia and later mental retardation, *Am. J. Clinical Nutr.*, 69(1), 4, 1999.

53. Hill, J. M., Distribution of iron in the brain, in *Brain Iron Neurochemistry and Behavioural Aspects,* Youdim, M. B. H. (Ed), Taylor and Francis, London, 1989, 1–24.

54. Bruner, A. B, Joffe, A., Duggan, A. K., Casella, J. F., and Brandt, J., Randomised study of cognitive effects of iron supplementation in non-anemic iron-deficient adolescent girls, *Lancet,* 12, 348(9033) 992, 1996.

55. Ross, J. and Horton, S., *Economic Consequences of Iron Deficiency,* Micronutrient Initiative, Ottawa, 1998.

56. World Development Report 1993, World Bank, Washington, D.C., 329.

57. Scholl, T. O. and Reilly, T., Anemia, iron and pregnancy outcomes, *J. Nutr.*, 130(2S), 443, 2000.

58. Brabin, L. and Brabin, B. J., The cost of successful adolescent growth and development in girls in relation to iron and vitamin A status, *Am. J. Clinical Nutr.*, 55, 955, 1992.

59. Ramachandran, P., Nutrition in pregnancy, in *Women and Nutrition in India,* Gopalan, C. and Suminder, Kaur, Eds., Nutrition Foundation of India, New Delhi, 1989.

60. DeMaeyer, E. and Adiels-Tegman, M., The prevalence of anaemia in the world, *World Health Stat. Q.*, 38, 302, 1985.

61. Sachdev, H. P. S., Low birth weight in South Asia and malnutrition in South Asia — a regional profile, UNICEF, Regional Office of South India, ROSA Publication No. 5, 1977.

62. Beaton, G. H. and Patwardhan, V. N., Physiological and practical considerations of nutrient function and requirements, World Health Organization Monograph Series, 62, 445, 1976.

63. Mehta, M. N., Effectiveness of daily and weekly iron and folic acid supplementation in anemic adolescent girls. Final report of the UNICEF Research Project, Bombay, 1998.

64. Srikantia, S. G., Prasad, J. S., Bhaskara, C., Krishnamachari, K. A., Anaemia and immune response, *Lancet,* 1307, 1976.

65. Zimmermann, M., Adou, P., Torresani, T., Zeder, C. H., and Hurrell, R., Persistence of goiter despite oral iodine supplementation in goitrous children with iron deficiency anemia in Cote d'lvoire, *Am. J. Clinical Nutr.*, 71(1), 88, 2000.

66. Reddy, V., Dietary diversification to improve micronutrient status, Workshop on Working with Communities to Improve Nutrition And Food Security, Department of Women and Child Development, Government of India, and CARE, New Delhi, March 6–8, 2000.

67. Vir, S. and Yambi, O., Vitamin A project plan of action, in *Nutrition in Children in Developing Country Concerns,* Sachdev, H.P. and Chaudhary, P., Eds., Cambridge Press, Delhi, 545, 1994.

68. Information on Anaemia prepared by member countries of South Asia region (Bangladesh, Bhutan, India, Indonesia, Myanmar, Thailand), International Conference on Nutrition, 1992.

69. Seshadri, S., Sharma, K., Raj, A. E., Thakore, B, and Saiyed, F., Iron supplementation to control pregnancy anaemia, *Proc. Nutr. Soc. India,* 41, 131, 1994.

70. Kannani, S. and Agarwal, V., Reducing anaemia and improving growth in early adolescence — nutrition education alone can make a difference, paper presented at the 16th International Congress of Nutrition, Montreal, July–August, 1997.

71. Choudhary, P. and Vir, S., Prevention and strategies for control of iron deficiency anaemia, *Nutrition in Children — Developing Country Concerns,* Sachdev, H. P. and Choudhary, P., Eds., Cambridge Press, Delhi, 492, 1994.

72. Viteri, F., Control of iron deficiency anemia — new approach, *Bull. Nutr. Found. India,* 20(2), 1999.

73. Gopaldas, T., Kanani, S. J., and Raghava, R., A case for introducing nutrient inputs and deinfestation measures in the mid-day meal programme, *Proc. Nutr. Soc. India,* 29, 31, 1983.

74. Van Stuijvenberg, M. E., Kvalsvig, J. D., Faber, M., Kruger, M., Kenoyer, D. G., and Benade, A. J. S., Effect of iron, iodine, and β carotene-fortified biscuits on the micronutrient status of primary school children: a randomized controlled trial, *Am. J. Clinical Nutr.,* 69 (3), 497, 1999.

75. Van Stuijvenberg, M. E., Kvalsvig, J. D., Faber, M., Vorster, N., and Benade, A. J. S., Addressing micronutrient deficiencies in school children with fortified biscuits. The effect of a micronutrient fortified biscuit and cold drink on the micronutrient status and cognitive function of primary school children — a randomized controlled trial, a technical report, National Research Programme for Nutritional Intervention, June 1997.

76. Viteri, F. E., Iron supplementation for the control of iron deficiency in populations at risk, *Nutr. Rev.,* 55(6), 195, 1997.

77. Gillespie, S., Improving adolescent and maternal nutrition: An overview of benefits and options, Nutrition Series # 97-002, UNICEF, New York, 1997.

78. Preventing iron deficiency in women and children: background and consensus on key technical issues and resources for advocacy, planning and implementing national programmes, Technical Workshop, UNICEF, New York, October 7–9, 1998.

79. Agarwal, K. N., Assessment of the prevalence of anemia and iron stores in response to daily and weekly iron and folic acid supplementation in adolescent girls (10–18 years) from urban slums of northeast Delhi, UNICEF Project Report, 1998.

80. Seshadri, S., Oral Iron Supplementation to Control Anemia in Adolescent Girls, M.S. thesis, University of Baroda, India, 1998.

81. Beaton, G. H. and McCabe, G. P., Efficacy of intermittent iron supplementation in the control of iron deficiency anaemia in developing countries: an analysis of experience, Final report to the Micronutrient Initiative, GHB Consulting, Toronto, 1999.

82. Parivar Seva Sansthan, UNICEF (India) project on social marketing of iron tablets (personal communication), 1997.

83. Sharma, A., Prasad, K., and Rao, K. V., Identification of an appropriate strategy to control anemia in adolescent girls of poor communities, *Indian Pediatr.,* 17(3), 261, 2000.

84. Wright, R. O., The role of iron therapy in childhood plumbism, *Curr. Opin. Pediatr.,* 11(3), 255, 1999.

85. Gujral, S. and Choudhary, A., The essentiality of faecal examination for worm infestation in supplementary feeding programme, *Indian J. Nutr. Diet.,* 14, 341, 1977.

7 Functional Consequences of Nutritional Anemia in Adults

John L. Beard

CONTENTS

7.1 INTRODUCTION

On a world wide basis, iron deficiency anemia is by far the most prevalent nutritional anemia in adults with estimates of as high as 50% of reproductive age women and 70% of pregnant women being iron deficient in developing countries.[1] In adults, the primary cause of a nutritional anemia is the lack of sufficient iron to meet daily iron needs. The resulting hypoproliferative anemia is characterized by decreased cell size (microcytosis) and decreased numbers of red cells. Increased RBC protoporphyrin, and decreased plasma Fe, decreased transferrin saturation are indications of iron deficient erythropoiesis (see Chapter 3). In contrast, deficiencies in folic acid and vitamin B_{12} result in maturational defects of erythrocytes with resulting megaloblastosis and a decrease in red cell number due to the decreased synthesis of thymidine and DNA. The prevalence and causes of nutritional anemias, their assessment, and functional consequences during pregnancy and childhood have been described in the preceding chapters. The objective of this chapter is to review the functional consequences of nutritional anemias in adults.

0-8493-8569-5/01/$0.00+$.50
© 2001 by CRC Press LLC

The first section is a brief description of the general clinical manifestations including the evolution of anemia as a function of nutrient depletion. The second section addresses specific functional consequences that have been documented in adults and include a range of physiologic functions that may be impaired, namely, immune function, physical and mental performance, and thermoregulation.

7.2 GENERAL CLINICAL MANIFESTATIONS

The overt physical manifestations of iron, folate, and B_{12} deficiency include the generic symptoms of anemia which are tiredness, lassitude, and general feelings of lack of energy. More specific clinical manifestations for iron deficiency are glossitis, angular stomatitis, koilonychia (spoon nails), blue sclera, esophageal webbing (Plummer-Vinson syndrome), and microcytic anemia. Manifestations of folate and B_{12} deficiency include paresthesia, diarrhea, anorexia, glossitis, neurologic damage, and of course anemia. Behavioral disturbances such as pica (which is characterized by abnormal consumption of nonfood items such as dirt (geophagia) and ice (pagophagia) are often present in iron deficiency. The physiological manifestations of iron deficiency have also been noted in immune function, thermoregulatory performance, energy metabolism, and exercise or work performance.[2] The literature is less complete for folate or B_{12} deficiency with regard to these specific outcome variables. For instance, B_{12} and folate are required for the proper metabolism of homocysteine since the enzymes methylene reductase, methionine synthase, and cystathionine synthase require these vitamins. However, anemia due to lack of intrinsic factor and a resulting B_{12} induced anemia do not produce increased incidence of heart disease despite the known relationship of elevated homocysteine and heart disease.[3]

7.2.1 TISSUE DEPLETION AND ANEMIA

Depletion of the storage iron pool is generally without influence on physiologic function with a few exceptions.[4,5] In those studies, correlations were noted between electroencephalogram asymmetry (a CNS abnormality) and plasma ferritin within the iron adequate range. Nonetheless, since nearly all functional consequences are strongly related to the severity of human anemia, the challenge of separating O_2 transport events from tissue iron deficits still looms large. This is largely an academic question because tissue iron deficits occur simultaneously with deficits in oxygen transport in iron deficiency anemia. Good examples are the decreases in muscle myoglobin content, cytochrome oxidase activity, and electron transport in muscle with iron deficiency at the same time the subjects have decreased oxygen transport capacity due to anemia.[6] Victor Herbert has proposed a similar model for the staging of effects of B_{12} deficiency with its few consequences until holotranscobalamine II levels begin to drop and the initial stages of B_{12} and folate deficient erythropoiesis begin.[7] Thereafter, clear metabolic abnormalities associated with B_{12} deficiency are poor myelination, elevated homocysteine levels, and elevations in methymalonate.[8-10] Well known consequences of depletion of iron stores, folate, and B_{12} are the declines in hemoglobin concentration, the decrease in mean Hb concentration, a change in the size and volume of new red cells, and reduced activity of cellular enzymes.

Diffusion of dioxygen from Hb into tissue becomes limited in this situation because of fewer erythrocytes packed close together in capillaries, increased membrane diffusivity, and decreased tissue myoglobin concentration. The heterogeneity of distribution of mitochondria around and adjacent to capillary walls is well known but is not well studied in the iron deficient individual or animal model. The delivery of red cells to tissue is subject to complex regulation by both systemic and local regulatory features. While not a part of this review, the reader is urged to consider that the matching of oxygen delivery to tissue needs for oxygen are the ultimate goals of these regulators. In severe anemia, oxygen transport is clearly limiting to tissue oxidative function at anything but the resting condition despite a significant right shifting of the Hb–O_2 dissociation curve (decreased affinity) and an increase in cardiac output in an attempt to increase TaO_2.[5] Tissue extraction of oxygen is increased by this compensation and mixed venous PO_2 is significantly lower in anemic individuals. While Hb–O_2 affinity compensation is reasonable at sea level, the opposite direction of compensation occurs in anemic individuals at high altitudes (4000 M). The Hb–O_2 dissociation curve is left-shifted in these hypobaric hypoxic conditions to increase O_2 loading in the lung at the expense of tissue delivery. The very significant decrease in myoglobin and other iron containing proteins in skeletal muscle in iron deficiency anemia contributes significantly to the decline in muscle aerobic capacity.[6]

Animal studies have assisted in our understanding of the tissue biology of iron, folate, and B_{12} and functional outcomes. For example, ^{31}P NMR spectroscopy was used to examine the functional state of bioenergetics in iron deficient and replete rat gastrocnemius muscle[11] at rest and during active muscle contraction. Muscles of iron deficient animals had a clear increase in phosphocreatine breakdown and a decreased reserve of high energy phosphate groups after exercise. Decreases in muscle iron containing enzymes during iron repletion experiments have been described.[6] Pyruvate and malate oxidase were decreased to 35% of normal in iron deficient muscle. What seems to determine the amount of decline in activity with iron deprivation is the rate of turnover of that particular iron containing protein during cellular deprivation of iron. Thus, the fundamental production of energy and utilization of energy substrates are likely altered by iron deficiency. In B_{12} dependent metabolism, only two enzymes are involved: methylmalonyl CoA mutase and methionine synthase. Manifestations of deficiency are found almost entirely in the hematopoiesis system and the nervous system.[12]

7.3   PHYSIOLOGICAL CONSEQUENCES

7.3.1   Impaired Immune Function

Most pathogens require iron and other micronutrients and have evolved sophisticated strategies for acquiring these micronutrients; iron, folic acid, and transcobolamine are also required by the host in order to mount an effective immune response. In a conceptual model of nutritional immunity, the host must effectively sequester iron away from pathogens and at the same time provide a supply of iron that is not limiting to its immune system.[13] New evidence for a common lineage of metal transporters shared by both bacteria and humans for the internalization of iron suggests that transport of iron is key to the survival of many pathogens as well as the host organism.[14] Extreme experimental manipulation of dietary iron may perturb the delicate balance between these two processes and may give results unrelated to those likely found in free-living humans. Additionally, the reduction in energy intake accompanying micronutrient deficiencies may contribute to immune dysfunction and the confounding presence of multiple nutritional deficiencies and unsanitary conditions limit what can be said about immune function in the large number of clinical or intervention studies.[15] There is clear evidence from cell and molecular biology that bacterial virulence is associated with the genes that code for iron acquisition by both *E. coli* and *Vibrio*.[16,17] In addition, provision of iron in rodents increases the pathogenicity of a number of bacteria.[18] Human data indicating that this is also the case are far less convincing. An often quoted study of Murray et al.[19] examined Somali nomads with iron deficiency anemia. Oral iron therapy led to a 12-fold increase in infections compared to controls. Replication of such a powerful effect of iron status has not been seen in other studies.[20]

In adult animals or humans with intact immune systems, nonspecific, cell-mediated, and humoral immunity are affected (to varying degrees) by iron deficiency. Experimental and clinical data suggest an increased risk of infection during iron deficiency, although a small number of reports indicate otherwise. Hershko urges caution in the interpretation of many studies as the confounding issues of poverty, generalized malnutrition, and multimicronutrient deficiencies are often present in those reports.[15] The molecular and cellular defects responsible for immune deficiency are complex since almost every effector of the immune response is limited in number or action by experimental iron deficiency. Development of the immune system is retarded, sometimes irreversibly, by iron deficiency.[21]

Folate and vitamin B_{12} are intimately involved in immune system functionality.[22] In a recent report on lymphocyte functioning in patients with B_{12} deficiency, Tamura and colleagues demonstrated a decreased number of lymphocytes, a decreased ratio of CD8+/CD4+ cells, and suppressed NK cell activity.[23,24] Treatment with B_{12} resulted in a correction of these abnormalities. In contrast, antibody dependent cell-mediated cytotoxicity, stimulated lymphocyte blast formation, and levels of immunoglobulins were unaffected by B_{12} status. Pernicious anemia results in abnormal response to stimulation of lymphocytes that is somewhat dependent on the folate status and the methyl group salvage pathways.[25] In some patients with rheumatoid arthritis, B_{12} treatment of cells improves the response of CD4+ and CD8+ cells to stimulation. However, a demonstration of B_{12} deficiency in rheumatoid arthritis is lacking.[26] These descriptive studies suggest specific effects of cobolamine on the immune system but details are lacking at this time. Nonetheless, these studies note an immunomodulatory role for methyl-B_{12} that had not been previously described. In addition, these studies confirm that the presence of multiple micronutrient deficiencies is likely to have multiple, independent and perhaps, synergistic effects on immune function.

Nonspecific immunity is affected by iron deficiency. Macrophage phagocytosis is generally unaffected by iron deficiency although the bactericidal activity of macrophages is limited.[27] Neutrophil function is also altered in iron deficiency, and may be due to reduced activity of the iron-containing enzyme, myeloperoxidase, which

produces reactive oxygen intermediates responsible for intracellular killing of pathogens. Decreases in both T lymphocyte numbers and T lymphocyte blastogene-
sis/mitogenesis in iron deficiency are largely correctable with iron repletion.[28] Recent
studies of T lymphocytes in iron deficiency note that protein kinase C activity and
translocation of both splenic and purified T cells are altered by iron deficiency.[29]
Others have found normal T lymphocyte proliferative responses to mitogens.[30]
Humoral immunity appears to be less affected by iron deficiency than is cellular
immunity. In iron deficient humans, antibody production in response to immuniza-
tion with most antigens is preserved.[27,28]

Several possible mechanisms could explain the effects of iron deficiency on the
immune system. DNA synthesis, initiated by the iron-containing enzyme ribonucleotide reductase, is a rate limiting factor in cellular replication and may be limited
by iron deficiency. In addition, Galen reported that in iron deficient subjects there
is a reduction in interleukin-2 (IL-2) production by activated lymphocytes.[31] IL-2 is
a key regulatory molecule in the immune system. A number of cytokines have a
profound effect on the metabolism of iron and its availability to pathogens as well
as host cells.[15] Tumor necrosis factor, TNF-α, IL-1, and interferon-δ work in a
coordinated fashion to reduce the size of the intracellular labile iron pool by a
reduction in the amount of TfR on the cell surface, an increased synthesis of ferritin
for iron storage, and activation of nitric oxide systems.[32-36] Since the sequestration
of iron seems important, several studies have given a potent iron chelator, desferrioxamine, to humans to examine the potential antimalaria impact.[37-40] In all cases,
the iron chelator treatment improved the recovery rate from active malaria and may
provide an additional route for the treatment of infectious diseases.

7.3.2 IMPAIRED MENTAL FUNCTION

There is a long history relating effects of poor folate and B_{12} status to psychiatric
illness, depression, and cognitive changes.[41] Folic acid deficiency is often related to
depression while cobolamine deficiency may be causally related to psychotic epi-
sodes. There is also some speculation regarding folate and amyotrophic lateral
sclerosis.[42] These studies often focus on older adults with geriatric dementias (where
specific aspects of memory are affected in the very old,[43] the elderly,[44-49]) and on
those with dementia of various causes.[50] Most of the observation and intervention
studies observed some differences in cognition as a function of folate or B_{12} status.
Cobolamine and folate deficiencies are associated with alterations in myelin production due to deficiencies in s-adenosylmethionine and oligodendrocyte functioning.[51,52] This vacuolar myelopathy may be related to DNA damage secondary to
folate and B_{12} deficiency states.[53] DNA breaks or misincorporations of uracil may
be related to these alterations in folate and B_{12} in the elderly with dementias although
not all dementias are responsive to treatment with either of these nutrients.[50,54] The
inhibition of methionine synthase activity in B_{12} deficiency is associated with an
accumulation of homocysteine and adohomocysteine and with a reduction in
methionine and adomethionine synthesis. The resulting hypomethylation potential
of the oligodendrocytes results in a decrease in myelin basic protein synthesis and
altered production of myelin.

Several reviews have covered the growing research relating iron status to cognition and behavior.[55-57] The studies reviewed in these articles demonstrate that iron deficient children have alterations in attention span, lower intelligence scores, and some degree of perceptual disturbance. Importantly, the recent studies using auditory evoked potentials demonstrate delayed nerve conduction velocity in iron deficient anemic children.[58] A much more limited database exists in the adult human literature. The perception exists that the brain is resistant to changes in brain iron content and distribution within normal variations in iron status of individuals although this has never been demonstrated in man.[59] Iron is heterogeneously distributed in the brain and the pattern is not the same in adult brains and the brains of children.[57,60] Iron is accumulated through childhood and into adulthood. A particular distribution is achieved in adulthood where substantial nigra, globus pallidus, and deep cerebellar nuclei are particularly rich in iron, while other regions, like cortex, contain far less iron. The role of iron in these brain regions is likely to be for oxidative metabolism, synthesis and degradation of neurotransmitters, and myelin repair. There is little direct evidence in the absence of neurological disease that iron distribution is significantly altered by iron deficiency in adulthood although MRI data would suggest that iron content is diminished. Restless Legs Syndrome (RLS) is a recently described clinical syndrome in which afflicted individuals have frequent recurring uncontrolled movements of their extremities, usually at night.[61] The prevalence of iron deficiency anemia in this clinical population is 2 to 4 times greater than in a more general clinical population and suggests an involvement of iron deficiency. We have recently described alterations in the CSF iron and ferritin concentrations in a sample of these patients, which suggest abnormal movement of iron across the blood-brain barrier.[62] Added stimulus for understanding iron entry and distribution in the brain is provided by current studies of the role of iron in neurologic pathology.[60] A large body of literature reviewed recently suggests that iron accumulation in adulthood may be related to Parkinsonian syndromes, Alzheimer's disease, and perhaps multiple sclerosis.[57,60] Oxidative damage as the result of iron participation in free radical production in this highly oxidative organ is quite feasible as a mechanism of action, although the regional specificity regarding these diseases and brain iron metabolisms is still poorly described.

Within the spectrum of normal iron status, two reports[63,64] covering adult subjects who had serum ferritin concentrations in the normal ranges demonstrated cortical asymmetry in electroencephalograph patterns that was related to the plasma ferritin concentration. The biochemical or biological alterations that occur in the brain and result in these EEG abnormalities is however unknown. While many animal studies have been conducted to probe the effects of iron deficiency anemia on brain neurotransmitter metabolism and behavior, nearly all studies have imposed this nutrient deficiency in either a lactational or post-weanling model and hence direct evidence for adulthood based effects are lacking. Nonetheless, numerous case studies and clinical reports of dialysis patients receiving rEPO and iron demonstrate that mental functioning can be improved with better iron status.[65]

The mechanisms of causality of decreased cognition by iron deficiency however remain unknown but much discussed. The key unresolved questions are: (1) How does one differentiate the effects of acute iron deficiency from the effects of chronic iron deficiency? (2) What role does the severity of iron deficiency have in these relationships? (3) Is there a proven biologic and/or psychosocial causal model that will explain these relationships? and (4) What is the effect of age on the neurologic effects of iron deficiency anemia?[66]

7.3.3 IMPAIRED PHYSICAL PERFORMANCE

7.3.3.1 Muscle Metabolism and Energy Utilization

Observations of lethargy, apathy, and listlessness are frequent symptoms of severe iron deficiency anemia and perhaps anemia in general. However, it has been known for some time that iron deficiency is associated with decreased physical capacity and that folate and B_{12} deficiencies will also result in altered physical performance.[67-69] The mechanisms of this effect have been thoroughly investigated in rodent models and showed clear distinctions between effects of diminished oxygen transport and oxidative capacity of muscle.[6] The animal studies demonstrate that depletion of essential body iron has profound effects on skeletal muscle with a significant decrease in mitochondrial iron-sulfur content, mitochondrial cytochrome content, and total mitochondrial oxidative capacity. The activity of tricarboxylic acid cycle enzymes and oxidative capacity of mitochondria in other organs is less strongly affected and appears to be readily reversible with iron repletion. Taken together, these studies illustrate that tissue iron is associated with endurance performance at submaximal workloads, while Hb associated iron plays an important role in oxidative capacity and maximal aerobic work performance. Detailed studies of muscle metabolism in folate or B_{12} deficient exercise trained animals provide little experimental evidence that dissociates tissue limitations on metabolism and muscle contractions apart from effects of anemia on oxygen transport.

One area of considerable interest has been the study of alterations in glucose metabolism in iron deficiency anemia.[6,70] The studies discussed in the two cited reviews consistently show elevations in fasting blood glucose, increased production of lactate, increased use of the Cori cycle, and metabolic adaptation in glucose metabolism to increase metabolic utilization of this substrate. While these studies were performed in rodent models of iron deficiency, recent studies in humans show a relationship of iron status to diabetes.[71,72] Increased insulin sensitivity in iron deficient rats is a related observation.[73,74] These studies using euglycemic clamps as well as radioisotope clearance methods demonstrate a clear preference for glucose oxidation to lactate in iron deficient and anemic animals. These studies have not been replicated in man to our knowledge and the role of altering insulin sensitivity in humans is unclear but deserving of a thorough examination.

Many reviewers of the scientific literature conclude that iron, folate, and B_{12} status are marginal or inadequate in a large number of individuals, particularly females, who engage in regular physical exercise.[69,75-77] Many authors argue that dietary intake patterns of these individuals are suboptimal with reduced intakes of a number of micronutrients.[69,78] Fogelman recently published a meta-type summary analysis of 18 studies of iron status in athletes and reached the conclusion that definitions of depleted nutrient status, rather than true deficiency, modify the reported amount of prevalence of nutrient deficiency in athletic populations.[76] The low storage iron pool often reported results from a negative iron balance that may have persisted for years. In their review of the literature on exercise and iron status, Weaver and Rajaram estimated that daily iron losses increase to 1.75 mg/d in male athletes and to 2.3 mg/d in female athletes with prolonged training.[77] This is in contrast to a whole body loss of iron of approximately 1 mg/d in males beyond puberty and 1.45 mg/d in menstruating females. A negative iron balance may exist in a number of young individuals engaged in large amounts of physical activity because of the higher iron requirement of growth coupled with either increased iron losses or limited absorbable dietary iron. A recent review article suggests that "exercising elderly may be at risk for B_{12}, B_6, calcium, and vitamin D deficiencies" due to changing nutrient needs.[78] While this might be prudent advice, there is scant data to support the conclusion that B_{12} and folate requirements change with exercise training or large increases in physical activity in adults.

Whole body iron turnover studies provide direct information regarding the rate of iron losses from the body and would provide direct proof of the hypothesis that exercise training alters the daily requirement for iron. Ehn and coworkers applied the approach of whole body radio-iron losses to calculate body iron turnover[79] and found that the biologic half-life of body iron was only approximately 1000 days in highly trained long distance runners. This is significantly shorter than the 1300 and 1200 days for male and female nonexercisers, respectively. While the causes of the increased iron losses were not clear from that study, a number of reviewers of this topic conclude that increased fecal losses and perhaps sporadic hematuria contribute to depressed iron stores in athletic segments of the population.[75,76,80,81] A recent training study of previously unfit young women failed to demonstrate any impact of moderate physical training on iron status. Thus the level of physical activity necessary to modify nutrient requirements might be considerable.[82]

There is some evidence that exercise training in humans will impair the absorption of iron, but not folate or B_{12}. The difference in absorption between runners and nonrunners was not significant and was likely confounded by differences in iron status.[75] A recent study using an imprecise method of determining iron absorption claims a 40% increase in the absorption of 100 mg of ferric citrate due to 1 hour of cycling exercise.[83] This dose of iron is quite large and not a form of iron normally consumed by humans. Iron intakes of runners and nonrunners are frequently similar, except for heme iron intakes as meat intake differs.[84] Considerable B_{12} and iron reserves in liver storage pools may provide a sufficiently large savings account to compensate for micronutrient poor intakes for a prolonged period of time. Consideration of the size of the storage pool when estimating costs of exercise needs to be implemented. Highly controlled studies on folate and B_{12} metabolism in exercise are lacking in humans and it remains uncertain if people eating specialized diets are truly at greater risk for nutritional anemias.

There is a significant reduction in hematologic parameters that could have been the result of increased intra-vascular hemolysis of red cells. Smith and colleagues demonstrated an increased rate of red cell turnover and red cell fragility in athletes.[85,86] A single bout of high intensity exercise was sufficient to increase the susceptibility of red cells to peroxidative damage and osmotic stress. Anemia, however, should not exist as long as red cell production can match an increased rate of red cell destruction. In fact, a younger red cell population may offer a distinct advantage with regard to oxygen delivery. Weight et al. demonstrated an increased rate of hemolysis of red cells by using ^{51}Cr labeled red cells.[87] Mean red cell lifetimes of male and female runners were significantly less (67 ± 7 days versus 72 ± 8 days) than those of nonrunners of the same sex (113 ± 10 days and 114 ± 9 days respectively). There was no correlation between red cell life span and iron status, body mass, or indices of training. Haptoglobin concentrations were somewhat decreased and consistent with accelerated erythropoietic drive and red cell turnover rate. Other studies using more moderate levels of exercise demonstrate some influence of exercise on circulating hematologic parameters although overt studies of iron metabolism have not been conducted.[88]

In summary, several mechanisms by which iron balance could be affected by intense physical exercise have been advanced.[81,89] These explanations include increased gastrointestinal blood losses following running, and hematuria as a result of erythrocyte rupture within the foot during running. Hematuria is not a consistent finding and is unlikely to lead to a great increase in body iron losses with exercise training.[90] Losses in sweat can likely be ignored since the iron content of sweat is quite small once careful data collection techniques are utilized.

7.3.3.2 Consequences of Poor Iron Status

Many investigations cited so far fail to demonstrate that a fall in plasma ferritin is detrimental to the physical performance of the athlete. That is, as long as no overt anemia is present, there is no consequence of the poor iron status. Exceptions to this are the studies of Zhu and Haas[91] and an earlier study by Lamanca and Haymes.[92] These authors demonstrated a lower VO_2 max in iron depleted but not anemic young women when compared to equally trained but not iron depleted controls. During a prolonged exercise event, the iron depleted, but not anemic, women required slightly less energy to complete the time after iron repletion than before. Since most organs show morphological, physiological, and biochemical changes with iron deficiency in a manner related to the turnover of iron and essential iron-containing proteins it is not surprising that with careful study, a drop in physical functioning could be demonstrated.[6]

Human subjects research documents the importance of adequate hemoglobin concentration to work performance.[93] Arterial oxygen content, oxygen delivery bound to Hb, and cardiac output are all key determinants of the amount of work that exercising muscles can do. In two separate studies, Gardner evaluated the physical work capacity and metabolic stress in iron deficient workers of a tea farm in Sri Lanka. In one study, 13 men and 16 women with Hb levels of 4.0 to 12.0 g/dL were divided into iron treatment or placebo groups.[94,95] Hematologic, cardiorespiratory, and exercise performance data were collected and 15% more O_2 was delivered per pulse in the iron treated group and peak exercise heart rates were reduced after iron treatment. In a second study, Gardner evaluated exercise performance in 75 female subjects with Hb levels from 6.1 to 15.9 g/dL. When performance time to exhaustion was measured, the lower Hb groups had the lowest exercise tolerance.[95]

Edgerton suggested that the decrement in work performance in iron deficient anemic subjects was a reflection of the level of anemia rather than other biochemical changes not related to Hb. When iron deficient subjects were re-transfused, work tolerance was the same as in subjects who had the same posttransfusion Hb levels.[96] Unlike the data of Perkkio, these studies suggested a more linear relationship between Hb and work performance and thus, do not necessarily support the presence of an Hb threshold phenomenon. These studies illustrate the importance of Hb for aerobic work performance where delivery of oxygen to metabolic tissues is limiting at high intensity workloads.

Cross-sectional studies in Indonesia and Guatemala have also demonstrated associations between iron deficiency anemia and work productivity.[97-101] Li et al. showed significant reductions in mean heart rate at work (95.5 to 91.1 beats/min) and improved production efficiency (ratio of productivity to energy expenditure) in nonpregnant iron deficient female cotton mill workers in China, following iron supplementation for 12 weeks.[102] What one must critically consider is whether a decrement in serum ferritin to levels indicative of a clinically defined deficiency (<12 µg/l) or higher would have a deleterious effect upon athletic performance in the absence of overt anemia. Several studies probe this issue.

Studies of VO_2 max levels of iron deficient women who demonstrate anemia illustrate that although circulating lactic acid is reduced following iron supplementation, no change in VO_2 max is observed.[103-104] Newhouse and Clement illustrated that raising the serum ferritin from 12.3 to 37.7 µg/l did not enhance maximal work capacity.[105] Lukaski investigated the effects of depletion and repletion of iron stores upon maximal work capacity, without the induction of overt anemia.[106] Serum ferritin was reduced from 26 µg/l to 6 µg/l by repeated venisection. These studies illustrated no change in VO_2 max at the reduced serum ferritin concentration (Hb 12 ± 2 g/dl), while increased CO_2 production and elevated post exercise lactate were observed. While a number of laboratories have demonstrated equivocal results in maximal work performance with iron supplementation[107-109] a singular study by Rowland[104] illustrated that increasing serum ferritin can enhance endurance performance. This study seems to stand alone. What remains to be consistently verified is whether endurance performance at workloads of, say, 35 to 65% of VO_2 max would be detrimentally affected by iron deficiency without anemia. A titration of serum ferritin values in the 5 to 50 µg/l range versus work time to exhaustion at submaximal exercise intensities has yet to be performed by any laboratory and could shed light on this unresolved yet important issue.

7.3.4 IMPAIRED THERMOREGULATION

7.3.4.1 Fundamentals of Thermoregulation in Homeotherms

Heat production is a product of metabolism, the transfer of chemical energy to work and heat. Because it is an aerobic process, a dependency on oxygen transport and level of nutritional anemia is expected. To date, nearly all studies of thermoregulation and nutritional anemia have investigated iron deficiency anemia, but not megaloblastic anemias due to folate or B_{12} deficiency. Metabolic heat in mammals comes from the following sources: basal metabolism, postprandial thermogenesis, diet induced thermogenesis, and shivering and nonshivering thermogeneses. Shivering and nonshivering thermogeneses represent the main sources of heat production utilized during cold exposure. Both of these processes are under hypothalamic control and serve as the primary thermoregulatory effectors for mammals. Humans and other large mammals depend mainly on shivering to maintain body temperature in the cold, whereas rats and other rodents augment shivering with nonshivering thermogenesis to provide heat.[110] Shivering can increase metabolic rate four to five times that of resting metabolic rate.

Heat production by metabolic processes that do not require muscular contraction is termed nonshivering thermogenesis. Nonshivering thermogenesis occurs primarily in brown adipose tissue, a type of fat tissue that produces heat via uncoupling oxidative phosphorylation in mitochondria. In addition to providing heat for temperature regulation, brown adipose tissue also expends excess energy from overabundant caloric intake, termed diet induced thermogenesis, and is related to our ability to buffer variations in energy intake.[111] Brown adipose tissue is the main organ for nonshivering thermogenesis in rodents and newborn mammals, but most adult mammals, including adult humans, have only small amounts of detectable brown adipose tissue. Thyroid hormone increases cellular metabolism and subsequent heat production, mainly by increasing iron pumping across the plasma membrane.[112] In addition to increasing heat production in the cold, primarily through shivering and nonshivering thermogenesis, homeotherms can thermoregulate by decreasing heat loss.[113]

7.3.4.2 Human Studies with Iron Deficiency Anemia

Iron deficiency anemia alters the ability of humans to maintain body core temperature during acute cold exposure.[114-116] Investigations have documented clear alterations in thermoregulation, the thyroid system, and the sympathetic nervous system. Extensive reviews of this literature have been recently published.[117,118]

Iron deficient anemic (IDA) humans have significantly greater losses of core body temperature when cold stressed than controls even when body fatness is accounted for in experimental settings.[115] Those carefully controlled studies utilized both cold air and cold water baths to thermally stress the subjects. Additionally, the iron deficient subjects had lower plasma thyroid hormone concentrations[115] and higher catecholamine responses to cold.[114,116] After repletion with iron supplements, the previously iron deficient human subjects showed improved ability to maintain body temperature in the cold.[115,116] Anemia plays a key role in this defect as nonanemic rats and nonanemic humans thermoregulate adequately despite tissue iron depletion. It is now well established from extensive animal studies that thyroid hormone metabolism is altered by iron deficiency anemia. There is reason to believe central regulation, thyroid gland functioning, and peripheral conversion of thyroxine to triiodothyronine are all altered by iron deficiency.

Anemic humans and rats have low plasma thyroid hormone concentrations (T_3) and rats have blunted thyroid stimulating hormone (TSH) responses to thyroid releasing hormone or cold challenge if anemic.[119,120] This does not occur if they are nonanemic. In addition, there is a decrease in activity of the peripheral production of T_3 from thyroxine and utilization of this hormone. Recently published studies in rodents note that iron deficiency anemia slows thyroid hormone kinetics.[119] This relationship of thyroid metabolism and iron has real significance for much of the developing world because of the large overlap in populations that may be simultaneously iodine and iron deficient. Recent data from an intervention study in West Africa demonstrates that the effectiveness of iodine supplementation in treating goiter is attenuated by coexisting iron deficiency.[121]

Peripheral catecholamine metabolism appears to be dramatically altered in iron deficiency. Elevated levels of norepinephrine in urine of iron deficient children[120] and adults are well documented.[114,115] In these studies, however, the level of epinephrine appears to be unaffected. Early studies suggested that decreased monoamine oxidase activity was causal to these observations although it is more likely that increased spillover into plasma is a significant contribution. The implications of these alterations in peripheral monoamine metabolism are unclear at this time although alterations in blood flow, nutrient flow, and organ perfusion may be affected by this neurotransmitter.

7.3   CONCLUSION

The brief review provided in this chapter documents that nutritional anemia in adults has profound influences on many aspects of functioning. While many of the consequences are likely directly related to the severity of anemia, others are not and are more tightly associated with cellular needs and requirements for iron, folic acid, and vitamin B_{12}. It is evident that relatively little scientific work has been conducted regarding the potential or real impact of B_{12} and folate deficiency on physical and mental functioning. This is somewhat surprising given the likelihood of deficiencies of these two micronutrients in selected portions of the world's population. Many aspects of the metabolism and effects of iron deficiency anemia are known and well described. Other aspects are just now emerging. For example, we have often assumed that the cognitive effects of iron deficiency anemia are developmentally bound relationships. Several studies of cognitive functioning in renal dialysis patients before and after treatment with rEPO and iron suggest that correction of iron deficiency anemia in these patients will improve cognitive skills and capacities. Specific mental alterations in nutritional anemias may not occur solely in young children and infants. We should all be encouraged as scientists to explore these relationships in adults and to utilize new technologies to re-examine previously assumed truths.

REFERENCES

1. Strategic approach to operationalizing selected end-decade goals: reduction of iron deficiency anemia by one-third of the 1990 levels, Report of WHO/UNICEF Joint Committee on International Health Policy, 30th Session, Geneva, 2000.
2. Beard, J. L. and Dawson, H., Iron, in *Handbook of Nutritionally Essential Elements*, Sunde, R. and O' Dell, B., Eds., Marcel Dekker, New York, 1996.
3. Green, R. and Jacobsen, D. W., Clinical implications of hyperhomocysteinaemia, in *Folate in Health and Disease*, Bailey, L. B., Ed., Marcel Dekker, New York, 75, 1995.

4. Hillman, R. S. and Finch, C. A., *Red Cell Manual*, 5th ed., F. A. Davis Company, Philadelphia, 1985.

5. Ekblom, B., Micronutrients: effects of variation in [Hb] and iron deficiency on physical performance, *World Rev. Nutr. Diet*, 82, 122, 1997.

6. Dallman, P. R., Biochemical basis for the manifestations of iron deficiency, *Annu. Rev. Nutr.*, 6, 13, 1986.

7. Herbert, V., Vitamin B_{12}, in *Present Knowledge in Nutrition,* 7th ed., Ziegler, E. and Filer, L. Eds., ILSI Press, Washington, D.C., 1996.

8. Frenkel, E. P., Abnormal fatty acid metabolism in peripheral nerves of patients with pernicious anemia, *J. Clinical Invest.,* 52, 1237, 1973.

9. Nygard, O. and Vollset, S. E., Refsum, H., Total plasma homocysteine and cardiovascular risk profile, The Hordaland Homocysteine Study, *J. Am. Med. Assn.*, 274, 1526, 1995.

10. Stabler, S. P., Allen, R. W., and Savage, D. W., Clinical spectrum and diagnosis of cobalamin deficiency, *Blood*, 76, 871, 1990.

11. Thompson, C. H., Green, U. S., Ledingham, J. G., Radda, G. K., and Rajagopalan, B., The effect of iron deficiency on skeletal muscle metabolism of the rat, *Acta Physiol. Scand.,* 147, 85, 1993.

12. Savage, D. G. and Lindenbaum, J., Neurological complications of acquired cobalamin deficiency: clinical aspects, *Bailliere's Clinical Haema.,* 8, 657, 1995.

13. Weinberg, E. D., Iron withholding: a defense against infection and neoplasia, *Physiol. Rev.,* 64, 65, 1984.

14. Canonne-Hergaux, F., Gruenheid, S., Govoni, G., and Gros, P., The Nramp 1 protein and its role in resistance to infection and macrophage function, *Proc. Assoc. Am. Physicians*, 111(4), 283, 1999.

15. Hershko, C., Iron and infection, in *Iron Nutrition in Health and Disease,* Hallberg, L. and Asp, N., Eds., John Libbey and Co., London, 1996, 231.

16. Ike, K., Kawahara, K., Danbara, H., and Kume, K., Serum resistance and aerobactin iron uptake in avian *Escherichia coli* mediated by conjugative 100-megadalton plasmid, *J. Vet. Med. Sci.,* 2992, 54, 1091.

17. Crosa, J. H., The relationship of plasmid mediated iron transport and bacterial virulence, *Annu. Review Microbiol.,* 38, 69, 1984.

18. Sussman, M., Iron and infection, in *Iron in Biochemistry and Medicine,* Jacobs, A. and Worwood, M., Eds., Academic Press, New York, 649, 1974.

19. Murray, M. J., Murray, A. B., Murray, M. B., and Murray, C. J., The adverse effect of iron repletion on the course of certain infections, *Br. Med. J.*, 2, 1113, 1978.

20. Damsdaran, M., Naidu, A. N., and Sarma, K. V. R., Anemia and morbidity in rural preschool children, *Indian J. Med. Res.,* 69, 448, 1979.

21. Hallquist, N. A., McNeil, L. K., Lockwood, J. F., and Sherman, A. R., Maternal iron deficiency effects on peritoneal macrophage and peritoneal NK cell cytotoxicity in rat pups, *Am. J. Clinical Nutr.,* 55, 741, 1992.

22. Das, K. C., Mohanty, D., and Garewal, G., Cytogenetics in nutritional megaloblastic anaemia: prolonged persistence of chromosomal abnormalities in lymphocytes after remission, *Acta Haema.,* 76, 146, 1986.

23. Tamura, J., Kubota, K., Murakami, H., Sawamura, M., Matshshima, T., Tamura, T., Saitoh, T., Kurabayashi, H., and Naruse, T., Immunomodulation of vitamin B_{12}: augmentation of CD8+ T lymphocytes and NK cell activity in vitamin B_{12} deficient patients by methyl-B_{12} treatment, *Clinical Exp. Immunol.,* 116, 28, 1999.

24. Kubota, K., Kurabayashi, H., Kawada, E., Okamoto, K., and Shirakura, T., Restoration of abnormally high CD4/CD8 ratio and low NKC activity by vitamin B_{12} therapy in a patient with post-gastrectomy megaloblastic anemia, *Intern. Med.,* 31, 125, 1992.

25. Katka, K., Immune function in pernicious anemia before and during treatment with vitamin B$_{12}$, *Scand. J. Haema.,* 32, 76, 1984.

26. Ueda, Y., Murakawa, Y., Takeno, M., Miki, T., and Sakane, T., Abnormalities in autologous mixed lymphocyte activation cascade in rheumatoid arthritis and their possible correction by methyl-B$_{12}$, *Ryumachi,* 30, 350, 1990.

27. Chandra, R. K. and Saraya, A. K., Impaired immunocompetence associated with iron deficiency, *Indian J. Pediatr.,* 86, 899, 1998.

28. Baliga, B. S., Kuvibidila, S., and Suskind, R. M., Effect of iron deficiency on the cell mediated immune response, *Indian J. Pediatr.,* 49, 431, 1982.

29. Kuvibidila, S. R., Kitchens, D., and Baliga, B. S., *In vivo* and *in vitro* iron deficiency reduces protein kinase C activity and translocation in murine splenic and purified T cells, *J. Cell Biochem.,* 1, 74(3), 468, 1999.

30. Krantman, H. J., Young, S. R., Jank, B. L., O'Donnell, C. M., Rachelefsky, G. S., and Stiehm, E. R., Immune function in pure iron deficiency, *Nutr. Rep. Int.,* 26, 862, 1982.

31. Galan, P., Thibault, H., Preziosi, P., and Hercberg, S., Interleukin 2 production in iron-deficient children, *Biol. Trace Elem. Res.,* 32, 421, 1992.

32. Konijn, A. M. and Hershko, C., Ferritin synthesis in inflammation: I. Pathogenesis of impaired iron release, *Brit. J. Haema.,* 37, 7, 1977.

33. Fahmy, M. and Young, S. P., Modulation of iron metabolism in monocyte cell line U937 by inflammatory cytokines: changes in transferrin uptake, iron handling and ferritin mRNA, *Biochem. J.,* 296, 175, 1993.

34. Byrd, T. F. and Horwitz, M. A., Interferon gamma-activated human monocytes down-regulate transferrin receptors and inhibit the intracellular multiplication of *Legionella pneumophila* by limiting the availability of iron, *J. Clinical Invest.,* 83, 1457, 1989.

35. Lane, T. E., Wu-Hsieh, B. A., and Howard, D. H., Iron limitation and the gamma interferon-mediated anthihistoplasma state of murine macrophages, *Infect. Immunol.,* 59, 2274, 1991.

36. Lancaster, J. R. and Hibbs, J. B., EPR demonstration of iron-nitrosyl complex formation by cytotoxic activated macrophages, *Proc. Natl. Acad. Sci. U.S.A.,* 87, 1223, 1990.

37. Traore, O., Carnevale, P., and Kaptue-Noche, L., Preliminary report on the use of desferrioxamine in the treatment of Plasmodium falciparum malaria, *Am. J. Hematol.,* 37, 206, 1991.

38. Bunnag, D., Poltera, A. A., and Viravan, C., Plasmodicidal effect of desferrioxamine B in human vivax and falciparum malaria from Thailand, *Acta Trop. Basel,* 52, 59, 1992.

39. Gordeuk, V. R., Thuma, P. E., and Brittenham, G. M., Iron chelation with desferrioxamine B in adults with asymptomatic Plasmodium falciparum parasitemia, *Blood,* 79, 308, 1992.

40. Gordeuk, V. R., Thuma, P., and Brittenham, G. M., et al., Effect of iron chelation therapy on recovery from deep coma in children with cerebral malaria, *New Engl. J. Med.,* 327, 1473, 1992.

41. Hutto, B. R, Folate and cobalamin in psychiatric illness, *Compr. Psychiatry,* 38, 305, 1997.

42. Yoshino, Y., Possible involvement of folate cycle in the pathogenesis of amyotrophic lateral sclerosis, *Neurochem. Res.,* 9, 387, 1984.

43. Hassing, L., Wahlin, A., Winblaad, B., and Backman, L., Further evidence on the effects of vitamin B$_{12}$ and folate levels on episodic memory functioning: a population-based study of healthy very old adults, *Biol. Psychiatry,* 45, 1472, 1999.

44. Rosenberg, I. H. and Miller, J. W., Nutritional factors in physical and cognitive functions of elderly people, *Am. J. Clinical Nutr.,* 55, 1237S, 1992.

45. Kwok, T., Tang, C., Wo, J., Lai, W. K., Law, L. K., and Pang, C. P., Randomized trial of the effect of supplementation on the cognitive function of older people with subnormal cobalamin levels, *Int. J. Geriatr. Psychiatry.,* 13, 611, 1998.

46. Riggs, K. M., Spiro, A., Tucke, K., and Rush, D., Relations of vitamin B_{12}, B_6, folate, and homocysteine to cognitive performance in the Normative Aging Study, *Am. J. Clinical Nutr.,* 63, 306, 1996.

47. LaRue, A., Koehler, K. M., Wayne, S. J., Chiulli, S. J., Haaland, K. Y., and Garry, P. J., Nutritional status and cognitive functioning in a normally aging sample: a 6-yr assessment, *Am. J. Clinical Nutr.,* 65, 20, 1997.

48. Ortega, R. M., Requejo, A. M., Andres, P., Lopez-Sobaler, A. M., Quintas, M. E., Rdondo, M. R., Navia, B., and Rivas, T., Dietary intake and cognitive function in a group of elderly people, *Am. J. Clinical Nutr.,* 66, 803, 1997.

49. Ebly, E. M., Schaefer, J. P., Campbell, N. R., and Hogan, D. B., Folate status, vascular disease and cognition in elderly Canadians, *Age and Aging,* 27, 485, 1998.

50. Bell, I. R., Edman, J. S., Morrow, F. D., Marby, D. W., Perrone, G., Kayne, H. L., Greenwald, M., and Cole, J. O., Vitamin B_1, B_2, and B_6 augmentation of tricyclic antidepressant treatment in geriatric depression with cognitive dysfunction, *J. Am. Coll. Nutr.,* 11, 159, 1992.

51. Hirono, H. and Wada, Y., Effects of dietary folate deficiency on developmental increase of myelin lipids in rat brain, *J. Nutr.,* 108, 766, 1978.

52. Chatterjee, A., Yapundich, R., Palmer, C. A., Marson, D. C., and Mitchell, G. W., Leukoencephalopathy associated with cobalamin deficiency, *Neurology,* 46, 832, 1996.

53. Blount, B. C., Mack, M. M., Wehr, C. M., MacGregor, J. T., Hiatt, R. A., and Wang, G., Wickramaasinghe, S. N., Everson, R. B., and Ames, B. N., Folate deficiency causes uracil mis-incorporation into human DNA an chromosome breakage; implications fro cancer and neuronal damage, *Proc. Natl. Acad. Sci. U.S.A.,* 94, 3290, 1997.

54. Reidel, W. J. and Jorissen, B. L., Nutrients, age and cognitive function, *Curr. Opin. Clinical Nutr. Metab. Care,* 1, 579, 1998.

55. Lozoff, B., Behavioral alterations in iron deficiency, *Adv. Pediatr.,* 35, 331, 1988.

56. Pollitt, E., Iron deficiency and cognitive function, *Annu. Rev. Nutr.,* 13, 521, 1993.

57. Beard, J. L., Connor, J. R., and Jones, B. C., Iron in the brain, *Nutr. Rev.,* 51, 157, 1993.

58. Roncagliolo, M., Garrido, M., Walter, T., Peirano, P., and Lozoff, B., Evidence of altered central nervous system development in infants with iron deficiency anemia at 6 mo: Delayed maturation of auditory brain stem responses, *Am. J. Clinical Nutr.,* 68, 683, 1998.

59. Dallman, P. R. and Spirito, R. A., Brain iron in the rat: Extremely slow turnover in normal rat may explain the long-lasting effects of early iron-deficiency, *J. Nutr.,* 107, 1075, 1977.

60. Connor, J. R., Proteins of iron regulation in the brain in Alzheimer's disease, in *Iron and Human Disease,* Lauffer, R. B., Ed., CRC Press, Ann Arbor, 365, 1992.

61. Sun, E. R., Chen, C. A., Ho, G., Earley, C. J., and Allen, R. P., Iron and restless legs syndrome, *Sleep,* 21, 371, 1998.

62. Earley, C. J., Connor, J. R., Beard, J. L., Malecki, W., Epstein, D., and Allen, R. P., Abnormalities in CSF concentrations of ferritin and transferrin in Restless Legs Syndrome, *Neurology,* submitted.

63. Tucker, D. M., Sandstead, H. H., Spectral electroencephalographic correlates of iron status: tired blood revisited, *Physiol. Behav.,* 26, 439, 1981.

64. Tucker, D. M., Sandstead, J. J., Swenson, R. A., Sawler, B. G., and Penland, J. G., Longitudinal study of brain function and depletion of iron stores in individual subjects, *Physiol. Behav.,* 29, 737, 1982.

65. Pickett, J. L., Theberge, D. C., Brown, W. S., Schweitzer, S. U., and Nissenson, A. R., Normalizing hematocrit in dialysis patients improves brain function, *Am. J. Kidney Dis.,* 33, 1122, 1999.

66. Beard, J. L., One person's view of iron deficiency, development, and cognitive function, *Am. J. Clinical Nutr.,* 62, 709, 1995.

67. Edgerton, V. R., Gardner, G. W., Ohira, Y., Gunawardena, K. A., and Senewiratne, B., Iron-deficiency anemia and its effect on worker productivity and activity patterns, *Br. Med. J.,* 2, 1546, 1979.

68. Ekblom, B., Iron deficiency, anemia and physical performance, in *Iron Nutrition in Health and Disease*, Hallberg, L. and Asp, N., Eds., John Libbey and Co., London, chap. 19, 1996.

69. Matter, M., Stittfall, T., Graves, J., Myburgh, K., Adams, B., Jacobs, P., and Noakes, T. D., The effect of iron and folate therapy on maximal exercise performance in female marathon runners with iron and folate deficiency, *Clinical Sci.,* 72, 415, 1987.

70. Brooks, G. A., Iron deficiency and physical performance: experimental studies, in *Iron Nutrition in Health and Disease*, Hallberg, L. and Asp, N., Eds., John Libbey and Co., London, chap. 18, 1996.

71. Moirand, R., Adams, P. C., Bicheler, V., Brissot, P., and Deugnier, Y., Clinical features of genetic hemochromatosis in women compared with men, *Ann. Intern. Med.,* 15, 127(2), 105, 1997.

72. Brandhagen, D. J., Fairbanks, V. F., Batts, K. P., and Thibodeau, S. N., Update on hereditary hemochromatosis and the HFE gene, *Mayo Clinical Proc.,* 74(9), 917, 1999.

73. Farrell, P. A. Beard, J. L., and Druckenmiller, M., Increased insulin sensitivity in iron-deficient rats, *J. Nutr.,* 118, 1104, 1988.

74. Borel, M. J., Beard, J. L., and Farrell, P. A., Hepatic glucose production and insulin sensitivity and responsiveness in iron-deficient anemic rats, *Am. J. Physiol.,* 264, E662, 1993.

75. Cook, J. D., The effect of endurance training on iron metabolism, *Semin. Hematol.,* 31, 146, 1994.

76. Fogelman, M., Inadequate iron status in athletes: an exaggerated problem? *Sports Nutr.,* 8, 81, 1995.

77. Weaver, C. M. and Rajaram, S., Exercise and iron status, *J. Nutr.,* 122, 782, 1992.

78. Hawley, J. A., Dennis, S. C., Lindsay, F. H., and Noakes, T. D., Nutritional practices of athletes: are they sub-optimal? *J. Sports Sci.,* 13, S75, 1995.

79. Ehn, L., Carlmark, B., and Haglund, S., Iron status in athletes involved in intense physical activity, *Med. Sci. Sports Exercise,* 12, 61, 1980.

80. Newhouse, I. J. and Clement, D. G., The efficacy of iron supplementation in iron depleted women, in Sports Nutrition: *Minerals and Electrolytes*, Kies, C. V. and Diskell, J. A., Eds., CRC Press, Boca Raton, 47, 1995.

81. Sacheck, J. M. and Roubenoff, R., Nutrition in the exercising elderly, *Clinical Sports Med.,* 18, 565, 1999.

82. Bourque, S. P., Pate, R. R., and Branch, J. D., Twelve weeks of endurance exercise training does not affect iron status measures in women, *J. Am. Diet Assoc.,* 97, 1116, 1997.

83. Schmid, A., Jakob, E., Berg, A., Russmann, T., Konig, D., Irmer, M., and Keul, J., Effects of physical exercise and vitamin C on absorption of ferric sodium citrate, *Med. Sci. Sports Exercise,* 28, 1470, 1996.

84. Lyle, R. M., Veaver, C. M., and Sedlock, D. A., Iron status in exercising women: the effect of oral iron therapy vs. increasing consumption of muscle foods, *Am. J. Clinical Nutr.,* 56, 1049, 1992.

85. Smith, J. A., Exercise, training and red blood cell turnover, *Sports Med.,* 19(1), 9, 1995.

86. Smith, J. A., Kolbunch-Braddon, M., Gillam, I., Telford, R. D., and Weidemann, M. J., Changes in the susceptibility of red blood cells to oxidative and osmotic stress following submaximal exercise, *Eur. J. Appl. Physiol.,* 70(5), 427, 1995.

87. Weight, L. M., Byrne, M. J., and Jacobs, P., Haemolytic effects of exercise, *Clinical Sci.,* 81, 147, 1991.

88. Hegenauer, J., Strause, L., Saltman, P., Dann, D., White, J., and Green, R., Transitory hematologic effects of moderate exercise are not influenced by iron supplementation, *Eur. J. Appl. Physiol.,* 52(1), 57, 1983.

89. Magnusson, B., Hallberg, L., Rossander, L., and Swolin, B., Iron metabolism and "sports anemia." I. A study of several iron parameters in elite runners with differences in iron status, *Acta Med. Scand.,* 216, 149, 1984.

90. Nachtigall, D., Nielsen, R., Fischer, R., Engelhardt, R., and Gabbe, E. E., Iron deficiency in distance runners. A reinvestigation using Fe-labeled and non-invasive liver iron quantification, *Int. J. Sports Med.,* 17, 473, 1996.

91. Zhu, Y. and Haas, J. D., Iron depletion with anemia and physical performance and in young women, *Am. J. Clinical Nutr.,* 66, 334, 1997.

92. Lamanca, J. J. and Haymes, E. M., Effects of low ferritin concentration on endurance performance, *Int. J. Sport Nutr.,* 2, 376, 1992.

93. Roach, R. C., Loskolou, M. D., Calbet, J. A., and Saltin, B., Arterial oxygen content and tension in regulation of cardiac output and leg blood flow during exercise in humans, *Am. J. Physiol.,* 276, H438, 1999.

94. Gardner, G. W., Edgerton, V., Barnard, R. J., and Bernaucer, E. H., Cardiorespiratory, hematological and physical performance responses of anemic subjects to iron treatment, *Am. J. Clinical Nutr.,* 28, 982, 1975.

95. Gardner, G. W., Edgerton, V., Senewiratne, B., Barnard, R., and Ohira, Y., Physical work capacity and metabolic stress in subjects with iron deficiency anemia, *Am. J. Clinical Nutr.,* 30, 910, 1977.

96. Edgerton, V. R., OHira, Y., Hettiarachi, J., Senewiratne, B., Gardner, G. W., and Barnard, R. J., Elevation of hemoglobin and work tolerance in iron-deficient subjects, *J. Nutr. Sci. Vitaminol.,* 27, 77, 1981.

97. Perkkio, M. V., Jansson, L. T., Brooks, G. A., Refino, C. J., and Dallman, P. R., Work performance in iron deficiency of increasing severity, *J. Appl. Physiol.,* 58, 1477, 1985.

98. Basta, S. S., Soerkirman, Karyadi, D., and Scrimshaw, N. S., Iron deficiency anemia and the productivity of adult males in Indonesia, *Am. J. Clinical Nutr.,* 32(4), 916, 1979.

99. Scholz, B. D., Gross, R., Schultink, W., and Sastroamidjojo, S., Anaemia is associated with reduced productivity of women workers even in less-physically-strenuous tasks, *Br. J. Nutr.,* 77(1), 47, 1997.

100. Viteri, F. E. and Torun, B., Anemia and physical work capacity, in *Clinics in Hematology,* Vol. 3, Garby, L., Ed., W. B. Saunders, London, 609, 1974.

101. Davies, C. T. M., Chukweumeka, A. C., and van Haaren, J. P. M., Iron-deficiency anemia: its effect on maximum aerobic power and responses to exercise in African males aged 17-40 years, *Clinical Sci.,* 44, 555, 1973.

102. Li, R., Chen, X., Yan, H., Deurenberg, P., Garby, L., and Hautvast, J. G., Functional consequences of iron supplementation in iron-deficient female cotton mill workers in Beijing, China, *Am. J. Clinical Nutr.,* 59(4), 908, 1994.

103. Shoene, R. B., Escaourrou, P., Robertson, H. T., Nilson, K. L., Parsons, J. R., and Smith, N. J., Iron repletion decreases maximal exercise lactate concentrations in female athletes with minimal iron-deficient anemia, *J. Lab. Clinical Med.,* 102, 306, 1983.

104. Rowland, T. W., Deisworth, M. B., Green, G. M., and Kelleher, J. F., The effect of iron therapy on the exercise capacity of non anemic iron-deficient adolescent runners, *Am. J. Dis. Child.,* 142, 165, 1988.

105. Newhouse, I. J., Clement, D. B., Taunton, J. E., and McKenzie, D. C., The effects of prelatent and latent iron deficiency on physical work capacity, *Med. Sci. Sports Exercise,* 21, 3, 263, 1989.

106. Lukaski, H. C., Hall, C. B., and Siders, W. A., Altered metabolic response of iron-deficient women during graded, maximal exercise, *Eur. J. Appl. Physiol.,* 63, 140, 1991.

107. Fogelhman, M., Jaakola, L., and Lampisjarvi, T., Effects of iron supplementation in female athletes with low serum ferritin concentration, *Int. J. Sports Med.,* 13, 158, 1992.

108. Powell, P. D. and Tucker, A., Iron supplementation and running performance in female cross-country runners, *Int. J. Sports Med.,* 12, 462, 1991.

109. Bourque, S. P., Davis, J. M., and Sargent, R. G., Effect of supplementation on endurance capacity in iron-depleted women, *Med. Sci. Sports Exercise,* 24, 819, 1992.

110. Himms-Hagen, J., Nonshivering thermogenesis, brown adipose tissue, and obesity, in *Nutritional Factors: Modulating Effects on Metabolic Processes,* Beers, R. F. and Bassett, E. G., Eds., Raven Press, New York, 85, 1981.

111. Rothwell, N. J. and Stock, M. J., Diet-induced thermogenesis, in *Mammalian Thermogenesis,* Girardier, L. and Stock, M. J., Eds., Chapman & Hall, London, 208, 1983.

112. Guernsey, D. L. and Edelman, I. S., Regulation of thermogenesis by thyroid hormones, in *Molecular Basis of Thyroid Hormone Action,* Oppenheimer, J. H., and Samuels, H. H., Eds., Academic Press, New York, 293, 1983.

113. Grayson, J., Responses of the microcirculation to hot and cold environments, in *Thermoregulation: Physiology and Biochemistry,* Schonbaum, E. and Lomax, P., Eds., Pergamon Press, New York, 221, 1990.

114. Beard, J. L., Borel, M. J., and Derr, J., Impaired thermoregulation and thyroid function in iron-deficiency anemia, *Am. J. Clinical Nutr.,* 52, 813, 1990.

115. Martinez-Torres, C., Cubeddu, L., Dillmann, E., Brengelmann, G. L., Leets, I., Layrisse, M., Johnson, D. G., and Finch, C., Effect of low temperature on normal and iron-deficient subjects, *Am. J. Physiol.,* 246, R380, 1984.

116. Lukaski, H. C., Hall, C. B., and Nielsen, F. H., Thermogenesis and thermoregulatory function of iron-deficient women without anemia, *Aviation Space Environ. Med.,* 61, 913, 1990.

117. Rosenzweig, P. H. and Volpe, S. H., Iron, thermoregulation, and metabolic rate, *Crit. Rev. Food Sci. Nutr.,* 39, 131, 1999.

118. Brigham, D. E. and Beard, J. L., Thermoregulation in iron deficiency anemia in *Crit. Rev. Food Sci. Nutr.,* 36, 747, 1996.

119. Beard, J. L., Brigham, D. E., Kelly, S., and Green, M., Plasma thyroid hormone kinetics is altered in iron deficient anemic rats, *J. Nutr.,* 128, 1401, 1998.

120. Voorhees, M. L., Stuart, M. J., Stockman, J. A., and Oski, F. A., Iron deficiency anemia and increased urinary NE excretion, *J. Pediatr.,* 86, 542, 1975.

121. Zimmermann, M., Adou, P., Torresani, T., Zeder, C., and Hurrell, R., Persistence of goiter despite oral iodine supplementation in goitrous children with iron deficiency anemia in Côte d' Ivoire, *Am. J. Clinical Nutr.,* 71, 88, 2000.

8 Supplementation for Nutritional Anemias

Eva-Charlotte Ekström

CONTENTS

8.1 INTRODUCTION

The provision of iron supplements during pregnancy as a strategy for the prevention and control of nutritional anemias is the oldest and most common supplementation activity which was established in the 1960s. Iron supplementation has reappeared as the difficulties in developing effective programs have become apparent. For many years, folic acid has been provided to pregnant women in combination with iron, but it has received much less attention; little is known about the relative importance of folic acid for nutritional anemia. The first guideline for routine supplementation of young children with iron and folic acid was recently published and discussions on the importance of providing supplements to adolescents, including vitamin A for utilization of iron stores, have just begun.

Nutrient supplementation may only be efficacious in preventing and controlling anemia if the anemia is due to deficiency of the supplemented nutrient(s). Unfortunately, the etiology of anemia is not well mapped and previous underlying assumptions that a major part of anemia is due to iron deficiency and, consequently, that iron supplementation may control all levels of anemia is increasingly being questioned.[1-4] The limited knowledge on the prevalence of nutritional anemia may confuse interpretation of results from nutrient supplementation studies. For example, efficacy and effectiveness of iron supplementation have often been evaluated by use of hemoglobin concentration. In populations where other types of anemia are prevalent, this practice may have lead to an underestimation of the efficacy and effectiveness of the supplementation. In these situations, what really has been assessed is the impacts of iron supplementation on anemia (Figure 8.1). It is possible that supplementation has been fully successful, i.e., all iron deficiency anemia has been controlled, but the impact on anemia has been limited due to high prevalence of other types of anemia. The same logic applies in assessing the effect of supplementation on different types of health and development outcomes.

This chapter will address efficacy and effectiveness of supplementation of iron, folic acid, and vitamin A. The first section discusses issues related to efficacy of supplementation including aim, health benefits, timing, and dosage of supplementation. The second section addresses important issues and experiences related to effectiveness of supplementation in anemia prevention and control programs.

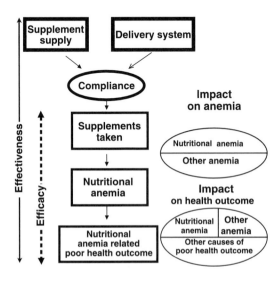

FIGURE 8.1 Efficacy, effectiveness of supplementation, and impact of nutrient supplementation programs on anemia and poor health outcome.

8.2   EFFICACY OF SUPPLEMENTATION

"Efficacy" — the extent to which a specific intervention, procedure, regimen, or service produces a beneficial result under ideal conditions.[6]

Despite the large variability in the prevalence of anemia and the proportion attributable to various nutrient deficiencies, there are some population groups in which supplementary iron generally is regarded as beneficial. Pregnant women and young children are at increased risk for iron deficiency due to the increased demands of rapidly growing tissue. These groups also have an increased demand for folic acid. In addition to the increased nutrient requirements of these population groups, a disadvantaged setting is often associated with higher prevalence of risk factors for iron and other nutrient deficiencies (see Chapter 2).

8.2.1   AIM OF IRON SUPPLEMENTATION

The ultimate aim of supplementation is to prevent or reduce negative health or developmental consequences of nutrient deficiencies. It would be logical to evaluate adequacy of a supplementation activity on the basis of achieved reduction in the negative effects. As most experiences of supplementation come from iron supplementation studies among pregnant women, they will be used as an example in discussing the aim of supplementation.

While there are numerous studies demonstrating a positive effect of iron supplementation on hemoglobin concentration and iron status, the limited evidence of a positive effect on pregnancy outcomes is controversial and has raised many questions.[3,7-10] In these debates, it is important to distinguish between the lack of impact and a paucity of well-designed studies addressing the issue. Part of the problem is designing a study where biologic efficacy is evaluated. Many studies have not controlled supplement intake or provided valid measures of compliance. The possibility exists that rather than estimating the biologic efficacy, a measure of effectiveness influenced by limited compliance has been obtained. The design of choice would be to randomize the placebo and intervention, and then compare indicators of micronutrient status as well as functional outcomes between the two groups. However, randomization is no longer an ethical option for some of the micronutrients (for example, iron) complicating the design of studies evaluating efficacy. Other factors such as nutrient deficiencies other than iron, chronic infection, and diseases may further limit the biologic efficacy of supplementation. Any selected poor functional outcome can have a number of different causes, and nutrient deficiencies may be one of many determinants. The impact of supplementation on a particular functional outcome may thus be small. A large sample size is required to detect small changes and to control for several potential determinants making such studies logistically difficult and expensive. In summary, limited understanding of the relation between change in iron status and anemia on the subsequent change in negative pregnancy outcome has led to difficulties in establishing the aim of supplementation and deciding on indicators for evaluation. Three different aims may be discussed.

TABLE 8.1

Different Options for Aims of Iron Supplementation Activities in Terms of Hemoglobin Concentration (Hb)

Aim	Whom to Supplement	Programmatic Implications	How to Evaluate Aim	Advantages	Disadvantages
Reach full Hb potential (prevent and treat)	All	Routine supplementation of all women		All who may benefit receive supplement	Low effectiveness
Prevent low Hb level	Those at risk for low Hb level	Routine or screening	% above low Hb level	Moderate effectiveness?	Uncertainty of cut-off levels, difficulties in screening?
Treat low Hb level	Those below low Hb level	Screening low level	% above low Hb level	High effectiveness	Uncertainty of cut-off levels, difficulties in screening?

The first aim is that supplementation should allow development to full potential of hemoglobin concentration (Table 8.1). The Institute of Medicine states that "an acceptable goal for iron nutrition during pregnancy is simply to avoid progression beyond low iron stores (first stage of depletion) to the stages of impaired hemoglobin production (second stage) or iron deficiency (third stage)."[11] The underlying assumption is that as long as there is a need for iron there will be a hemoglobin response and the effect on functional outcome is only optimized when full potential is reached. Furthermore, when requirements are met there will be no further increase in hemoglobin. Even if the increased risk associated with mild or moderate anemia may be smaller than that of severe anemia, mild and moderate anemia can have a larger public health importance due to the higher prevalence. The programmatic implication is routine supplementation to all pregnant women and the aims are prevention and treatment. Evaluation is difficult because absolute levels of hemoglobin concentration and their changes will vary in different populations (due to the prevalence of nutritional anemia). Effectiveness may be low as many individuals receive supplementation without requiring it.

The second option is prevention of a low level of hemoglobin concentration, where a low level needs to be defined and justified. The women who should be targeted to receive supplements are those at risk for developing low levels. Unless all women are considered at risk there will be a need of an indicator to screen for women at risk of progressing below the cut-off; such a predictive indicator has to be defined and justified. In this case the extent to which the aim has been achieved can be evaluated by measuring the proportion of individuals above the low level after supplementation. Screening usually increases effectiveness and this approach may be more effective than routine supplementation. A difficulty is the limited knowledge of appropriate cut-off levels for low hemoglobin as well as the prediction of later low levels of hemoglobin.

The third aim focuses on pregnant women below a given cut-off level of hemoglobin concentration, most frequently those with severe anemia. The rationale is that only hemoglobin concentration below this level will have any negative effect on pregnancy outcome. This approach implies a curative strategy where pregnant women, who already have pathologic hemoglobin concentrations, should be supplemented. What supports this approach is the established increased risk associated with severe anemia and the possibility of greater effectiveness if individuals at highest risk are selected. Limited resources may best be used in a selected population. Another argument for this approach is the possible negative effect of iron supplements if distributed unnecessarily. This approach may pose programmatic difficulties in constructing a delivery system that will effectively detect severe anemia, treat it, and limit the time an individual is exposed to a severely low hemoglobin concentration.

This theoretical discussion has been limited to hemoglobin concentration. The difficulties with using hemoglobin concentration as a measure of iron nutrition adequacy are well known as is the contributing difficulty in interpretation due to hemodilution. However, this type of discussion also applies to other iron status measures that may be more valid indicators of iron status.

8.2.2 Timing of Iron Supplementation

Apart from establishing aims of iron supplementation, it is necessary to decide on the appropriate timing of intervention. When should a supplementation activity start in order to produce optimal effect on functional outcome? The concern is that there might be a window of opportunity for supplementation. There might be a limited time for reversing exposure to low level of hemoglobin before a negative functional effect is manifested, or, in case the negative consequence is not reversible to prevent an exposure. The two most important periods in the lifecycle during which routine supplementation has been recommended are pregnancy and early childhood.

8.2.2.1 Pregnancy

The estimated need for iron in pregnancy is high. Due to the low absorption of dietary iron, it is doubtful whether it can provide the required amount of iron. This high requirement may warrant the large dose of iron which supplements provide. The question regarding timing is whether it matters if an improvement in iron status is achieved early in pregnancy or is sufficient if it is reached closer to delivery. Epidemiological studies of anemia during pregnancy and risk of preterm birth found an increased risk for preterm delivery among women who had anemia during the second trimester.[12-14] No association was found between anemia during the third trimester and risk of preterm delivery[4,14] indicating that iron supplementation should be introduced early in pregnancy to be efficacious. The lack of evidence of an effect of late anemia may in part be due to the difficulties in differentiating low hemoglobin concentration associated with hemodilution from low levels due to a deficiency.

8.2.2.2 Infants and Young Children

Infants and young children are growing rapidly and have an increased demand for iron. The highest prevalence of iron deficiency anemia is found among premature infants who have limited stores and among children between 6 and 24 months, when the iron stores they are born with have become depleted. The potential impairment of mental and psychomotor development as a consequence of iron deficiency anemia is a major concern (see Chapter 6). The risk that permanent damages occur strongly supports a preventive approach at an early age.[8] In populations where iron fortified complementary foods are not widely and regularly consumed by young children, iron supplements are recommended in the first year of life.[15] Low birth weight infants may develop iron deficiency anemia earlier and should start to receive iron supplements at 2 months of age.

8.2.3   DOSAGE OF IRON SUPPLEMENTS

Limited knowledge of the relation between dose of iron and subsequent effect on hemoglobin concentration and functional outcome have made it difficult to judge which dose of iron should be recommended. The dosage recommendation has frequently been revised and the recent trend is a lowering of the dose. As more understanding is gained about the relation between iron dose and outcome and thus the aims of supplementation become clearer, it is likely the recommendations may be revised.

8.2.3.1   History of Iron/Folic Acid Dose Recommendations for Pregnant Women

In the seminal work to estimate how much additional iron pregnant women required, a factorial approach was used. Based on iron content of blood and tissue the iron needed for growth of the fetus and the maternal red cell expansion was calculated and it was estimated that 1000 mg of additional iron was needed to be accumulated during the second and third trimesters.[16] Thus, an extra 6 mg iron per day should be absorbed.[11] Studies showed that on average 5% of iron was absorbed from a diet with a low iron bioavailability common in many developing countries.[16] It may have been that this rate of absorption was applied to iron supplements suggesting that a dose of 120 mg of iron would be required. Several supplementation trials have tested 120 mg of iron, as well as multiples of it (60 and 240 mg) and assessed response as a change in hemoglobin concentration. A review of results from trials conducted and published between 1966 and 1989 showed average increases in hemoglobin concentration of 10, 12 and 16 g/l when doses of 60 to 90, 91 to 120, and ≥120 mg of iron, respectively, were used.[17] In the 1980s there was a large interest in iron supplementation trials and a monograph was also published with detailed instructions on design and analyses of iron supplementation studies.[18]

   The development of recommendations for iron supplementation is summarized in Figure 8.2. In 1968, WHO recommended at least 60 mg of elemental iron to be given daily during the second and third trimesters of pregnancy.[19] Although the importance of folate for nutritional anemia was acknowledged, no specific recommendation was made on dose. Folate requirement was estimated to be 800 µg per day but later revised and lowered to 400 µg per day.[20] In 1977, INACG issued

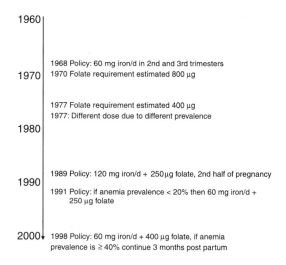

1960

1968 Policy: 60 mg iron/d in 2nd and 3rd trimesters
1970   1970 Folate requirement estimated 800 µg

1977 Folate requirement estimated 400 µg
1977: Different dose due to different prevalence
1980

1989 Policy: 120 mg iron/d + 250 µg folate, 2nd half of pregnancy
1990
1991 Policy: if anemia prevalence < 20% then 60 mg iron/d +
        250 µg folate

2000   1998 Policy: 60 mg iron/d + 400 µg folate, if anemia
        prevalence is ≥ 40% continue 3 months post partum

FIGURE 8.2 History of recommendation for iron supplementation during pregnancy.

guidelines for the eradication of iron deficiency anemia. They included a study design to evaluate iron and folate supplementation among pregnant women, which suggested use of different doses of iron, based on anemia prevalence.[20] In 1989, new guidelines for supplementation of pregnant women were issued by WHO which recommended two tablets, each containing 60 mg of elemental iron and 250 µg folic acid throughout the second half of pregnancy.[21] Two years later, ACC/SCN modified the dose according to the anemia prevalence among pregnant women in the last trimester. If anemia prevalence was low (less than 20%), one tablet of 60 mg of iron and 250 µg folate was deemed sufficient for the prevention and treatment of mild anemia.[22] In 1995, the UNICEF/WHO Joint Committee on Health Policy endorsed iron/folic acid supplementation as the strategy of choice for pregnant women and recommended that when the prevalence of anemia during pregnancy exceeded 30% all women should receive supplements.[23] The latest guidelines that were issued in 1998 by INACG/WHO/UNICEF recommend 60 mg iron and 400 mg folic acid daily. One of the differences from previous recommendations is that instead of modifying the dose of iron according to anemia prevalence, the duration of the supplementation is modified.[15]

Several of the guidelines provide recommendations of dosage based on the prevalence of anemia. One can question the logic of modifying the doses for individuals on the basis of change in population prevalence, which suggests that each individual's requirement changes with the number of anemic individuals in society. Supposedly the assumptions are that an increase in prevalence of anemia is associated with a similar increase in prevalence of severe anemia, that the degree of severity is associated with degree of iron deficiency, and that a larger dose of iron is required for more severe iron deficiency. These assumptions are not well substantiated in the literature. On the contrary, there is some evidence that severe anemia may be a different problem from mild and moderate anemia.[2]

8.2.3.2 Current International Guidelines for Iron/Folate Supplements

The most current international guidelines for use of iron supplements were published in 1998 by INACG/WHO/UNICEF (Table 8.2).[15] These guidelines cover all age groups and have included young children and adolescents for the first time. In the case of pregnant women, a daily dose of one tablet containing 60 mg iron and 400 mg folic acid has been recommended for all except those who are severely anemic, in which case a higher dose of 120 mg iron is to be used. In areas where anemia prevalence is <40%, the duration of the supplementation should be 6 months. In other areas, the supplementation should continue 3 months postpartum. The dose of folic acid was increased to 400 µg, not because it is required to produce optimal hemoglobin concentration, but to reduce the risk of neural tube defects if provided at time of conception. It has been discussed whether iron supplementation in iron deficient populations is associated with increased risk of infections, in particular, of malaria in malaria endemic areas. The current consensus is that iron supplementation is a safe public health measure for women in all countries including those where HIV/AIDS and malaria are endemic and that the known benefits of iron supplementation outweigh any risk of an increase in malaria.[24]

8.2.3.3 Intermittent Iron Supplementation

Iron supplements are often associated with gastrointestinal side effects. Because it is assumed that side effects are major determinants of compliance, many efforts have aimed at reducing them. Side effects are dose dependent and the lowest dose possible is preferred. Recent research suggesting that an intermittent dosing of standard strength iron/folate supplements could be as efficacious as a daily dose schedule has generated considerable excitement, extensive discussions, and research in the international iron nutrition community.

Animal studies had suggested that weekly or biweekly doses of iron may be as efficient as daily dosage in improving hematologic status.[25,26] The hypothesized mechanism for the higher efficacy of weekly iron supplementation was related to the mucosal blockage theory, where a first dose of iron would load the gut mucosa and prevent absorption of further supplements. By matching dose frequency to mucosal turnover time, an optimal absorption would be gained from each supplement and a lower dose of iron would be required.[26] Apart from the hypothesized increased efficacy in absorption, an intermittent dosage of iron was also believed to produce fewer side effects and improve compliance and thus program effectiveness. However, some subsequent absorption studies in humans and in anemic rats suggested that intermittent dosage may produce slightly better absorption but the differences were small and could not explain the poor effectiveness of iron supplementation programs using daily dose schedules.[27,28]

A large number of iron supplementation studies have been conducted among pregnant women, adolescents, and children. A meta-analysis including 22 of these studies demonstrated that both weekly and daily supplementation are efficacious but daily produced a larger final hemoglobin concentration.[2] Although the average final

TABLE 8.2
Guidelines for Iron and Folic Acid Supplementation to Individuals without Severe Anemia

Anemic Subjects (%)	Daily Dose	Duration	Comments
Pregnant women			
<40%	60 mg iron + 400 µg folic acid	6 months in pregnancy	If 6-month duration cannot be achieved in pregnancy, continue for 6 months postpartum or increase iron dose to 120 mg. A supplement with less folic acid may be used where iron supplements containing 400 µg are not available.
≥40%	60 mg iron + 400 µg folic acid	6 months in pregnancy and 3 months postpartum	
Children 6–24 months			
<40%	12.5 mg iron + 50 µg folic acid	6–12 months for normal birth weight; 6–24 months for birth weights <2500 g	If the prevalence of anemia is not known, assume it is similar to prevalence among pregnant women in the same population. Iron dosage is based on 2 mg/kg body weight/d.
≥40%	12.5 µg iron + 50 µg folic acid	6–24 months for normal birth weight and 2–24 months for birth weights <2500 g	
Children 2–5 years	20–30 mg iron		Dosage based on 2 mg/kg body weight
Children 6–11 years	30–60 mg iron		
Adolescents and adults	60 mg iron		If the population group includes females of reproductive age, 400 µg folic acid should be included.

Source: Modified from Stolzfus, R.J. and Dreyfuss, M.L., INACG/WHO/UNICEF, Washington, D.C., 1998. With permission.

hemoglobin concentration was only 2.17 g/l lower in the weekly group, it was associated with a significant increased risk of anemia (relative risk 1.34, 95% CI 1.20–1.49). Furthermore, the degree of control of tablet intake in the studies was inversely positively associated with final anemia prevalence, suggesting that limited compliance may have influenced the effectiveness of the supplementation in some studies. The conclusions from the meta-analyses were that weekly supplementation should not be used among pregnant women, and that it may be effective in other population groups only if a high level of compliance can be assured. Another concern with weekly supplementation is the delay in hematologic response that may pose difficulties in timing of the required hematologic response and make it potentially useful only for strictly preventive purposes.

A study among pregnant women in Bangladesh provides information that may explain the small difference in final hemoglobin concentration observed between daily and weekly supplementation.[29,30] Compliance was monitored in this study by using a pill bottle equipped with an electronic counting device, which recorded date and time whenever the pill bottle was opened; it was possible to know the number of supplements consumed by each subject. Hemoglobin response per tablet consumed was similar in both groups, implying that efficacy was not improved in the weekly group. When final hemoglobin concentration was modeled as a function of tablet intake, the results suggested that most of the hemoglobin response was produced by the first 20 tablets taken. When 40 tablets had been consumed, there was no further benefit of additional supplements. A weekly supplementation for 12 weeks provides 24 tablets and, thus, produces a large part of the expected response. This may explain why final hemoglobin concentration in the weekly group was only 2.2 g/l lower than that of the daily group in this study. It is reasonable to assume that if duration of supplementation increased, the response produced by weekly doses would have approached the response from daily doses. Relatively long supplementation periods may explain the limited difference in hemoglobin concentration observed in the studies.

8.2.4 OTHER MICRONUTRIENTS

Iron supplementation has historically received most attention in prevention and control of anemia; it can be questioned whether this emphasis has led to a neglect of other causes of anemia, both nutritional and non-nutritional. Other nutrients of potential public health significance for nutritional anemia are folic acid, vitamin A, and to some extent B_{12}.

The relative contribution of folic acid deficiency to anemia prevalence is not well documented but its importance has been acknowledged by including folic acid in iron supplements for pregnant women for a long time. The most recent guidelines for use of iron supplements have issued dose recommendations of folic acid for young children (Table 8.2). Although vitamin B_{12} deficiency is also associated with macro-cytic anemia, it occurs mainly among strict vegetarians and takes a long time to develop. It is not common among Western vegetarians but has been observed in population groups from the Indian sub-continent and of African origin.[31,32] Vitamin B_{12} is provided along with iron and folate supplements for pregnant women in India. A high prevalence of Vitamin B_{12} deficiency has been reported in Mexico where it is believed to be due to malabsorption, possibly in combination with low dietary intake.[33]

Experimental studies have shown that vitamin A supplementation may have a positive effect on hemoglobin concentration and iron status in several disadvantaged population groups.[34-37] Although the primary justification for vitamin A supplementation is not to control nutritional anemias, it may in some populations improve the efficacy of iron supplementation. WHO, in collaboration with Micronutrient Initiative, has issued recommendations for vitamin A dosage during pregnancy.[38] In populations with endemic vitamin A deficiency, a daily supplement not exceeding 10,000 IU vitamin A (3,000 µg RE) is considered safe at any time of pregnancy. Vitamin A supplementation for infants and children has almost exclusively focused on periodic distribution of high doses of vitamin A. Distribution of a low dose (8000 IU) on a weekly basis may be effective and may provide advantages as it could safely be managed by a community system.[39] If weekly supplementation of low dose of vitamin A among children is implemented it could be coordinated with weekly preventive iron supplementation.

The population groups most often affected by nutritional anemia may also have other nutrient deficiencies associated with impaired health and development. A multimicronutrient supplement has been developed to be used instead of iron/folate supplements in trials among pregnant women in developing countries.[40] The supplement contains 15 micronutrients including iron (30 mg), folic acid (400 µg), Vitamins A (800 µg RE), and B_{12} (2.6 µg). The benefits of combining a range of nutrients seem obvious. However, biological and chemical interactions between the nutrients may both increase and decrease the efficacy observed in single nutrient trials. Efficacy needs to be evaluated before multimicronutrient supplements can be recommended as a substitute for iron/folate supplements.

8.3   EFFECTIVENESS OF SUPPLEMENTATION PROGRAMS

"Effectiveness" — the extent to which a specific intervention, procedure, regimen, or service, when deployed in the field, does what it is intended to do for a defined population.[6]

Much knowledge has been gained from iron and folate supplementation during pregnancy. While efficacy in terms of reducing anemia prevalence has been established in trials, programs have often been accused of poor effectiveness. While this may be true, it is also possible that other non-nutritional factors have contributed to the anemia problem. Rather than assessing the effectiveness of the program, a measure of impact has been obtained (Figure 8.1). To have realistic expectations as to what can be achieved, it is crucial to know the extent of nutritional deficiencies by supplementation.

A number of true constraints for program effectiveness have been reported. Many developing countries have launched national programs to prevent and control anemia and they appear to share similar reasons for lack of success. This section will address the components in supplementation programs as well as discuss some of the problems encountered and some measures which have been proposed for improvement in effectiveness.

8.3.1   SUPPLEMENTATION POLICY

The first step to an effective supplementation program is the adoption of a supplementation policy. Many countries have a policy for supplementation of pregnant women and several cover other population groups, such as infants and young children.

TABLE 8.3
Status of Iron/Folic Acid Supplementation Programs Reported by UNICEF
Field Offices in 57 out of 163 Countries

Program/Policy	Number of Countries (%)
Pregnant women	
Policy on routine supplementation for all women	49 (86)
Policy on supplementation only for anemic women	8 (14)
Daily doses of 60 mg iron + 250 µg folic acid	43 (76)
Weekly dosing in combination with prepregnancy supplementation	5 (9)
Weekly dosing without prepregnancy supplementation	3 (5)
Supplementation post partum	4 (7)
Coverage estimated to be above 50%	29 (51)
Coverage estimated to be above 80%	11 (19)
Preschool and school aged children	
Policy of supplementation	23 (40)

Source: From UNICEF, Progress towards improving iron/folate supplementation programs, New York, 1997. With permission.

In 1997, UNICEF conducted a survey among their 163 field offices on the status of programs for prevention and control of iron deficiency;[41] completed questionnaires were returned from 57 (35%) countries (Table 8.3). Most of the countries replying had a policy of routine supplementation of pregnant women and reported the use of 60 mg iron and 250 µg folic acid per day, which has been recommended to prevent and treat mild anemia in areas of low anemia prevalence.[22] Five countries used a weekly schedule in combination with prepregnancy supplementation. Some countries included different nutrients; Mexico used only iron, India recommended iron, folate, and B_{12}, and Cuba and Honduras used multivitamin mineral supplements.[42]

While most developing countries follow recommendations issued or endorsed by WHO, the recommendations adopted by industrialized countries are less homogenous. The observed variation reflects a current debate whether a routine or selective approach should be used.[43] Even in countries with similar anemia prevalence such as Sweden, Norway, and Denmark, the recommendations are quite different. In Sweden, the recommendation of 100 mg of iron daily for all women from midpregnancy,[44] is quite high and a revision has been suggested.[45] A selective approach has been suggested in Norway where the proposed recommendations of iron supplementation are based on an assessment of S-ferritin early in pregnancy. If ferritin is >60 µg/l then additional iron is deemed as not required, if S-ferritin is 20 to 60 µg/l supplementation should start week 20, and if S-ferritin < 20 µg/l supplementation should start week 12 to 14.[46] The dose, which is recommended, is 30 to 50 mg iron per day. In Denmark, routine iron supplementation has been reintroduced after being interrupted for some years. All women are advised to take 50 to 70 mg iron per day from week 20.[47,48] The issue of selective or routine supplementation of pregnant women has been addressed in other countries, for example, England[49,50] and Finland.[51,52] In the U.S., a policy issued in 1998[53] recommends 30 mg of iron daily starting at time of first prenatal visit until delivery. If a woman is diagnosed as anemic by use of cut-off criteria for specific stage of pregnancy, she receives a higher dose, 60 to 120 mg, and her response is monitored.

8.3.2 SUPPLY OF SUPPLEMENTS

Many programs have been reporting that the logistics of tablet supply is a major constraint.[22] Supplements have been reported to be available infrequently and in limited amounts, resulting in too few tablets distributed to each individual or some not receiving any supplements at all.

In India, an evaluation of the National Nutritional Anemia Prophylaxis Program was carried out in Andhra Pradesh after 15 years of operation. The program aimed at prophylactic supplementation of pregnant and lactating women and children under 12 years of age by supplying iron/folic acid supplements at the household level. The evaluation showed that among the pregnant women who had received supplements, there had been a problem with continuous supply, and 79% reported that they had discontinued the use of supplements because they did not receive any more tablets.[54] India is not the only country from which there are reports of limited supply and poor coverage. Similar problems have been reported in programs in Indonesia,[55] Malawi,[56] Thailand, and Burma.[22]

Inadequate supply can be due to a number of factors, such as incorrect estimation of the quantities of supplements needed, lack of financial resources for procurement of the supplement, competing demands of other pharmaceuticals resulting in low priority for supplements, or lack of awareness of the anemia problem by policymakers leading to limited funds available for supplementation activities.

8.3.3 DELIVERY SYSTEM

A major concern for program effectiveness is the delivery system used for distributing iron supplements. The potential public health impact of the supplementation activity is greatly dependent on the magnitude of the proportion of the intended target population covered by the delivery system. If attendance is limited, the program will have minimal effect on reducing the overall anemia prevalence in the area. In the survey of UNICEF's field stations, about 50% of the countries estimated that they covered less than half of the pregnant women.[41] Only 20% of the programs reach more than 80% of the target population. For example, India reported 19% coverage of pregnant women.[54]

Another concern is that utilization of health services may be influenced by the socioeconomic situation. If social stratification of participation is associated with better health and nutrient status, the group reached may be in less need for supplements. Because the group in greatest need is not covered, the program will have limited effectiveness. It is of great importance to know the characteristics of the population reached by a particular delivery system. In settings where supplements are not free of charge the cost may prevent women from buying them.

The delivery system must provide an opportunity for supplementation when it has the most potential effect. A classic approach has been to use primary health care systems such as antenatal care service. Late registration in antenatal service has been reported as a problem in many programs and can reduce the effect iron supplementation may have on pregnancy outcome. This was the case in Indonesia, where a limited use of iron supplements was considered to be mainly due to late registration for antenatal care.[57] A problem with late registration of pregnant women and few antenatal visits has also been seen in a refugee population in the Near East.[58]

Alternative delivery systems can improve effectiveness. Delivery of supplements at "door step" by a community health worker may increase the coverage of the target population. It may also have a favorable effect on compliance as community health workers often have a good rapport with the community. Several systems outside the formal health services have been proposed and tested, e.g., traditional birth attendants and healers, schools, religious groups, workplaces, and women's groups. The positive experience of using traditional birth attendants as distributors of iron supplements in the community has been recognized in Indonesia. When traditional birth attendants distributed the supplements the coverage of pregnant women increased from 51 to 92% and the mean number of supplements consumed from 23 to 64.[59]

A more recent approach is aiming at the identification of a delivery strategy for newly wed women, which would enable supplementation before conception. A similar aim is underlying efforts to supplement adolescent girls.[60,61]

8.3.4   COMPLIANCE OF SUPPLEMENT USERS

Limited compliance on the part of women has often been considered a major reason for ineffective supplementation programs.[1,21,62-64] This problem has been reported in industrialized [65-67] and developing countries.[55,68-70] In many programs that have been severely constrained by poor supply of iron supplements, it has not been possible to judge the extent to which compliance is a problem. The main factors that have been associated with compliance by the supplement users are discussed in this section.

8.3.4.1   Side Effects

Gastro-intestinal side effects are often blamed to be the main reason for limited compliance[21,69,71] but this view has been challenged by others.[72] Actual information on the prevalence of side effects in supplementation programs and their impact on compliance is limited. A study in Tanzania showed that women experiencing side effects reduced their tablet intake by one-third, but a large part of noncompliance remained to be explained when the impact of side effects had been taken into account.[70]

Side effects are dose dependent and a lower dose reduces the risk of side effects.[11,73] The current trend of a lower dosage of iron is favorable for compliance. However, even weekly doses of 120 mg iron have been reported to produce side effects among as many as 30% of pregnant women.[74] Modifying the dosages may not completely prevent side effects. Appropriate counseling on what to expect in terms of side effects can counteract their negative effect on compliance.[75]

The prevalence of side effects reported in iron supplementation trials shows a great variation even with similar doses. It is not clear if this is a real difference in occurrence of side effects, an effect of difference in compliance, or a consequence of different definitions and methods of assessments. Side effects do not appear to be affected by the type of iron compound used. No difference has been observed between ferrous-sulfate, fumarate, gluconate, or glycine sulfate.[76,77] Dividing a daily dosage into two administrations or taking supplements with a meal may reduce side effects,[69] but absorption of iron is reduced in the latter case.[78,79]

Side effects are dependent on type of iron preparation. The so-called sustained-release preparations where granules coated with iron gradually dissolve during the passage through the gastro-intestinal system produce fewer side effects than conventional iron preparations.[80] These preparations may be associated with less absorption,[77,82] as they expose the upper part of duodenum, the site where most of iron is absorbed, [81] to a smaller amount of iron. A reduced local concentration of iron in the upper part of intestine without a compromise in absorbability of the iron compound has been achieved in preparations in which the ferrous sulfate is mixed with a wax matrix.[83] The matrix floats on the stomach content delivering the iron to the upper part of the intestine over a longer time period. In supplementation trials, the gastric delivery system has been associated with a substantially higher absorption and fewer side effects than conventional preparations.[70,84] A major constraint is the high cost of sustained-release iron preparations, a comparison of cost effectiveness between the supplement preparations is needed before deciding which to use in a program. The gastric delivery system preparation is currently not available on the market.

8.3.4.2 Appearance and Quality

Iron supplements, which disintegrate and emit odors, will not be consumed. Coating of the tablets increases their stability and is particularly important in humid climates.[15] Colors and shapes may also have a meaning and imply the strength the drug has, thereby raising expectations which can influence compliance.[85] Red tablets may be more suitable because of their similarity in color to blood.[86] Whenever an iron supplementation program is initiated, there is need to determine whether color is important and if so, which is the appropriate one. Coating also reduces the metallic taste of the supplements. The packaging of tablets influences their stability. In developing countries supplements are often provided in a small plastic bag, which is likely to reduce their ability to withstand humidity. The use of plastic bags may also increase the risk that children ingest the bags, resulting in potentially serious intoxications. Although other types of packaging such as pill bottles and blister charts are more expensive, they may prove to be more cost effective.

8.3.4.3 Understanding and Motivation

Poor compliance to medical regimens may occur because the clients do not know how to take the supplement.[87,88] This has also been suggested as a reason for limited use of iron supplements among pregnant women.[22,89] A lack of understanding could be due to poor information given by the supplement distributor. Although understanding of the regimen is necessary to enable good compliance, it is not sufficient to produce it. There are many reasons why women could be poorly motivated to use iron supplements. Apart from gastro-intestinal side effects issues related to perceptions of need of supplement, expected health effects and cultural barriers may affect compliance.

Anemia does not have unique symptoms that are unmistakable and it is difficult to discern its magnitude and recognize it as a health problem. Although many women identify weakness or weak blood as a condition of pregnancy, there is often little knowledge about anemia and it is often not perceived as a major health problem.[72,90,91] This may even be true among anemic women, explaining their limited motivation for taking iron supplements. Among women without any symptoms of anemia, it may be even more difficult to encourage the use of supplements. Preventive health behavior demands action before symptoms appear and it requires that women accept the possibility of illness before there is evidence for it. This may be difficult and may explain poor response to preventive measures.[92,93] The extent to which the preventive health concept is internalized is likely to vary in different sociomedical settings and in some areas there may be a need to introduce the concept.

Women may have expectations that the supplements will treat a number of symptoms. The noticeable effects may be subtle and fail to meet women's expectations thereby reducing their incentive to continue taking the supplements.[72,94] In Tanzania, pregnant women receiving iron supplements were asked how long a time they thought it would take for an effect to occur. Many women expected the effect within some hours and most of them within 1 to 2 days suggesting that unless realistic expectations are raised there is considerable risk for disappointment in the supplements.[95]

There may be cultural barriers when supplement use does not fit in the prevailing sociomedical system. In several parts of Africa a fear that iron supplements may cause the women to have "too much blood" has been expressed.[56,96] This has also been noted in Brazil.[97] A common belief in Thailand and India is that the use of an iron supplement will make the baby big and cause a difficult labor.[98,99] Other fears women may have include spontaneous abortions. This may be based on the belief that health is maintained by keeping a balance between hot and cold. Foods, physiologic conditions, and illnesses are classified according to this continuum to be hot/heating or cold/cooling. Hot substances may cause the womb to be too hot and cause abortion. In a study in south India, iron supplements were rejected because they were thought to produce too much heat and thus a risk for losing the baby.[99] At times mothers are concerned that the iron supplement may be some other drug. A particular worry seems to be that it is a contraceptive; reduced acceptance of iron supplements due to this reason has been reported in India.[100]

The reasons for poor motivation are many and their relative importance will vary with setting. Commonly, research has been limited to descriptions of anecdotal character and with few exceptions, motivational factors have not been addressed in experimental research. There is a need for intervention studies to evaluate different strategies to improve compliance to supplementation.

8.3.4.4   Interaction between Supplement, Providers, and Users

Programs have often given priority to supplies and delivery system of supplement, disregarding the importance of interaction between supplement providers and users and the need for information, education, and communications (IEC) to promote use of supplements.[101] Supplement providers, whether they are health workers or not, play a key role; it is of great importance to ensure that they are well trained and highly motivated.

Problems with limited promotion of iron supplements have been reported in developing and industrialized countries. A study in Guatemala indicated that only about 60% of the women were advised to take iron supplements by the health workers.[102] Similarly, studies in Sweden and Norway have shown that many health workers do not advise pregnant women to take iron supplements according to current recommendations, resulting in their limited use.[67,103,104] It has also been reported that iron tablets are one of the drugs that most frequently pile up at health centers receiving essential drug kits suggesting limited prescription of them.[105] Evaluations of unsuccessful programs have shown that health care personnel may need as much education about anemia as those who are going to use the supplement.[15,72]

The information provided in IEC should be adapted to its sociomedical setting. There may be a need to collect information on existing beliefs and fears regarding anemia, its causation, and expected effects of iron supplementation, both positive and negative. Before implementing an IEC activity on a large scale, it is recommended to evaluate its effectiveness in smaller intervention trials.

Positive effects of counseling on compliance have been reported from several countries;[69,75,98] counseling should always be a component in distribution of supplements. In Indonesia, following an IEC campaign which complemented a government program, coverage among pregnant women increased from 51 to 86% and the average number of supplements taken from 24 to 48 tablets.[57,59] When IEC activities were combined with community based distribution of supplements by traditional birth attendants an even larger effect on compliance was observed. The number of tablets taken increased to 66. IEC activities need to include not only the users of supplements but also close relatives, such as husbands and mothers-in-law, as they may greatly influence a woman's decision in use of supplements.[90,91,106]

8.4   CONCLUSIONS

This chapter has focused on supplementation as a means to control and prevent nutritional anemia. Issues related to efficacy, effectiveness, and impact have been addressed to identify strengths and limitations in current supplementation efforts; the main findings including the different actions for follow-up are summarized in this section. Although supplementation may remain as the most effective option in some population groups and in some settings, care should be taken that the efforts to develop effective supplementation programs do not distract attention from addressing the underlying causes of nutritional deficiencies.

Efficacy:

This is the part of supplementation program where most research has been focused. Efficacy of supplementation in reducing nutritional anemia is established. Still, the effect on other functional outcomes remains a topic of scientific discussion. Because there is limited knowledge on association between level of severity of nutritional anemia and health outcome, it is difficult to set unequivocal hematological aims for supplementation. Although considerable research has addressed dosages there are still uncertainties even regarding optimal dose of iron. Furthermore, there is a need to gain more information on nutritional and nonnutritional factors limiting response to supplementation.

Effectiveness:

It is clear that all program components; supplement supply, delivery system, and compliance have suffered from constraints. All are required for an effective program. More attention needs to be paid to efforts to increase coverage of delivery systems and to improve compliance. Exploring alternative delivery systems and addressing factors that limit motivation to take nutritional supplement may have the largest potential toward improving program effectiveness.

Impact:

The proportion of anemia that may be prevented and controlled by nutrient supplementation depends on the number of cases attributable to nutrient deficiencies. The proportion is likely to vary with population groups, socioeconomic, and geographical settings. The negative health outcomes of anemia may also have other causative factors. Multiple interventions, nutritional and non-nutritional, may be required to make a substantial impact on health outcomes.

REFERENCES

1. Hughes, A., Prevention and treatment of severe anaemia in pregnancy, Background paper for discussion, a meeting of technical working group on prevention and treatment of severe anemia in pregnancy, World Health Organization, Geneva, 1991.
2. Beaton, G. H. and McCabe, G. P., Efficacy of intermittent iron supplementation in the control of iron deficiency anemia in developing countries: an analysis of experience. Final report to the Micronutrient Initiative, GHB Consulting, Toronto, 1999.
3. Rush, D., Nutrition and maternal mortality in the developing world, Paper prepared for Opportunities for Micronutrient Interventions, Washington, D.C., 1998.
4. Scholl, T. and Hediger, M., Anemia and iron-deficiency anemia: compilation of data on pregnancy outcome, *Am. J. Clinical Nutr.,* 59(Suppl.), 492s, 1994.
5. Habicht, J.-P., Epidemiology for scientific and programmatic decision-making, in *Beyond Nutritional Recommendations: Implementing Science for Healthier Populations,* Proceedings from the 14th annual Bristol/Myers Sqibb/Mead Johnson Nutrition Research Symposium, Garza, C., Haas, J., Habicht, J.-P., and Pelletier, D., Eds., Cornell University, Ithaca, NY., 1995.
6. Last, J. M., *A Dictionary of Epidemiology,* Oxford University Press, Oxford, 1988.
7. Allen, L. H., Pregnancy and iron deficiency: unresolved issues, *Nutr. Rev.,* 55, 91, 1997.
8. Institute of Medicine, *Iron Deficiency Anemia. Recommended Guidelines for the Prevention, Detection, and Management of Iron Deficiency Anemia among U.S. Children and Women of Childbearing Age,* National Academy of Science Press, Washington, D.C., 1993.
9. Ramakrishnan, U., Manjrekar, R., Rivera, J., Gonzales-Cossio, T., and Martorell, R., Micronutrients and pregnancy outcome: a review of literature, *Nutr. Res.,* 19, 103, 1999.

10. de Onis, M., Nutritional interventions to prevent intrauterine growth retardation: evidence from randomized controlled trials, *Eur. J. Clinical Nutr.,* 52, s5, 1998.

11. Institute of Medicine, *Nutrition during Pregnancy,* National Academy Press, Washington, D.C., 1990.

12. Scholl, T. and Reilly, T., Anemia, iron and pregnancy outcome, *Am. J. Clinical Nutr.,* 130, 443S, 2000.

13. Scholl, T. O., Hediger, M. L., Fischer, R. L., and Shearer, J. W., Anemia vs. iron deficiency: increased risk of preterm delivery in a prospective study, *Am. J. Clinical Nutr.,* 55, 985, 1992.

14. Klebanoff, M., Shiiono, P., Selby, J., Trachtenberg, A., and Graubard, B., Anemia and spontaneous preterm birth, *Am. J. Obstet. Gynecol.,* 164, 59, 1991.

15. Stolzfus, R. J. and Dreyfuss, M. L., *Guidelines for the Use of Iron Supplements to Prevent and Treat Iron Deficiency Anemia,* International Anemia Consultative Group, World Health Organization, United Nations Children's Fund, Washington, D.C., 1998.

16. *Requirements of Vitamin A, Iron, Folate and Vitamin* B_{12} Food and Agriculture Organization and World Health Organization, Rome, 1988.

17. Sloan, N., Jordan, E., and Winikoff, B., *Does Iron Supplementation Make a Difference?* MotherCare, Arlington, 1992.

18. The design and analyses of iron supplementation trials: a report from the International Nutritional Anemia Consultative Group, International Anemia Consultative Group, The Nutrition Foundation, Washington, D.C., 1984.

19. Conquest of deficiency diseases: achievements and prospects, World Health Organization, Geneva, 1970.

20. Guidelines for the eradication of iron deficiency anemia: a report of the International Nutritional Anemia Consultative Group, The Nutrition Foundation, Washington, D.C., 1977.

21. DeMaeyer, E., Preventing and controlling iron deficiency anemia through primary health care. A guide to health administrators and programme managers, World Health Organization, Geneva, 1989.

22. Controlling iron deficiency, World Health Organization, Geneva, 1991.

23. Third report on the world nutrition situation, World Health Organization, Geneva, 1997.

24. Preventing iron deficiency in women and children: background and consensus on key technical issues and resources for advocacy, planning, and implementing national programmes, International Nutrition Foundation, Micronutrient Initiative, New York, 1998.

25. Wright, A. J. and Southon, S., The effectiveness of various iron-supplementation regimens in improving the Fe status of anemic rats, *Br. J. Nutr.,* 63, 579, 1990.

26. Viteri, F., Xunian, L., Tolomei, K., and Martin, A., True absorption and retention of supplementatal iron is more efficient when iron is administered every three days rather than daily to iron-normal and iron-deficient rats, *J. Nutr.,* 125, 82, 1995.

27. Cook, J. D. and Reddy, M. B., Efficacy of weekly compared to daily iron supplementation, *Am. J. Clinical Nutr.,* 62, 117, 1995.

28. Benito, P., House, W., and Miller, D., Influence of iron supplementation frequency on absorption efficiency and mucosal ferritin in anaemic rats, *Br. J. Nutr.,* 78, 469, 1997.

29. Ekström, E.-C., Hyder, Z., Habicht, J.-P., and Persson, L.-Å., Iron repletion achieved with lower doses of iron than expected among pregnant women in rural Bangladesh, *FASEB J.,* 13, A698, 1999.

30. Ekström, E.-C., Hyder, Z., Chowdhury, A. M. R., Chowdhury, S., Habicht, J.-P., Lönnerdal, B., and Persson, L.-Å., Efficacy of weekly iron supplement: new evidence from a study among pregnant women in rural Bangladesh, *FASEB J.,* 13, A698, 1999.

31. Gomber, S., Kumar, S., Rusia, U., Gupta, P., Agarwal, K. N., and Sharma, S., Prevalence and etiology of nutritional anaemias in early childhood in an urban slum, *Indian J. Med. Res.,* 107, 269, 1998.

32. Cooper, B. A., Nutritional macrocytic anemia, in *Nutritional Anemias,* Vol. 30, Fomon, S. J. and Zlotkin, S., Eds., Vevye Raven Press, New York, 1992.

33. Allen, L., Rosade, J., Casterline, J., Martinez, H., Lopez, P., Munoz, E., and Black, A., Vitamin B_{12} deficiency and malabsorption are highly prevalent in rural Mexican communities, *Am. J. Clinical Nutr.,* 62, 1013, 1995.

34. Bloem, M., Wedel, M., Egger, R., Speek, A., Schrivjer, J., Saowakontha, S., and Schreurs, W., Iron metabolism and vitamin A deficiency in children in northeastern Thailand, *Am. J. Clinical Nutr.,* 50, 332, 1989.

35. Mejia, L. A. and Chew, F., Hematological effect of supplementing anemic children with vitamin A alone and in combination with iron, *Am. J. Clinical Nutr.,* 48, 595, 1988.

36. Muhilal, Permeisih, D., Idjradinata, Y. R., Muherdiyantiningsih, and Karyadai, D., Vitamin A -fortified monosodium glutamate and health, growth and survival of children: a controlled field trial, *Am. J. Clinical Nutr.,* 48, 1271, 1988.

37. Suharno, D. and Muhilal., Vitamin A and nutritional anemia, *Food Nutr. Bull.,* 17, 7, 1996.

38. Safe vitamin A dosage during pregnancy and lactation, World Health Organization, Geneva, 1998.

39. Underwood, B. A., Prevention of Vitamin A deficiency, in *Prevention of Micronutrient Deficiencies. Tools for Policy Makers and Public Health Workers,* Howson, C. P., Kennedy, E. T., and Horwitz, A., Eds., National Academy Press, Washington, D.C., 1998.

40. Composition of a multi-micronutrient supplement to be used in pilot programs among pregnant women in developing countries. Report from a UNICEF/WHO/UNU workshop, New York, 1999.

41. Progress toward improving iron/folate supplementation programs. First draft, UNICEF, New York, 1997.

42. Huffman, S. L., Baker, J., and Shuman, J., The case for promoting multiple vitamin/mineral supplements for women of reproductive age in developing countries, Academy of Educational Development, Washington, D.C., 1998.

43. Villar, J. and Bergsjo, P., Scientific basis for the content of routine antenatal care. I. Philosophy, recent studies and power to eliminate or alleviate adverse maternal outcome, *Acta Obstet. Gynecol. Scand.,* 76, 1, 1997.

44. Halso-overvakning vid normal graviditet [Routine antenatal care], *ARG Rapport,* 21, 37, 1991.

45. Halsovard fore, efter och under graviditet [Health care before, after and during pregnancy], *Socialstyrelsen Rapport,* 7, 1996.

46. Borch-Iohnsen, B., Halvorsen, R., Andrew, M., Forde, R., and Toverud, E.-L., Trenger vi nye retningslinjer for bruk av jerntilsudd i svangerskapet? [Need for new recommendations on iron supplementation during pregnancy?] *Tidsskrift for Norske Laegeforening,* 113, 2414, 1993.

47. Milman, N., Bergholt, T., Eriksen, L., Ahring, K., and Graudal, N. A., Iron requirements and iron balance during pregnancy. Is iron supplementation needed for pregnant women? *Ugeskr Laeger,* 159, 6057, 1997.

48. Vejledning om jerntilskud til gravide [Guidelines for iron supplementation during pregnancy], Sundhetsstyrelsen, Denmark, 1992.

49. Hibbard, B., Iron and folate supplements during pregnancy: supplementation is valuable only in selected patients, *Br. Med. J.,* 297, 1324, 1988.

50. Horn, E., Iron and folate supplements during pregnancy: supplementing everyone treats those at risk and is cost-effective, *Br. Med. J.,* 297, 1325, 1988.

51. Hemminki, E. and Merilainen, J., Long-term follow-up of mothers and their infants in a randomized trial on iron prophylaxis during pregnancy, *Am. J. Obstet. Gynecol.,* 173 1995.

52. Hemminki, E. and Rimpela, U., A randomized comparison of routine versus selective iron supplementation during pregnancy, *J. Am. Coll. Nutr.,* 10, 3, 1991.

53. Recommendations to prevent and control iron deficiency in the United States, *MMWR,* 47, 1, 1998.

54. Vijayaraghavan, K., Brahmam, G., Nair, K., Akbar, D., and Prahald Rao, N., Evaluation of National Nutritional Anemia Prophylaxis Programme, *Indian J. Pediatr.,* 57, 183, 1990.

55. Schultink, W., Iron supplementation programmes: Compliance of target groups and frequency of tablet intake, *Food Nutr. Bull.,* 17, 22, 1996.

56. Sibale, C., Williams, L., Cousens, S., Semo, L. and Franco, C., Determining the prevalence and risk factors for anaemia in women of reproductive age in Thyolo, Malawi, in *Improving the Quality of Iron Supplementation Programs, The Mother-Care Experience,* Galloway, R., Ed., MotherCare, Arlington, 1997.

57. Hessler-Radelet, C., Utomo, B., Budiono, T., Achadi, E., Sloan, N., and Moore, M., Improving the coverage of compliance with iron-folate supplementation in the Indramayu regency of Indonesia, in *Improving the Quality of Iron Supplementation Programs, The MotherCare Experience,* Galloway, R., Ed., MotherCare, Arlington, 1997.

58. Pappagallo, S. and Bull, D. L., Operational problems of an iron supplementation programme for pregnant women: an assessment of UNRWA experience, *Bull. World Health Organ.,* 74, 25, 1996.

59. Achadi, E., Reducing maternal anemia, Indonesia, *Mothers Child.,* 14, 11, 1995.

60. Kurz, K. and Galloway, R., Improving adolescent iron status before childbearing, *J. Nutr.,* 130, 437S, 2000.

61. Lynch, S. R., The potential impact of iron supplementation during adolescence on iron status during pregnancy, *J. Nutr.,* 130, 448S, 2000.

62. *Iron Supplementation during Pregnancy: Why are not Women Complying?* World Health Organization, Geneva, 1990.

63. Cook, J., Letter to the editor, *Am. J. Clinical Nutr.,* 63, 610, 1996.

64. Viteri, F. E., Weekly compared with daily iron supplementation, *Am. J. Clinical Nutr.,* 63, 610, 1996.

65. Bonnar, J., Goldberg, A., and Smith, J., Do pregnant women take their iron?, *Lancet,* 457, 1969.

66. Porter, A., Drug defaulting in a general practice, *Br. Med. J.,* 1, 218, 1969.

67. Ekström, E.-C. and Wulff, M., Kvalitetssäkring inom modrahålsovården, graviditet och jarnsupplementering. Foljs rekommendationerna? Preliminår rapport, Umeå University, Umea, 1997.

68. Schultink, W., van, d.-R. -. M., Matulessi, P., and Gross, R., Low compliance with an iron-supplementation program: a study among pregnant women in Jakarta, Indonesia, *Am. J. Clinical Nutr.,* 57, 135, 1993.

69. Charoenlarp, P., Dhanamitta, S., Kaewvichit, R., Silprasert, A., Suwanaradd, C., Na, N.-S., Prawatmuang, P., Vatanavicharn, S., Nutcharas, U., Pootrakul, P. et al., A WHO collaborative study on iron supplementation in Burma and in Thailand, *Am. J. Clinical Nutr.,* 47, 280, 1988.

70. Ekström, E.-C., Kavishe, F., Habicht, J.-P., Frongillo Jr, E., Rasmussen, K., and Hemed, L., Adherence to iron supplementation during pregnancy in Tanzania: determinants and hematologic consequences, *Am. J. Clinical Nutr.,* 64, 386, 1996.

71. Afifi, A., Banwell, G., Bennison, R., Boothby, K., and Griffiths, P., A simple test for ingested iron in hospital and domiciliary practice, *Br. Med. J.,* 1, 1021, 1966.

72. Galloway, R. and McGuire, J., Determinants of compliance with iron supplementation: supplies, side-effects, or psychology, *Soc. Sci. Med.,* 39, 381, 1994.

73. Sölvell, L., Oral iron therapy side-effects, in *Iron Deficiency: Pathogenesis, Clinical Aspects, and Therapy,* Hallberg, L., Harwerth, H. G., and Vannotti, A., Eds., Academic Press, London, 1970.

74. Bobrow, E. A., Young, M. W., and Van der Haar, F., Compliance and side-effects in a supplementation trial in pregnant women in rural Malawi, International Anemia Consultative Group Meeting, Durban, 1999.

75. Galloway, R. and McGuire, J., Daily versus weekly: How many pills do pregnant women need? *Nutr. Rev.,* 54, 318, 1996.

76. Hallberg, L., Ryttinger, L., and Sölvell, L., Side-effects of oral iron therapy: A double-blind study of different iron compounds in tablet form, *Acta Med. Scand.,* Suppl. 459, 23, 1967.

77. Hallberg, L. and Sölvell, L., Succinic acid as absorption promoter in iron tablets: absorption and side-effect studies, *Acta Med. Scand.,* 23, 1967.

78. Cook, J., Lipschitz, D., and Skikne, B., Absorption of controlled-release iron, *Clinical Pharmacol. Ther.,* 32, 531, 1982.

79. Ekenved, G., Arvidsson, B., and Sölvell, L., Influence of food on the absorption from different types of iron tablets, *Scand. J. Haema.,* 28(Suppl.), 79, 1976.

80. Sjöstedt, J., Manner, P., Nummi, S., and Ekenved, G., Oral iron prophylaxis during pregnancy: a comparative study of different dosage regimens, *Acta Obstet. Gynecol. Scand.,* Suppl., 60, 3, 1977.

81. Conrad, M., Regulation of iron absorption, in *Essential and Toxic Trace Elements in Human Health and Disease: An Update,* Wiley-Liss Inc., New York, 1993, 203.

82. Bothwell, T., Charlton, R., Cook, J., and Finch, C., Eds., *Iron Metabolism in Man,* Blackwell Scientific Publications, Oxford, 1979.

83. Brock, C., Curry, H., Hanna, C., Knipfer, M., and Taylor, L., Adverse side-effects of iron supplementation: a comparative trial of a wax-matrix iron preparation and conventional ferrous sulfate tablets, *Clinical Ther.,* 7, 568, 1985.

84. Cook, J. D., Carriaga, M., Kahn, S. G., Schalch, W., and Skikne, B. S., Gastric delivery system for iron supplementation, *Lancet,* 335, 1136, 1990.

85. Buckalew, L. and Sallis, R., Patient compliance and medication perception, *J. Clinical Psychol.,* 42, 49, 1986.

86. Bledsoe, C. and Goubaud, M., The reinterpretation and distribution of Western pharmaceuticals: an example from the Mende of Sierra Leone, in *The Contexts of Mediciens in Developing Countries,* van der Geest, S. and Whyte, S., Eds., Kluwer Academic Press, Dordrecht, Holland, 1985, 253.

87. Kristeller, J. and Rodin, J., A three stage model of treatment continuity: compliance, adherence, and maintenance, in *Handbook of Psychology and Health,* Baum, A., Taylor, S., and Singer, J., Eds., Lawrence Erlbaum Associates, London, 1984, 85.

88. DiNicola, D. and DiMatteo, M., Practitioners, patients, and compliance with medical regimens: a social psychological perspective, in *Handbook of Psychology and Health,* Baum, A., Taylor, S., and Singer, J., Eds., Lawrence Erlbaum Associates, London, 1984, 55.

89. Raina, N., Gupta, A., Sharma, M., Verma, M., and Dhingra, K., Operational study on nutritional anemia in pregnant women, lactating women and adolescent girls in a rural community in India, in *Improving the Quality of Iron Supplementation Programs. The MotherCare Experience,* Gallloway, R., Ed., MotherCare, Arlington, 1997.

90. Moore, M., Riono, P., and Pariani, S., A qualitative investigation of factors influencing use of iron folate tablets by pregnant women in West Java: a summary of findings, MotherCare, Arlington, 1991.

91. *MotherCare Matters,* 6, MotherCare, Guatemala, 14, 1997.

92. Kanani, S., Combatting anemia in adolescent girls: a report from India, *Mothers Child.,* 13, 1, 1994.

93. Rosenstock, I., The Health Belief Model: explaining health behavior through expectancies, in *Health Behavior and Health Education,* Glanz, K., Lewis, F., and Rimer, B., Eds., Jossey Bass, San Francisco, 1991, 39.

94. Murmu, L. R., Supplementation study compliance and the role of health care staff, *Am. J. Clinical Nutr.,* 59, 433, 1994.

95. Ekström, E.-C., Unpublished results from iron supplementation study among pregnant women in Tanzania, 1995.

96. Ekström, E.-C., Iron Supplementation during Pregnancy in Tanzania: Determinants and Hematologic Consequences of Adherence, Ph.D. thesis, Cornell University, Ithaca, 1995.

97. Atkinson, S. J. and Farias, M. F., Perceptions of risk during pregnancy amongst urban women in northeast Brazil, *Soc. Sci. Med.,* 41, 1577, 1995.

98. Valyasevi, A., Delivery system for iron supplementation in pregnant women: Thailand experience, in INACG Workshop on Maternal Nutritional Anemia, Geneva, 1988.

99. Nichter, M. and Nichter, M., The ethnophysiology and dietetics of pregnancy: a case study from South India, *Hum. Organ.,* 42, 235, 1983.

100. Evaluation of the National Nutritional Anaemia Prohylaxis programme, Indian Council of Medical Research, New Delhi, 1989.

101. Report of the meeting of the working group on iron deficiency, World Health Organization, Geneva, 1998.

102. Grajeda, R., Hurtado, E., Bocaletti, E., and Recinos, S., Knowledge and practice regarding anemia and iron supplementation during pregnancy of health personnel in Guatemala, in *Improving the Quality of Iron Supplementation Programs. The MotherCare Experience,* Galloway, R., Ed., MotherCare, Arlington, 1997.

103. Eskeland, B. and Malterud, K., Iron supplementation in pregnancy. General practitioners' compliance with official recommendations, *Scand. J. Prim. Health Care,* 11, 263, 1993.

104. Rytter, E., Forde, R., Andrew, M., Matheson, I., and Borch-Ionsen, B., Graviditet og jerntilskud: blir offisielle retningslinjene fulgt? [Pregnancy and iron supplements: are the national recommendations followed?] *Tidsskrift for Norske Laegeforening,* 113, 2416, 1993.

105. Haak, H. and Hogerzeil, H., Essential drugs for ration kits in developing countries, *Health Policy Plann.,* 10, 40, 1995.

106. Homedes, N. and Ugalde, A., Patient's compliance with medical treatments in the third world. What do we know? *Health Policy Plann.,* 8, 291, 1993.

9 Fortification

Tomás Walter, Manuel Olivares, Fernando
Pizarro, and Eva Hertrampf

CONTENTS

9.1   INTRODUCTION

Over 2 billion people are affected by iron deficiency worldwide; nearly half have the most severe form, iron deficiency anemia (IDA). It is highly prevalent in most of the developing world and probably the only nutritional deficiency of consideration in industrialized countries.[1] For physiological reasons seen in previous chapters, the most commonly affected groups are infants, preschool children, adolescents, and women of childbearing age. While infants and women of reproductive age are affected in many developing countries, in industrialized countries, IDA is present mainly in women due to the additional iron requirements imposed by menstruation and pregnancy.

The common strategies to prevent and control nutritional anemias are to increase iron intake and absorption by changing dietary habits, providing medicinal iron (supplementation), or by adding iron to the diet (fortification). Iron supplementation can be directed to those populations at greatest risk and has the advantage of targeting the high risk groups such as pregnant women and infants. These efforts are usually hampered due to the difficulty in sustaining the motivation of the participants, who may be discouraged by the common occurrence of gastrointestinal side effects, which may be mitigated by intermittent schedules recently developed.[2] Supplementation requires an effective system of health care delivery and is relatively costly to maintain.[3] It is the most widely used strategy to prevent iron deficiency during pregnancy when a relatively short period of time is required, individuals are easily recognizable, motivated, and usually accessible to the health care providers. Additionally, the enormous increase in iron requirements imposed by pregnancy cannot be met by the usual diet alone. Folic acid is commonly integrated into this strategy for iron.

On the other hand, fortification is generally accepted as the best all around approach for combating iron deficiency. It can be tailored to reach all sectors of the population, does not require the cooperation of the individual, the initial cost is relatively small, and the maintenance expense is less than that of supplementation. However, there are technical and other policy hurdles in fortifying the diet with iron. For example, the selection of the food vehicle and fortificant iron source are important considerations that have been recently reviewed.[4,5] An overview of the key issues related to iron fortification which include technical aspects, quality control, and demonstration of effectiveness is presented in the first section of this chapter. This is followed by a critical review of the experience and lessons learned specifically in Chile and other Latin American countries which serve as excellent case studies for other parts of the world, where fortification remains to be implemented successfully as a strategy to combat nutritional anemias.

9.2   DEVELOPMENT OF A FORTIFICATION PROGRAM

The several steps that need to be carried out for the successful development and implementation of a fortification program are outlined in Table 9.1[6] and are:

- Prevalence studies are needed at the onset to establish that iron deficiency is sufficiently widespread to warrant a national intervention program.
- Having already determined the need for fortification, dietary surveys are indispensable to characterize the original diets with respect to content of

---

TABLE 9.1
Steps in Planning a Regional Fortification Program

Evaluate prevalence of iron deficiency
Select target groups
Study diets and dietary habits
Measure dietary content of heme and nonheme iron
Evaluate the absorption of dietary iron in typical diets
Select vehicle and iron fortificant
Select the necessary fortification level
Estimate absorption enhancers, if necessary
Study absorption of iron from fortified food (bioavailability)
Study acceptability of fortified food in the laboratory
Study biologic effect and acceptability via field trial
Study biologic effect, acceptability, and feasibility under original
   conditions of distribution and consumption via field trial
Plan future evaluation of impact

---

heme and nonheme iron as well as factors that may enhance or inhibit iron absorption.

- It is important to measure the actual iron absorption from the original diets in human subjects. This is usually accomplished using the extrinsic radio-iron method and in more recent years utilizing stable nonradioactive-isotopes of iron. Dietary surveys and absorption studies are needed for determining whether the major problem is limited iron intake, low bioavailability, or a combination, and for estimating the level of iron fortification that will be required to reduce the prevalence of iron deficiency. This exercise has been performed for typical Latin American diets.[7]

- A major requirement in the selection of a vehicle-fortificant combination is centralized processing in a facility that will permit the controlled addition of the fortificant. The addition cannot affect organoleptic characteristics of the product or shorten shelf life.

- After all these appraisals have been completed and the selection of fortificant and the vehicle have been adequately studied, a costly and time consuming but necessary step before the development of a national fortification program is conducting a field trial to establish its efficacy in a carefully controlled situation.

9.2.1 SELECTION OF THE VEHICLE

Rice, corn, and wheat and their derivatives like flours and meals, are the preferred vehicles for fortification because these are the most widely consumed staple foods in many developing countries. On a global basis, cereals provide half of all calories consumed and are also major contributors of protein in the whole form or in derivative products such as breads, pastas, and biscuits. Technical advances have enabled flour fortification technology to be transferred to a number of developing countries. New micronutrient premix powders offer the nutritional value, cost, and stability that ensure that fortified flour will look, feel, taste, and smell like unfortified flour. Initiatives in rice fortification are also overcoming barriers of incompatible consumer habits, cost, and diversity of small village based processors.

Wheat is the most widely consumed cereal. China and Russia grow the most wheat and consume most of what they produce. Most countries import much of their wheat, usually from the major wheat exporting countries, Canada, U.S., Argentina, Australia, and France. The importation of wheat is often under government control and involves large, multinational companies that generally own and operate flour mills and have been involved in fortification of flour for decades. A few countries obtain wheat through aid programs but most imports are commercial transactions. Wheat consumption is particularly high in the Middle East and per capita consumption ranges from 300 to 600 g/day. While many countries in this region grow significant amounts of wheat, imports are still needed to meet consumption. Egypt and Syria import more than half their requirements. While overall consumption in Asia is lower, trends indicate a rise in consumption in many nations. For example, on a per capita basis, from 1992 to 1996, wheat consumption was up 44% in Indonesia and about 33% in Thailand.

Rice is the second most consumed cereal and is the dominant staple in Asia, where it represents 50 to 75% of the caloric intake. In Latin American countries, rice constitutes about 20% of the total calories consumed. Although there are many different varieties, the three basic types of products are brown rice, white or polished rice, and rice flour. Corn or maize is used heavily in Africa and Latin America. In Malawi, Zambia, Zimbabwe, and Kenya, maize products represent 40 to 60% of the caloric intake. In many Latin American countries, nixtamalized corn flour is used in tortillas and chips.

All cereals are processed or milled before they are consumed. Milling of wheat and maize separates inner starchy endosperm from the bran covering and the germ and the endosperm becomes flour. This process results in the loss of several micronutrients present in the aleurone layer between the endosperm and the bran. The extraction rate is the flour yield or percent of flour that the miller extracts from the whole wheat and is related to the micronutrient content of the flour. Wheat contains approximately 82% endosperm, which would be the theoretical maximum extraction rate. Since mills are not totally efficient, the actual extraction rate is often lower, usually in the 72 to 76% range. As the extraction rate decreases, micronutrient levels increase. The final content of iron and zinc in flour is about a third of what was contained in the wheat, and phytic acid, which impairs the absorption of micronutrients like iron, is also partially lost in the milling process.

While the Green Revolution has greatly increased cereal production, providing billions of people with adequate energy and protein intakes, diets high in milled cereals have low micronutrient contents compared to their former diets. This problem can be readily dealt with by enrichment or fortification. The terms "fortification" or "enrichment" are often used interchangeably. It is important to recognize that enrichment means restoring nutrients lost in the milling process and fortification is the addition of micronutrients in amounts sufficient to combat demonstrated population wide micronutrient deficiencies. Bread and other flour products are attractive vehicles that can effectively carry micronutrients to deficient populations. In many settings, bread is consumed daily by all age groups and socioeconomic strata in relatively standard amounts and often with meals. Infants are exceptions and should be protected with other vehicles such as milk and weaning cereals.

From the point of view of achieving goals for the elimination of micronutrient malnutrition, the distinction between enrichment and fortification might arouse political reticence. It is often easier in many countries to establish an enrichment program rather than a true fortification program. The argument of adding back what was lost during processing is easier for some people to accept than explaining how a traditional food like bread can become a public health opportunity to end micronutrient malnutrition. One of the major concerns expressed by millers regarding the addition of micronutrients is whether the addition will affect or change the flour and products baked with the flour. These fears are unfounded. Based on many years of test baking field experience, we can say that the addition of iron, calcium, and vitamins to flour and bread, when done properly, does not alter the taste, color, appearance, or general baking properties. Fortification of wheat flour is truly invisible to the consumer.

9.2.2 FORTIFICANTS AND PROCESS TECHNOLOGY

Of all the nutrients added to food products, iron is the most needed and the cheapest. While there are many different types of iron are available, only two are used in wheat flour: ferrous sulfate and reduced or elemental iron. Ferrous sulfate ($FeSO_4$) is recommended because of its good bioavailability. Bakery flour made with an extraction rate above 72% and stored no longer than a few months, and semolina for use in pasta production, can be fortified with $FeSO_4$, depending on factors like humidity. All other types of wheat flour can be fortified with reduced iron. More recently, forms such as ferrous fumarate, amino chelate-iron, and iron-EDTA have been used for other cereals and food products such as soy sauce (see Section 9.3). The main issues related to the process technology of flour are summarized in this section.

Flour mills are continuous operations, while bakeries are batch operations. This means that the micronutrients, in the form of a single premix, must be continuously metered into the flour stream as it moves through the mill. The premix must contain the correct levels of nutrients to be uniform and free flowing. Many premix companies provide excellent quality products throughout the world which makes the premix readily available and cost competitive.

The premix is usually added to flour at the mill through a machine called a feeder or dosifier. Such machines have existed for half a century. The older ones use revolving disks or drums to deliver a constant rate of premix, whereas the new ones use screws run by adjustable speed motors. While the older units work well by manual adjustment, the newer equipment records continuous loss of weight in a feeder and transfers that data electronically to a device measuring the rate of flow of flour for continuous on-line adjustment.

Two basic methods are used for delivering the premix from the dosifier to the flour. One is to gravity feed the premix directly into a flour conveyor. The conveyor may collect and blend different flour streams or it may be dedicated to adding micro ingredients. An alternative is a pneumatic system, which involves blowing the premix from the dosifier to a pipe or conveyor carrying flour. Pneumatic systems have higher capital and upkeep costs than gravimetric systems

The cost of a basic dosifier is $2000 to $4000 (U.S.), but even this small capital cost which may be a constraint to mills wishing to fortify flour can be removed by having premix manufacturers assist in providing feeders to qualifying flour mills. More recently, additional assistance in the design, engineering, and installation of the dosifier and related equipment is available through the Micronutrient Initiative or other groups promoting micronutrient fortification of food staples. Many flour mills in the Americas and parts of Europe are accustomed to adding micro ingredients such as enzymes (malted barley flour or fungal alpha-amylase), bleaching agents, and oxidative dough improvers (ascorbic acid, potassium bromate, and azodicarbonamide) to flour. Many mills in Latin America, the Middle East, and the Far East are already set up for adding micro ingredients, including vitamins and iron, even if they are not currently fortifying flour.

9.2.3   QUALITY CONTROL AND STANDARDS

Iron standards vary greatly. For example, while restoration levels are in the 30 to 40 ppm range, the U.K. and Venezuela have lower standards. In contrast, the Institute of Nutrition for Central America and Panama (INCAP) recommends higher levels, which hopefully will be adopted throughout Central America. An enrichment standard is the level required in the final product. The actual amount of nutrient added is generally lower, because the natural content of the nutrient in flour is included to bring the total up to the standard. Current flour enrichment standards in the U.S. and Canada include five required nutrients. A folic acid standard was added recently to help reduce the incidence of neural tube birth defects. Calcium is optional in the U.S. and Canada has additional optional nutrients.

It is important to recognize that having enrichment standards does not mean that enrichment is mandatory and that standards are followed. Enrichment is not required in the U.S., but 33 states have laws requiring that only enriched cereal products can be sold. Similarly, Russia may also choose to require enrichment at a regional or city level rather than for the whole country.

Flour mills and regulatory agencies use a variety of methods for ensuring and ascertaining whether flour is properly fortified. One of the most critical aspects of fortification is to properly adjust the dosifier to deliver the proper level of premix based on the flow of flour. This assumes that the flour flow is both constant and known which is not always the case. Although analytical tests are available to test the levels of vitamins and minerals, most flour mills often use simple spot tests to assess whether the flour has been enriched and to make sure it is not grossly under or over treated. Mills may then do occasional quantitative tests, as may government agencies regulating the program.

9.2.4   COSTS

The actual cost of cereal fortification is very low, but the contribution it makes to the diet and the resultant health benefits are very large. For example, the cost of flour fortification increases the price of a 50 kg bag that normally costs anywhere from $10 to $20 by only a few cents. The increase is included in the price the baker pays for the flour, and is only 10 cents per person per year in Venezuela. This cost represents a fraction of the normal fluctuation in the price of flour caused by normal variations in the price of wheat.

Bakers and millers may quite naturally object to the burden placed on their industry by the increase in the price of flour. Consequently, during the initial stages, governments may identify ways to intervene in order to distribute the price increase over several years. This makes a small increase truly invisible. It is not a good idea for the government to totally absorb the cost because once the government stops the subsidies, fortification may stop. Cereal fortification must be sustainable which can only occur if the consumer eventually absorbs the cost. While a bag of flour may show a small price increase, a loaf of bread will not since the increase is too small to show up in the local monetary units. For example, if a mill charged ten cents more for a 50 kg bag of fortified flour, a 500 g loaf of bread made from that flour would contain 350 g of fortified flour, costing the baker 0.007 cents per loaf.

In summary, fortification of wheat flour, bread, and milled maize is a proven, cost effective way to deliver more iron and other micronutrients to the people who need them. Many countries have been doing this for half a century. The technology is available and can be applied to many developing countries where the need for more micronutrients in the diet is great. For more details, a comprehensive review of wheat fortification published by Ranum[8] is recommended.

9.2.5 BIOAVAILABILITY STUDIES

The first step in choosing the appropriate fortificant is to conduct bioavailability studies, which can be done both *in vitro* and *in vivo*. *In vitro* studies measure the extent of ionization (or solubility) of the fortificants when subjected to conditions that simulate the gastrointestinal environment during digestion and the results represent the extent of the fortificants' participation in the common pool of nonheme iron in the diet. Although these estimates of bioavailability do not provide actual amounts, they are useful to rank different combinations of vehicles and fortificants, which in turn permits the selection of the best combinations for *in vivo* studies, thus saving time and money.

In vivo bioavailability is usually estimated by using radioactive absorption measurements. Iron bioavailability from an iron chemical form in the amount estimated to provide 30 mg of elemental iron per kg of flour prepared as bread, and from a reference dose of ferrous ascorbate, can be established using a double isotopic method with radioactive iron isotopes. The label $^{59}Fe\ Cl_3$ is used as the tracer in the reference dose of ferrous ascorbate and another tracer such as $^{55}Fe\ Cl_3$ is used to evaluate the absorption of the iron form selected. The theory behind this methodology is that all the forms of soluble iron form a common pool in the gut and that a small amount of radioactive tracer will behave identically with this pool: the information of the absorption of the tracer will express the total absorption of iron. On day 15 after each isotope is given, venous blood samples are obtained to determine the radioactivity incorporated into erythrocytes. This allows for a precise estimate of the iron absorbed and the influence of the form of iron utilized, the vehicle, and the promoters or inhibitors of absorption. After the best combinations and proportions are established, the next step is testing under field conditions.

9.2.6 THE FIELD TRIAL

Field trials are required to ascertain the biological efficacy of the fortified product in solving the problem before fortification can be expanded and adopted to a large scale. The first step in determining the acceptability of the fortified product is to carry out studies in which the organoleptic qualities of the food products are tested by a panel of judges under controlled conditions. This can then be followed by a pilot field study that evaluates the acceptability and biological efficacy, and usually requires a few hundred individuals. The actual number of subjects will depend on the expected changes in hematological measurements in order to obtain statistically valid conclusions. During the second stage, the field trial needs to be planned to test the product's attributes, using the health infrastructure and the food delivery systems that normally operate for consumption of the foods to be fortified. This is a crucial step to determine program effectiveness and sustainability, since fortification of food products is intended as a long term approach. Once the effectiveness of the planned fortification has been tested under pilot and expanded field situations, provisions should be made to permit the long term evaluation of the program. Regions can be left unfortified or alternatively evaluated prospectively at periodic intervals.

Field studies may fail to demonstrate the beneficial effect of fortification for a variety of reasons. The fortification level may be too low, the bioavailability of fortification iron may be insufficient because of unforeseen inhibitory effects of the usual diet, consumer acceptance is poor, or errors may have occurred in the laboratory assessment of the iron status of the population. Often, the duration of the trial may be too short to assure a statistically significant effect, particularly in the case of populations with low or moderate prevalence of iron deficiency. The study may have been designed in a suboptimal fashion and prevents adequate statistical evaluation. Fortunately, the ability to detect small changes in iron nutrition in the population has been greatly improved in recent years by better employment of a battery of iron status measurements,[9] such as transferrin saturation, red cell protoporphyrin, and serum ferritin[10] and more recently, the serum transferrin receptor.[11,12] (see Chapter 3 for details.) These laboratory investigations must be carefully performed and adequately standardized to ensure reliable results. Investigation of other factors that may influence the reliability of results must be implemented, such as measurement of quantities of fortified products consumed (by dietary surveys) or by other means, such as the measurement of stool iron (a cumbersome but useful method in infants).[13] Morbidity, particularly for gastrointestinal disorders, is important when they are common in the target community, since it may influence iron absorption or increase iron losses, or may be inadvertently related to the fortified food. It is also possible that the community may wrongly attribute any symptom (diarrhea or constipation) to the introduction of the fortified food, thus limiting its acceptability. The anemia under investigation could be due to causes other than iron deficiency. It is important to identify the other causes such as parasitic infections (malaria and helminth infections), other nutrient deficiencies (folate, vitamin B_{12}) or non-nutritional causes such as hemoglobinopathy.

Field trials are expensive and require several years to design, conduct, and analyze. In countries where the costs of preliminary field trials are prohibitive or where the high prevalence of iron deficiency anemia dictates immediate action, it would seem reasonable to forego a field trial and proceed directly to a national fortification program. In this case, the efficacy of fortification must be assessed by monitoring iron status in the population, before and at periodic intervals after implementation of the program. The change of iron status may take several months or years to be detected. Many factors may contribute to changes in iron status in a given country so that evaluation of a nutritional intervention in the absence of data on predictable effects (such as would be available from a field trial and the studies leading to it) or an adequate baseline evaluation may hamper the effort to gauge the effect of the policy.

9.3 FIELD TRIALS OF FORTIFIED FOOD: THE CHILEAN EXPERIENCE

9.3.1 BREAST FEEDING AND USE OF WEANING CEREALS

9.3.1.1 Rationale

The duration and adequacy of breast feeding depends on a number of physiologic, nutritional, social, and cultural factors. The industrial revolution, urbanization, and the availability of alternate sources of infant milk have been implicated as causes for the decline in breast feeding all over the world. The proportion of Chilean children from the urban low class exclusively breast fed at 3 months of age remained similar in various studies performed between 1942 and 1977. The incidence ranges from 27 to 52%, with most figures lying between 30 and 42%.[14,15] In the last ten years, the tendency has reverted and over 60% of mothers breast feed exclusively up to 6 months and continue breast feeding up to a year (supplemented with solids and cow's milk) in 20 to 30% of those studied. This has been attributed to an intensive media campaign that firmly and permanently changed the breast feeding culture in Chile.

When breast milk becomes insufficient to sustain normal growth, the common practice is to introduce cow's milk supplements in a bottle, resulting in the rapid termination of breast feeding. In areas where prolonged breast feeding is prevalent, weaning cereals represent a good means of providing the necessary supplementary calories and iron starting at about 4 to 6 months of age. Cereals, fed with a spoon as a gruel, do not compete with sucking from the breast, thus contributing to the maintenance of successful lactation. It has become well recognized that around 4 to 6 months of age, caloric supplements must also be introduced in breast fed infants as spoon fed solids in such a way not to interfere with breast feeding.[16-18] Ideally, these solids should have high caloric density and adequate protein quality. Additionally, they should provide the iron needed by breast fed infants after about 4 to 6 months of age because the iron in breast milk is well absorbed but it will not confer adequate protection from iron deficit after that age[16,19] Supplementation is critical for preterm infants.[20,21]

9.3.1.2   Infant Cereal Fortified with Heme Iron

Our laboratory designed an extruded rice flour cereal fortified with 5% bovine hemoglobin concentrate that was prepared in an attempt to fulfill these requirements. This cereal provides a suitable gruel preparation at 20% dilution and also has improved protein quality. It provides 14 mg of hemoglobin iron per 100 g with an estimated 2.1 mg of bioavailable iron. It is designed to be started at 4 months of age and to be increased gradually to 40 g/d by 6 months of age, thereby providing 140 kcal and 0.84 mg of bioavailable iron.[22-24] The design and results of the field trial that examined the influence of this cereal on the duration and adequacy of breast feeding and on the iron nutriture of infants attending a NHS clinic in Santiago are described in this section.

Term infants (N = 255) who were breast fed at 3 months of age were admitted to the study. One group of 123 randomly assigned infants received 1.5 kg of the cereal per month beginning at 4 months of age. The other group received the routine recommendations of the NHS, i.e., introduction of fruits at 3 months of age; vegetable-meat soup at 4 months; eggs, cereals, and legumes at 6 to 7 months; and regular table food at 9 to 12 months. The follow-up at 12 months of age was completed for 88 infants in the fortified group and 108 infants in the control group. The duration of exclusive breast feeding was similar in both groups. At 6 months of age, 92% of all infants in the cereal group and 94% of those in the control group were still consuming breast milk as the only source of milk, and these figures were 73% and 69%, respectively, at 9 months of age. These figures were obtained during an active program of supplementary food distribution in which mothers received cow's milk to take home, indicating that the free cow's milk is not necessarily detrimental when accompanied by the promotion of and education about breast feeding.

At 12 months of age, there was a significant improvement of iron status in the supplemented group, and the prevalence of anemia was 8% and 19% among fortified and unfortified infants, respectively. These results show that under the conditions of a controlled field trial, a fortified infant weaning cereal can significantly decrease iron deficiency in breast fed infants without affecting duration of lactation. A major impact on prolonging breast feeding was accomplished by an active program of education and promotion of this practice by health personnel. It should be noted that the prevalence of anemia in this study was higher compared to only 1.6% in the fortified group in a previous trial using fortified milk. This may be explained by the fact that the fortified milk was introduced earlier (at 3 month of age) and was consumed in constant measurable amounts compared to cereal. The growth of the infants in both groups was similar.

9.3.1.3   Rice Cereal Fortified with Reduced Iron

According to the schema presented in Figure 9.1, we designed a field trial which included 5 groups of infants: two who were exclusively breast fed and three who were weaned early, and compared (1) an iron-fortified rice cereal to (2) unfortified

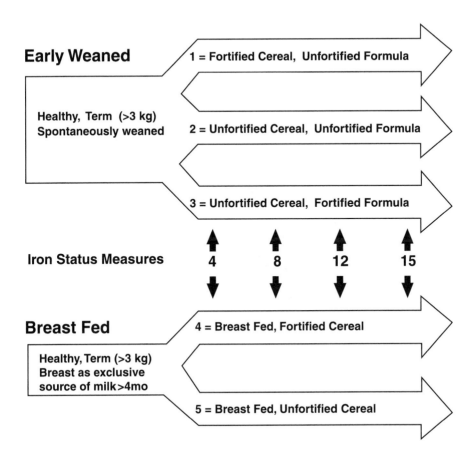

FIGURE 9.1 Study design of field trial of rice cereal fortified with reduced iron. (Walter, T., Dallman, P. R., Pizarro, F., et al., Effectiveness of iron-fortified infant cereal in prevention of iron deficiency anemia, *Pediatrics,* 91:976-982, 1993. With permission.)

rice cereal in those infants who were exclusively breast fed for more than 4 months; among infants who were weaned to formula before 4 months of age we compared; (3) iron-fortified formula (compared to unfortified cereal) versus two groups of infants with non fortified milk and either (4) with fortified cereal or (5) unfortified cereal. The design was double blind with respect to the presence or absence of fortification iron in the cereal or formula and included 515 infants who were followed on the protocol from 4 to 15 months of age. Rice cereal was fortified with 55 mg of reduced iron per 100 g of dry cereal and infant formula with 9 mg of ferrous sulfate per 100 g of dry powder, levels approximating those in use in the U.S. Measures of iron status were obtained at 8, 12, and 15 months. Infants with hemoglobin levels of <105 g/L at any point were excluded from the study and treated.[25]

Consumption of cereal reached plateaus at means of about 30 g/day after 6 months of age in the formula fed groups and 26 g/day after 8 months in the breast fed groups; these amounts are higher than the 19 g/d mean intake by the 73% of infants who consume such cereal in the U.S.[26] As shown in Figure 9.2, among the infants weaned

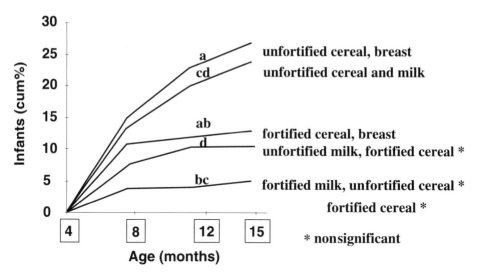

FIGURE 9.2 Prevalence of anemia by age among infants who received iron fortified and unfortified cereal. (Walter, T., Dallman, P. R., Pizarro, F., et al., Effectiveness of iron-fortified infant cereal in prevention of iron deficiency anemia, *Pediatrics*, 91:976-982, 1993. With permission.)

to formula before 4 months, the cumulative percentages of infants excluded for anemia by 15 months were 8%, 24%, and 4%, in the fortified cereal, unfortified cereal, and formula groups respectively (P <0.01 unfortified versus either fortified group; the difference between the two fortified groups was not significant). In infants breast fed for more than 4 months, the corresponding values were 13% and 27%, respectively, in the fortified and unfortified cereal groups (P <0.05). Mean hemoglobin level and other iron status measures were in accord with these findings. The prevalence of iron deficiency anemia at 8 months (Hb <105 g/l) is depicted in Figure 9.3.

This trial proves that iron-fortified infant rice cereal can contribute substantially to preventing iron deficiency anemia, provided it is consumed in the quantities described, i.e., above 25 g/day in the population of infants with very low alternative sources of iron. This group of infants obtain only about 5 mg/day of iron in the diet mostly from poorly bioavailable vegetable sources. In populations where other foods such as fortified milk, or larger intakes of meat are consumed, lower quantities of fortified cereal may foster the prevention of iron deficiency.

9.3.2 SCHOOL AGE CHILDREN: COOKIES FORTIFIED WITH BOVINE HEMOGLOBIN

9.3.2.1 Background

The government of Chile sponsors two programs that address the nutritional needs of school children, the Nursery School Feeding program and the School Breakfast/Lunch program. These national programs reach a significant proportion of the nutritionally vulnerable population, and have enjoyed long standing support. On any given day,

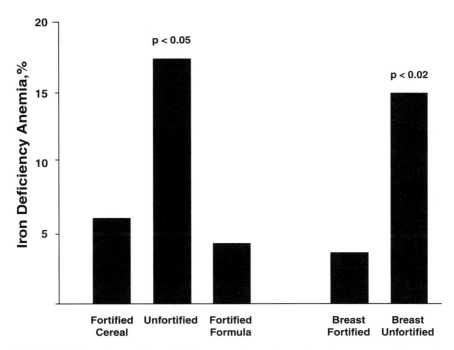

FIGURE 9.3 Prevalence of iron deficiency anemia at 8 months of age among infants who received iron-fortified and unfortified cereal. (Walter, T., Dallman, P. R., Pizarro, F., et al., Effectiveness of iron-fortified infant cereal in prevention of iron deficiency anemia, *Pediatrics,* 91:976-982, 1993. With permission.)

90% of the eligible school children participate. For many years, three or four cookies (10 g each) have been given with milk or milk substitutes to participating children. Since cookies represented a daily component of the children's diet, they seemed ideal food vehicles to fortify with iron. Previous studies proved ferrous sulfate and other inorganic iron substances were unsatisfactory in cookies because of undesirable color or taste at levels of fortification used. Until the investigations by Instituto de Nutricion y Technologia de los Alimentos (INTA), there had been little experience using hemoglobin iron as a fortificant in cookies.

The first step was to determine the absorption, stability, efficacy, and acceptability of hemoglobin iron as a fortificant. The amount of iron in foods and its bioavailability vary considerably. Studies have demonstrated that iron enters into two common pools, the so-called heme iron and the nonheme iron pool, and these pools have different absorption mechanisms. Heme iron, present in animal tissue, is well absorbed and its absorption is relatively unaffected by diet composition.[27] Unlike inorganic iron, heme iron is soluble in an alkaline medium, which makes the intestinal pH more favorable for its absorption, and it does not appear to be greatly affected by cooking.

Because the diets of Chilean children often consist chiefly of cereals and vegetables, it was considered that adding nonheme iron to their diets would not be beneficial, especially when limited to the amounts that could be satisfactorily incorporated into cookies. In contrast, it was hypothesized that an equivalent amount of hemoglobin iron would be more effective, based primarily on the characteristics of hemoglobin iron, and the relative poor absorption of nonheme iron fortificants.

Hemoglobin from animal blood is a relatively abundant source of iron and can be obtained through simple, low cost technology. In addition to the isolation of hemoglobin from blood, the process permits the isolation of other blood proteins, which can be used as protein supplements to the animal food. The key concern is to collect and process the blood in a sterile environment. Once dried, collected blood material is relatively safe for use.

In 1977, we initiated investigations oriented to the possible use of hemoglobin in food fortification in Chile.[28,29] Initially, the studies were focused on the fortification of milk. Three heme iron concentrates were obtained from bovine red cells: hemoglobin with stroma, hemoglobin without stroma, and hemin were tested separately. When added to milk in a concentration of 15 mg elemental iron per liter, there was no change in flavor and the color of the fortified milk was that of café-au-lait. Radioisotope absorption studies with intrinsic labeled hemoglobin preparation obtained from an Fe-labeled calf were conducted on 70 infants 6 to 18 months of age. Absorption of each of the three heme iron concentrates was similar, with a geometric mean of 18.8%. Absorption of hemin was significantly higher in milk than in water, indicating that milk probably protected hemin from forming insoluble macromolecular aggregates. Hemoglobin added to milk produced rapid rancidity of the product due to the oxidation of fat in the powdered milk. Hemoglobin fortification of milk was thus judged impractical. The lower fat content of cookies prompted studies of their use in heme fortification.

9.3.2.2 National Program

The National School Breakfast/Lunch program decided to introduce the bovine hemoglobin concentrate (BHC) fortified cookies. Officials in charge of the program concluded, on the basis of the initial absorption studies, that sufficient scientific justification for using the cookie in the school program existed. These studies demonstrated that the cookies would supply the required absorbable iron. Moreover, the protein quality of the fortified cookies was a marked improvement over the unfortified cookies. Several steps were necessary to develop a national program:

1. Definition and requisites of BHC for human consumption
2. Development of large scale production of BHC
3. Transfer of technology from small scale production at the university to large scale industrial production
4. Modification of contacts between governmental authorities and concessionaires in order to replace unfortified with fortified cookies and provide payment for additional cost involved

A set of norms was prepared on the basis of the studies performed at INTA. Entitled "Blood for Human Consumption — Dehydrated Concentrate of Corpuscular Fraction," the norms defined BHC as a "fine powder of dark-red color obtained by centrifugation and further dehydration of the corpuscular fraction of blood of slaughtered animals." It specified the requirements for quality of the raw materials, organoleptic characteristics, chemical and physiochemical characteristics, microbiological requisites, packaging, storing, and refrigeration.

Although there is an established market for bovine plasma, a product that is used in the meat industry, no market for red blood cells existed. The possibility of drying the red cells to produce BHC for the cookies fortification program made the project economically feasible.[22] The main technical problem was expanding the drying conditions used in the laboratory to an industrial level, and maintaining a suitable product that would comply with standards established by the norms. This was accomplished by close collaboration between INTA investigators and representatives of the new industry. In practice, most of the blood needed for the national program is obtained from the main slaughterhouse in Santiago. Processing entails initial collection of the blood in stainless steel containers, transfer of the product to fiberglass tanks, transport of the blood filled tanks at ambient temperature to the drying plant, separation of plasma from the red blood cells, and drying the red blood cells in a spray dryer at an entrance temperature of 160°C and exit temperature of 85°C. All the blood is processed and dried within 4 hours of collection.

Fortified cookies must conform to rigidly established norms. In addition to quality control procedures instituted by each manufacturer, random samples of fortified cookies from all the manufacturers were analyzed by INTA each month. Samples were subjected to microbiological analyses, physicochemical analyses (proximate analysis), and sensory evaluations.

To measure the impact on iron nutriture of the national programs, the province of Linares was left unfortified. The Chilean school lunch program, which serves one million children nationwide, provided three 10 g cookies fortified with 6% BHC, designed to provide 1 mg bioavailable iron per day. A survey of 1000 children was performed after 3 years, comparing the province of Linares (non fortified) with a contiguous province of similar socioeconomic characteristics. Significant differences in hemoglobin concentrations (Figure 9.4) were found in the children from the fortified versus the nonfortified children ($P < 0.01$). Low serum ferritin values were more prevalent in the nonfortified group ($P < 0.05$). These differences were seen despite the very low prevalence of anemia in this population. Of particular relevance was the improved iron status of menstruating girls, presumably to prepare them for the higher requirements of menstruation and eventually pregnancy (Figure 9.5). In summary, heme iron-fortified cookies represent a feasible and effective way to improve the iron status of school age children. In regions of high prevalence of iron deficiency anemia, the effect of a heme fortified cookie program should be even more important.[30] Obviously, the cultural acceptability of this product in some settings (e.g., South Asia) needs to be considered.

9.3.3 WHEAT FLOUR FORTIFICATION

In 1951, the Institute of Agriculture and Economy proposed the enrichment of wheat flour with vitamin B complex with the purpose of "improving nutrition status of the Chilean population through the enrichment of bread with vitamins and minerals."[31]

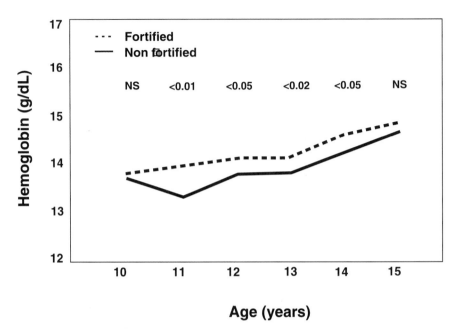

Age (years)

FIGURE 9.4 Comparison of mean hemoglobin levels among school age children receiving BHC fortified and unfortified cookies in the National School Breakfast/Lunch program in Chile. (Walter, T., Hertrampf, E., Pizarro, F., et al., Effect of bovine-hemoglobin-fortified cookies on iron status of schoolchildren: A nationwide program in Chile. © *Am. J. Clinical Nutr.*, 57: 190-194, 1993. American Society for Clinical Nutrition. With permission.)

This early effort was promoted by physicians who sought improvement of B complex nutritional status in alcoholic population groups. The only available source of these vitamins at the time was a premix of niacin, riboflavin, and thiamin plus iron and calcium. The recommendation was to add 6 mg of iron per 460 g of flour with no specification of the iron compound. The commercially available premix contained reduced iron. This initiative was enacted in 1951, establishing the addition of the premix to wheat flour processed in the mills. It is noteworthy that the addition of iron to the flour was not designed as part of a program to prevent iron deficiency. The Ministry of Health assumed evaluation of the quality control of adding this premix to wheat flour.

Data from the monitoring system from that time is not available. It is likely that the contribution of this early effort toward the dietary intake of absorbable iron was nearly nonexistent for the following reasons: (1) the amount of iron added was very low (12 mg/kg), corresponding neither to restoration nor enrichment levels; (2) the particles of the iron compound employed were much larger than the optimal size, so that they were caught on the screw conveyor during the milling process; and, (3) bioavailability of the small fraction ingested must have been very low due to the large size of the iron particles and the presence of calcium. On the other hand, this early attempt prompted the milling industry to introduce the equipment required for adding the premix. In 1967, the law was modified so that (1) the amount of iron in

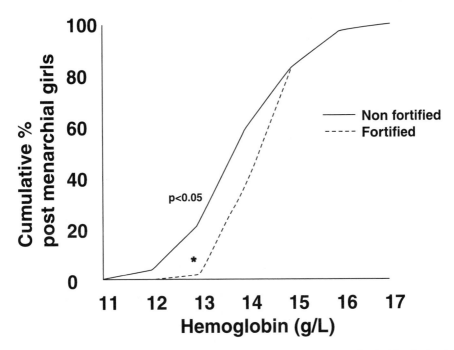

FIGURE 9.5 Comparison of mean hemoglobin levels among post-menarcheal girls of school age child receiving iron fortified and unfortified cookies in the National School Breakfast/Lunch program in Chile. (Walter, T., Hertrampf, E., Pizarro, F., et al., Effect of bovine-hemoglobin-fortified cookies on iron status of schoolchildren: A nationwide program in Chile. © *Am. J. Clinical Nutr.*, 57: 190-194, 1993. American Society for Clinical Nutrition. With permission.)

the premix added to the wheat flour was increased to 30 mg/kg (restoration level), (2) it became mandatory that the iron compounds used should be ferrous sulfate or pyrophosphate, and (3) calcium was removed from the premix.

The quality control of the fortification was commissioned to the Bromatology Laboratories of the National Institute of Public Health. Monitoring of the final product is done at the mills by obtaining random wheat samples and running quantitative tests on a regular basis. The Ministry of Health uses the information confidentially.

9.3.3.1 Wheat Flour Production and Consumption

Processed wheat in Chile is transformed into wheat flour with the extraction rate determined by law (75 to 80%). About 10% of mill production is used for pasta and other bakery products. There are 112 mills in Chile, located mainly in the central and southern regions. The largest 18 mills, which represent 40% of the country's milling capacity, are concentrated in the Santiago Metropolitan Area (around 5 million inhabitants). The total annual milling volume has been quite stable during the past two decades, hovering around 1,500,000 metric tons.[32] Wheat flour is used mainly for bread making and the turn around time is less than 60 days from the mill to the shelf.

9.3.3.2 Monitoring the Fortification Process

The addition of iron to flour during the milling process is monitored on a regular basis throughout the country by the Institute of Public Health (ISP). According to the sanitary food legislation, the iron fortificant used should be ferrous sulfate. The fortificant is purchased by the mills as a premix from two main providers: an international (Roche) and a national laboratory (Granotec S.A). According to government records, ferrous sulfate has been the compound sold since the late 1960s.[33] The amount of premix sold is quite stable, corresponding to what is needed for the milling process. Chemical determinations from the collected samples suggest that the legislation has been adequately implemented.[34]

9.3.3.3 Impact of Flour Fortification on the Prevalence of IDA

Two key questions that need to be answered to demonstrate that fortification has had an impact on iron status are (1) was there a decrease in the prevalence of IDA? (2) if the answer is yes, was the decrease due to the fortification of flour with iron? Answering the second question requires examining whether the fortification led to a significant increase of bioavailable iron in the same population groups which can be accomplished by analyzing bread consumption, iron content in bread, and its bioavailability. It is also important to examine whether the improvement in IDA could be explained by other factors such as decreased iron losses over the same period; increased iron intake produced by other programs, such as food fortification (other than bread), iron supplementation, or control of vitamin A deficiency; or improved intake of foods rich in iron.

9.3.3.3.1 Decrease in Prevalence of IDA

The decrease in prevalence usually requires measuring IDA before and after the implementation of the fortification policy. Reliable, representative data is available only in 1974, seven years after the improvement of flour fortification with iron and from 1975 to 1997 from isolated surveys, which are not necessarily representative of the whole population.[35-46] Anemia has gradually disappeared after 1974 in school children, decreasing from an already low figure of 7% in 1974 to less than 1% in 1987.[30] A similar process was observed in adolescents going from a low figure of 5% in 1974 to 1% in 1997. Pregnant, adolescent women with less than 22 weeks of gestation from a low income group showed only 1% of anemia, apparently because they were accumulating adequate reserves for their first pregnancy.[47] In adult, non-pregnant women, the prevalence of anemia was 7%, compared to 27% in Buenos Aires, Argentina,[48] where wheat flour is also highly consumed but is not iron fortified. In a sample of people, older than 65 y and living on their own, the prevalence of IDA was 1% in 1982. Incomplete as these data may be, they show that the prevalence of IDA in Chile was already low in 1974 and continued to decrease to present day. Still, there are two population groups with relatively high levels of anemia: infants 6 to 24 months, with a consistent range of prevalence of 28 to 31% of IDA and adult pregnant women with 8% of anemia in the first trimester and 20% at the third trimester.

9.3.3.3.2   Contribution of Fortification

Bread consumption: The mean intake of bread in Chile has varied little, between 247 and 318 g per capita per day during the last 20 years (INE/Central Bank). Bread is the main single source of energy for the population. Consumption is greater in school children and adolescents in whom the daily mean intake is 300 g and 400 g, respectively.[48] Iron content in french type bread, which represents 70% of the bread consumed in Chile, was measured in our lab during 1987. A total of 301 bakeries from Santiago and suburban areas were randomly sampled at the counter level. Iron content of bread was normally distributed with a mean of 2.4 mg/100g (SD 0.7). This figure is close to the expected value of 2.9 mg, derived from the native iron (approximately 1 mg/100 g of wheat flour) plus the fortification amount in 71g of flour needed to prepare 100 g of bread, using a mean of 27 mg of iron per kg of flour.

Bioavailability of iron in bread: Radioiron ^{55}Fe and ^{59}Fe absorption measurements were performed in healthy, non pregnant, volunteer women to assess the bioavailability of iron in french type bread. Iron absorption when bread was given alone was 10.5%, decreasing to 7.5% and 6.4% when it was consumed with milk or tea, respectively. Values were normalized to 40% absorption of the reference dose.[49] These results confirm prior work[50-51] indicating similar bioavailability of ferrous sulfate when it is used to fortify bread.

In conclusion, the consumption of bread, the content of iron in bread, and its bioavailability indicate that the iron added to flour is making an important contribution (about 75% of requirements, or approximately 1 mg per day) to the school children, adults, adolescents, and the elderly. No indication of iron overload has been found in the elderly.[52-54] However, no improvement in iron status has been achieved in 6- to 24-month old infants or in pregnant multiparous women during the third trimester of pregnancy.

9.3.3.3.3   Role of Other Factors

Decreased iron losses over the same period: The prevalence of intestinal worm infections such as *Ancylostoma duodenate* and *Necator americanus* is virtually non-existent in Chile because of the geography and weather conditions. The improvement in the coverage of running water and sanitation may have contributed in the decreased prevalence of other types of intestinal parasites and infectious diarrhea. Malaria was eradicated 50 years ago, and 6- to 24-month old infants have not shown intestinal parasitism except for endemic Giardiasis that is rarely massive enough to impair iron absorption. Thus, IDA seems to be caused by low iron intake of poor bioavailability.[55,56] Although improved access to water and sanitation could have contributed to the decrease in IDA, it cannot explain the impressively low prevalence of IDA in school children, adolescents, adults, and the elderly. In addition, it does not explain the high prevalence of IDA observed in the 6- to 24-month old group or in multiparous, pregnant women. Stekel and coworkers began research to find ways to decrease the high prevalence of iron deficiency anemia in children less than 24 months of age, and several options including iron fortification of milk[14-15,36-39,57-65] and of infant cereal were developed.[23] Nevertheless, until 1999, no program has been implemented as yet at the national level, for infants under 24 months and preschool children.

Iron supplementation: Iron supplements have been delivered free of cost to infants less than 1 year of age and to pregnant women during their prenatal visits, as part of routine maternal and child health care. Although there is no formal evaluation of compliance, the general impression among health personnel is that it is rather poor. In any case, these are the two groups in whom IDA prevalence has not decreased in the last 20 years. These actions cannot explain the decrease observed in IDA in the rest of the population.

Improved intake of foods rich in iron: Recent information suggests that an increase in the dietary intake of iron rich foods during the last four years may be occurring due to increased access to food brought on by a stronger economy. This fact would not explain the already low prevalence in IDA observed before 1992.

In summary, none of the proposed factors discussed could convincingly explain the decrease in IDA due to a significant increase of bioavailable iron intake (other than wheat flour) in the population consuming bread and not in infants, who do not eat bread. In conclusion, the results of this analysis indicate that: (1) there was a significant decrease in the prevalence of IDA, observed since 1974 and that has continued up to now; and, (2) it is highly probable that this effect was produced to a large extent by the fortification of flour with iron, particularly after 1967.

9.4 MEXICAN CORN-MASA TORTILLA CASE STUDY

9.4.1 INTRODUCTION

In the case of Mexico, the diet contains little iron, because the best source of iron, which is meat, is expensive and thus rarely consumed by the disadvantaged population. In addition, this population consumes large amounts of corn-masa flour bread "tortillas," from 300 to 500 g per person per day as their main staple food. The corn flour contains large amounts of inhibitors of iron absorption, so that the little iron they may consume cannot be absorbed and utilized. It is no surprise indeed that the prevalence of anemia is 20 to 40% in the general population, with even higher rates among infants and pregnant women. [66]

The best means to combat IDA is through dietary approaches. This requires changing dietary habits and/or improving food availability, which can be challenging and may take a long time to accomplish (see Chapter 10). Clearly, fortification of commonly consumed foods is a cost effective strategy in achieving the goal of improving the micronutrient status of populations. The obvious vehicle in this situation is corn flour which is consumed daily in large amounts (300 to 500 g/day) especially by the poor in Mexico and other Central American countries. Another advantage is that infants also receive a corn flour water mix as a weaning food called locally "atole," which provides an invaluable opportunity to reach this critical age group who are often left out of many fortification programs.

However, very little work has been done with corn flour. This product contains high concentrations of inhibitors of iron absorption that has challenged attempts to fortify this staple. Tortillas are typically consumed with legumes and vegetables which may further impair bioavailability. The first step is to identify the most suitable fortificant (chemical form of iron) that could be added to corn flour and would efficaciously improve iron status in the target population. Recent advances in the types of iron-fortificants and related bioavailability studies are discussed in this section. Specifically, the results of this experience may be useful for other countries that would like to fortify common staples and condiments with iron and other micronutrients.

The bioavailability of three forms of iron alone (ferrous fumarate, amino chelate iron, and iron EDTA) and a combination of at least two (ferrous fumarate and elemental iron with and without EDTA) in various proportions were considered. This was done in corn-masa tortillas. The best probable combinations were selected with laboratory tests of solubility *in vitro* that served to rank the best fortificant quantities and combinations. Once the best probable preparations were selected, radioiron bioavailability studies in human subjects were executed. The results of these studies also served to estimate the amount of iron that needs to be added to the corn flour to achieve an effective absorption of iron to cover a proportion of the daily iron requirements of a given population. A review of the literature on the different types of iron fortificants, followed by the results of bioavailability studies in corn-masa, and other recent efforts are presented in the following sections.

9.4.2 Iron Fortificants

9.4.2.1 Iron Salts

The fortificants ordinarily added to wheat flour are in the form of soluble iron salts such as ferrous sulfate or fumarate in Latin America and elemental iron in the northern hemisphere. It is unlikely that either can make a significant contribution to iron nutrition in the face of the large concentration of inhibitors in Mexican corn flour. The soluble iron salts, though theoretically bioavailable, may be unsuitable because they are pro-oxidant causing organoleptic changes that are unacceptable and shorten shelf life. Additionally, their solubility readily supports interaction with the inhibitors in the corn meal, thus bioavailability is low. Nevertheless, because of their low cost and the large body of experience in wheat flour, it is necessary to address the potential benefit of soluble iron salts as fortificants in Mexican flour.[67-69] Most of the iron bioavailability studies of corn flour have been performed on porridge showing absorption of an average of 3.7% in iron sufficient individuals and 3.8 to 6.8% in iron deficient subjects. Only one study addresses tortillas prepared with nixtamalized corn flour, in a meal with beans and rice characterized as a typical Mexican combination. Absorption was less than with maize alone at 2.6% (range 1.2 to 3.6%). Absorption increased when the meal was supplemented with ascorbic acid. This improvement in bioavailability with ascorbic acid comes as no surprise. The issue is the feasibility of the addition of this enhancer either in the manufacture or as a part of dietary modification. A recent field trial performed by Dr. Adolfo Chávez et al. using tortillas fortified with 40 mg of ferrous fumarate and 20 mg of elemental iron, showed lack of improvement in hematological measures after one year in a Mexican village.[67] This goes to show that the formulations used in Venezuela's "arepa" (bread), made also of corn flour, but manufactured with many fewer phytate inhibitors, cannot be applied to other products.

9.4.2.2   Influence of Vitamin A

Vitamin A has been shown to interact with iron absorption in a favorable way. Studies with iron deficient (and vitamin A deficient) populations in Indonesia show that the response to iron therapy is improved when given concomitantly with vitamin A.[70-74] A study in Venezuela demonstrated that the addition of fairly large doses of vitamin A to maize "arepa" bread fortified with iron (as ferrous fumarate) seems to overcome the inhibitory effect of coffee or tea and possibly also of phytates. Chemical studies suggest the formation of a chelate between vitamin A and the iron liberated during digestion that protects the iron from being trapped by inhibitors.[75,76] These findings indicated that vitamin A must be introduced as a factor in iron bioavailability studies in maize flour products.

9.4.2.3   Amino Chelates

The absorption of inorganic iron salts is strongly negatively influenced by compounds present in the diet such as phytates, polyphenols, and casein. Newer chemical forms using amino acid chelation of iron have overcome some major problems of soluble iron salts. Iron bis-glycine chelate (Ferrochel®) is formed by two glycine molecules bound to a ferrous cation, resulting in a double heterocyclic ring compound. The carboxyl group of glycine is linked with iron by an ionic bond, while the alpha-amino group is joined with the metal by a coordinate covalent bond.[77] This configuration presumably protects the iron from dietary inhibitors and prevents the prooxidant properties of iron. Studies performed[78,79] have shown that vitamin losses with storage of infants foods fortified with iron amino acid chelate were lower than when ferrous sulfate was the fortificant. However, recent studies have shown potent oxidant properties of iron bis-glycine chelate in a maize porridge that must be neutralized with the addition of antioxidants. The effectiveness of iron bis-glycine chelate in the treatment of iron deficiency anemia has been shown in humans.[80] Research from our laboratory has established that this compound is absorbed in water to a level comparable to ferrous ascorbate.[81] Iron amino acid chelate has been used as a fortificant of foods with a high content of inhibitors of inorganic iron absorption or a high fat content, such as milk, Petite Suisse® (a milk casein concentrate snack), and maize products.

Unmodified cow's milk has a marked inhibitory effect on the absorption of non-heme iron, due to its high content of inhibitors of iron absorption. When 10 to 15 mg/L of iron, as ferrous sulfate, is added to unmodified cow's milk, only 4 to 5% is absorbed. In our lab, we have shown a 2- to 2.5-fold higher iron absorption when iron bis-glycine replaces ferrous sulphate as the fortificant.[81,82] Iron absorption of this milk fortified alone with iron bis-glycine is comparable to that which we obtained in milk fortified with ferrous sulfate plus ascorbic acid.[83] Furthermore, bioavailability of iron bis-glycine in milk is further improved by adding ascorbic acid. However, iron amino acid chelate absorption is less favored by the action of this vitamin.

In Brazil,[84] Lost et al.[85] have shown in field trials the beneficial effect of a fluid cow's milk enriched with 3 mg/L of elemental iron, as iron bis-glycine, in reducing the prevalence of iron deficiency anemia among infants. Fisberg et al.[86] found in a field trial an improvement of iron status of preschool children who consumed daily 90 g of Petit Suisse containing 2 mg of elemental iron as iron bis-glycine chelate per serving. The absorption of maize porridge fortified with 1 mg of elemental iron as ferrous sulfate or iron bis-glycine chelate per 100 g was reported. The absorption of iron bis-glycine chelate was four times better than ferrous sulfate. Nevertheless, the percent absorption obtained was no higher than 6%.[87] A British study showed that iron amino acid chelation does not improve the iron bioavailability in the presence of dietary inhibitors. Iron absorption or iron bis-glycine chelate added to a vegetable-based infant food was absorbed as well as ferrous sulfate.[88] Furthermore, when the bioavailability of the two iron compounds added to a high whole grain cereal weaning food and lower phytate vegetable food was compared, iron bis-glycine chelate was inhibited by phytates to the same extent as ferrous sulfate.[88] It was postulated that the iron amino acid chelate could be absorbed like a peptide in the jejunum rather than as inorganic iron in the duodenum.[77,89] There was concern about the role of iron stores on the regulation of iron absorption from the chelate. Three independent investigators[82,87,88] showed that the absorption of iron amino acid chelate is regulated by iron stores. The alternative assumption for the mechanism of absorption is that at least part of the iron is released from the chelate in the gut and absorbed. This hypothesis is supported by the behavior of the iron in Ferrochel, being affected (inhibited or enhanced) by intraluminal contents, just as iron salts. Nonetheless, this remains to be proven. On the other hand, data from double isotope competing absorption studies show that it behaves apparently as if it were absorbed by a different route from that of ferrous sulphate. Further research is needed to elucidate the mechanism of intestinal absorption of iron amino acid chelates.

9.4.2.4   Iron EDTA

Another attractive chelate is iron-sodium ethylene di-amino-tetra-acetic acid (Na Fe EDTA) also called iron EDTA. It should be most efficacious when added to cereals due to the properties discussed below. Its safety has been supported by the approval given by the Joint FAO/WHO Expert Committee on Food Additives (JECFA). A comprehensive report on the properties of iron EDTA has been issued under the auspices of The International Nutritional Anemia Consultative Group.[90] Some of the relevant conclusions of this panel were:

1. When NaEDTA is added to food, some of the intrinsic food iron forms complexes with the EDTA to form NaFeEDTA in the stomach. When NaFeEDTA is added to food there is exchange between the iron moiety and other iron in the meal.
2. Iron bound to EDTA is released to physiological mechanisms at the intestinal cell surface with the amounts absorbed being controlled by the body's requirements. The EDTA then forms complexes with other metals in the intestinal lumen. Only a very small fraction (<1% of the iron administered as NaFeEDTA) is absorbed as the intact NaFeEDTA complex.

3. Up to 5% of the EDTA moiety in any meal is absorbed. This occurs regardless of the EDTA-metal complex administered and is an unregulated process. With NaFeEDTA, most of the EDTA is absorbed after exchange of the iron with other metals, such as zinc and copper. After absorption the EDTA-metal complex is completely eliminated unchanged in the urine within 24 to 48 hours.

4. Human absorption studies have shown that the iron in NaFeEDTA added to inhibitory meals is 2 to 3 times as well absorbed as iron added as ferrous sulphate. However, the absorption of iron NaFeEDTA is no better than that from ferrous sulphate when added to meals of high bioavailability that contain significant quantities of ascorbic acid or meat.

5. NaFeEDTA in the dose range proposed for food fortificants has no toxic side effects. When NaEDTA is present in food, NaFeEDTA is formed in the stomach. The widespread use of Na_2EDTA as additives by the food industry is not associated with any untoward effects.

As indicated above, iron and EDTA absorption from NaFeEDTA are independent processes. Sufficient information about the safety of both substances at proposed fortificant concentrations is already available to recommend the use of NaFeEDTA as a food fortificant. Further toxicological studies are not necessary. Concern has been expressed about the use of NaFeEDTA for prolonged periods of time because exchange of the metal moiety could theoretically lead to trace element depletion. Exchange of iron for zinc is probably the predominant reaction in the lumen of the small intestine. The effect of EDTA on zinc balance depends on the EDTA: zinc molar ratio in the diet. The use of NaFeEDTA in the fortification range proposed (10 mg iron, 67 mg EDTA/person per day) has no detrimental effect on zinc balance. Zinc absorption and zinc balance may actually be improved if the diet has a low zinc content or low zinc bioavailability. In summary, NaFeEDTA is an attractive option for delivering fortification iron because

- it is a light colored compound
- it can be added to several potential food vehicles without affecting the organoleptic properties of the vehicle
- it is a form of bioavailable fortification iron
- it promotes the absorption of the intrinsic food iron from low bioavailability meals, and
- its enhancing effect on iron absorption is not affected by storage conditions or food preparation

Three field trials have demonstrated that fortifying the diet with NaFeEDTA has a significant beneficial effect on iron status. The implementation of iron fortification with NaFeEDTA should not require extensive further research. Sufficient information about its potential benefit in various dietary situations is already available to allow for the selection of suitable food vehicles. It might be satisfactory under some circumstances to fortify foods with a soluble iron salt and Na_2EDTA or possibly $CaNa_2EDTA$, because NaFeEDTA would be formed in the stomach. The fortification would require that the iron salt be added to the food item without rendering it organoleptically unacceptable. It might also be necessary to add the EDTA chelate and the iron salt before processing to ensure adequate mixing. This could be an advantage, since preliminary evidence suggests that a EDTA: Fe molar ratio of 0.5:1 in diets results in maximal iron absorption in diets of low iron bioavailability. Furthermore, the use of a cheap, soluble iron salt together with a smaller quantity of the more expensive chelator may reduce the cost. There are no restrictions by JECFA in the use of Na_2EDTA or $CaNa_2EDTA$ which are used extensively in the food industry. The total dose of 2.5 mg/kg/day per person is a figure difficult to attain at the proposed fortification targets. JECFA has reached the conclusion that NaFeEDTA is safe used in supervised food fortification programs in iron-deficient populations and has given provisional approval for its use.

9.4.3 BIOAVAILABILITY STUDIES IN CORN FLOUR

The strong inhibitory characteristics of iron absorption of corn flour (masa) and the rigors of the preparation of tortillas (addition of water and heating for several minutes at 160 to 180°C) must be tested in human isotopic bioavailability studies. Only then can recommendations be given as to the form and amount of iron fortificants to add to effectively improve iron nutrition of the target population. Three *in vitro* studies show that iron salts (ferrous sulfate as well as fumarate) and bis-iron glycine are not solubilized in a satisfactory way. Utilizing NaEDTA in a 3:1 and 2:1 ratio increases dialyzability markedly. The highest solubility is achieved by a 1:1 ratio, i.e., NaFeEDTA (Figure 9.6A). *In vivo* radioiron bioavailability studies showed that intrinsic iron and ferrous fumarate were poorly absorbed, 0.7 and 0.8% respectively. When NaEDTA was added, fumarate's bioavailability increased threefold. The reduced iron was assumed to have the same bioavailability of intrinsic iron. The *in vitro* bioavailability with a molar ratio of 3:1 and 2:1 of iron to EDTA was 2.4 and

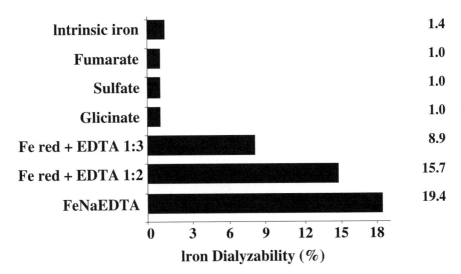

FIGURE 9.6A Dialyzability *in vitro* of iron in corn-masa tortilla.

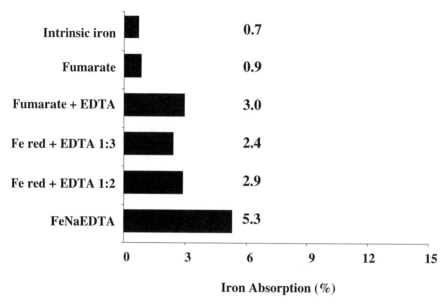

FIGURE 9.6B Bioavailability *in vivo* of iron from corn-masa tortilla.

2.9% respectively. A molar ratio of 1:1, i.e., iron-EDTA or NaFeEDTA was 5.3% (Figure 9.6B). The studies done with Mexican corn-masa flour confirm that this vehicle is extremely inhibitory for the absorption of iron. The best results are obtained with NaFeEDTA added in 3 ppm per kg of flour. The 5.3% absorption allows the absorption of about 0.4 mg of iron, if 300 g of tortilla are consumed. This would be a satisfactory amount for a successful program, however it is several times as expensive as iron salts. As an alternative, ferrous fumarate with a 2:1 molar ratio of iron to NaEDTA also reaches a 3% bioavailability and, though less iron is absorbed, it is threefold higher than iron without the ETDA molecule as enhancer. These studies need to be completed with shelf life and organoleptic evaluations in order to be applicable to a nationwide program.

9.5   CONCLUSIONS

Efforts are under way in many developing countries to promote the fortification of a wide range of food products (staples, condiments, industrially processed foods) with iron and other micronutrients such as vitamin A and folate. Although limited efficacy research has been carried out, when a widely consumed staple such as corn-masa flour can be fortified with iron, the invaluable opportunity to add additional micronutrients cannot be overlooked, particularly when the population is also deficient in these nutrients and its cost is very low. Vitamin A not only prevents blindness but reduces infant mortality. Folic acid may contribute to anemia, and more recently has been shown to reduce neural tube defects at birth. Zinc is an important mineral involved in immunity and may contribute to the high prevalence of stunting in many parts of the world. Adding a multivitamin, multimineral mix to a ton of corn flour costs from \$3 to \$5 (U.S.), an influence of less than 2% of the cost of flour or \$0.003 per kilo. The cost per person fortified is about \$0.70 per year and estimations by The World Bank show that every dollar spent in fortification has a return of \$80.

Attempts to utilize EDTA to enhance iron absorption have been made in Thailand adding it to fish sauce,[91] sugar in Guatemala,[92] and curry powder in South Africa.[93,94] Though these field trials have met certain degree of success, they have not been implemented in a large scale national study. China and Vietnam have conducted tests with iron EDTA added to soy and fish sauce, respectively and are currently undergoing extensive field trials with the prospect of implementing national scale fortification. Condiments such as fish or soy sauce provide an effective way of reaching these Asiatic populations since the fortification of home grown rice — their main staple diet — is impractical. Adding fortified fish or soy sauce not only will provide a form of bioavailable iron, but will also promote the absorption of other sources of iron in the diet. Another option that has a lot of potential and has been pursued for a long time is to double fortify salt with iron and iodine. Although, these efforts were hampered by several technical problems,[95-97] recent investigations in India have shown that this approach is feasible using ferrous fumarate and malto-dextrin-encapsulated potassium iodate to prevent iron catalyzed iodine losses.[98] Testing the effectiveness of this product in the field setting remains to be carried out.

REFERENCES

1. Second report on the world nutrition situation, Administrative Committee on Coordination: Subcommittee on Nutrition, World Health Organization, Geneva, 1992.
2. Berger, J. et al., Weekly iron supplementation is as effective as 5 day per week iron supplementation in Bolivian school children living at high altitude, *Eur. J. Clinical Nutr.,* 51(6), 381, 1997.
3. Yip, R., The challenge of improving iron nutrition: limitations and potentials of major intervention approaches, *Eur. J. Clinical Nutr.,* 51 (Suppl. 4), S16, 1997.
4. Hurrell, R. F., Bioavailability of iron, *Eur. J. Clinical Nutr.,* 51 (Suppl. 1), S4, 1997.
5. Hurrell, R. F., Prospects for Improving the Iron Fortification of Foods, *Nutritional Anemias,* 30, 193, 1992.
6. Cook, J. D. and Reusser, M. E., Iron fortification: an update, *Am. J. Clinical Nutr.,* 38(4), 648, 1983.
7. Cook, J. D. et al., Nutritional deficiency and anemia in Latin America: A collaborative study, *Blood,* 38(5), 591, 1971.
8. Ranum, P., Iron fortification of cereals, in *The Mineral Fortification of Foods,* Hurrell, R., Ed., Letterhead Publishing, Surrey, England, 1999, chap. 11, 237.
9. Cook, J. D., Finch, C. A., and Smith, N. J., Evaluation of the iron status of a population, *Blood,* 48(3), 449, 1976.
10. Cook, J., Dallman, P., Bothwell, D., et al., Measurements of iron status, International Nutritional Anemia Consultative Group, The Nutrition Foundation, Washington, D.C., 1985.
11. Skikne, B. S., Flowers, C. H., and Cook, J. D., Serum transferrin receptor: a quantitative measure of tissue iron deficiency, *Blood,* 75, 1870, 1990..
12. Cook, J. D., Baynes, R. D., and Skikne, B. S., The physiological significance of circulating transferrin receptors, *Annu. Rev. Med.,* 44, 63, 1993.

13. Pizarro, F., Amar, M., and Stekel, A., Determination of iron in stools as a method to monitor consumption of iron fortified products in infants, *Am. J. Clinical Nutr.,* 45, 484, 1987.

14. Dallman, P. R., Siimes, M. A., and Stekel, A., Iron deficiency in infancy and childhood, *Am. J. Clinical Nutr.,* 33, 86, 1980.

15. Stekel, A., Pizarro, F., and Olivares, M., Prevention of iron deficiency by milk fortification, *Acta Paed. Scan. Suppl.,* 38(6), 1119, 1988.

16. Fomon, S. J. and Strauss, R. G., Nutrient deficiencies in breast-fed infants, *New Engl. J. Med.,* 299(7), 355, 1978.

17. Nelson, S. E. et al., Gain in weight and length during early infancy, *Early Hum. Dev.,* 19(4), 223, 1989.

18. Guo, S. et al., Reference data on gains in weight and length during the first two years of life, *J. Pediatr.,* 119, 355, 1991.

19. Fomon, S. J., Requirements and recommended dietary intakes of protein during infancy [erratum appears in *Pediatr. Res.* 31(1), 21, 1992], *Pediatr. Res.,* 30(5), 391, 1991.

20. Lundstrom, U., Siimes, M. A., and Dallman, P. R., At what age does iron supplementation become necessary in low-birth-weight infants? *J. Pediatr.,* 91(6), 878, 1977.

21. Lundstrom, U. and Siimes, M. A., Red blood cell values in low-birth-weight infants: ages at which values become equivalent to those of term infants, *J. Pediatr.,* 96(6), 1040, 1980.

22. Asenjo, J. A. et al., Use of a bovine heme iron concentrate in the fortification of biscuits, *J. Food Science,* 50, 795, 1985.

23. Hertrampf, E. et al., Haemoglobin fortified cereal: a source of available iron to breast-fed infants, *Eur. J. Clinical Nutr.,* 44(11), 793, 1990.

24. Calvo, E. et al., Haemoglobin-fortified cereal: an alternative weaning food with high iron bioavailability, *Eur. J. Clinical Nutr.,* 43, 237, 1989.

25. Walter, T., Dallman, P. R., Pizarro, F., Velozo, L., Pena, G., Bartholmey, S. J., et al., Effectiveness of iron-fortified infant cereal in prevention of iron deficiency anemia, *Pediatrics,* 91(5), 976, 1993.

26. Bartholmey, S. J., Bioavailability of electrolytic iron, *Pediatric Basic,* 1, 1990.

27. Turnbull, A. et al., Iron absorption. IV. The absorption of hemoglobin iron, *J. Clinical Investigation,* 41, 1897, 1962.

28. Olivares, M. et al., Effect of a hemoglobin fortified cereal on morbidity in breast fed infants, *Colloque INSERM,* 197, 653, 1990.

29. Amar, M. et al., Utilizacion del hierro heminico en la fortificacion de alimentos, *Cuadernos Medico -Sociales,* 21, 85, 1980.

30. Walter, T. et al., Effect of bovine-hemoglobin-fortified cookies on iron status of schoolchildren: a nationwide program in Chile, *Am. J. Clinical Nutr.,* 57, 190, 1993.

31. David, J., Milling and baking news and world grain, Technical report, Milling Association of Chile, Santiago, 1987.

32. Annual Report of the National Institute of Statistics, Santiago, 1995.

33. Cori, H., Laboratories Roche, Gonzalez M, Granotec. personal communication.

34. Lladser, M., Chief of the Bromatology Dept., Instituto de Salud Publica, Santiago, personal communication, 1998.

35. Hertrampf, E. et al., Hemoglobin fortified cereal: its effect in the prevention of iron deficiency in breast fed infants, *Colloque INSERM,* 197, 647, 1990.

36. Hertrampf, E. et al., Nutrition de hierro y lactancia natural en lactantes chilenos, *Rev. Chilean Pediatr.,* 58, 193, 1987.

37. Stekel, A. Pizarro, F., Olivares, M., et al., Prevention of iron deficiency by milk fortification, Acta Paediatr. Scand., Suppl., 38(6) 1119, 1988.

38. Stekel, A., Pizarro, F., Olivares, M. et al., Prevention of iron deficiency by milk fortification, III., Effectiveness under the usual operational conditions of a nation-wide food program, *Nutr. Reports Int.,* 38, 1119, 1988.

39. Olivares, M. et al., Prevention of iron deficiency by milk fortification. The Chilean experience, *Acta Paediatr. Scand. Suppl.,* 361, 109, 1989.

40. Franco, E. et al., Nutricion de hierro en lactantes mapuches alimentados con leche materna (2a etapa), *Rev. Chilean. Pediatr.,* 61(5), 1990.

41. Hertrampf, E. et al., Iron-deficiency anemia in the nursing infant: its elimination with iron-fortified milk, *Rev. Med. Chil.,* 118(12), 1330, 1990.

42. Hertrampf, E., Olivares, M., and Walter, T., Anemia ferropriva en el lactante: errad-icacion con leche fortificada con hierro [Control of infant iron deficiency anemia: use of iron supplemented milk], *Rev. Med. Chile,* 118, 1330, 1990.

43. Hertrampf, E. et al., Iron nutriture in breast-fed infants from Chilean aborigenes (Mapuches), *Colloque INSERM,* 197, 323, 1990.

44. Walter, T., Olivares, M., and Hertrampf, E., Field trials of food fortification with iron: the experience in Chile, in *Iron Metabolism in Infants,* Lonnerdal, B., Ed., CRC Press, Boca Raton, Fl. 127, 1990.

45. Pena, G., Pizarro, F., and Hertrampf, E., Aporte del hierro del pan a la dieta Chilena, *Rev. Med. Chile,* 119, 753, 1991.

46. Pizarro, F. et al., Iron status with different infant feeding regimens: relevance to screening and prevention of iron deficiency, *J. Ped.,* 118, 687, 1991.

47. Hertrampf, E. et al., Situacion de la nutricion de hierro en la embarazada adolescente al inicio de la gestacion, *Rev. Med. Chile,* 122, 1372, 1991.

48. Calvo, E. and Sosa, E., Iron status in non-pregnant women of child bearing age living at Great Buenos Aires, *Eur. J. Clinical Nutr.,* 45, 215, 1991.

49. Hertrampf, E., Pena, G., and Pizarro, F., Dietary iron contribution of bread in Santiago, Chile, *Colloque INSERM,* 197, 641, 1990.

50. Cook, J. D. et al., Absorption of fortification iron in bread, *Am. J. Clinical Nutr.,* 26(8), 861, 1973.

51. El Guindi, M., Lynch, S. R., and Cook, J. D., Iron Absorption from fortified flat breads, *Br. J. Nutr.,* 59, 205, 1988.

52. Cook, J. D., Skikne, B. S., and Lynch, S. R., Estimates of iron sufficiency in the US population, *Blood,* 68, 726, 1986.

53. Cook, J. D., Dassenko, S. A., and Lynch, S. R., Assessment of the role of nonheme-iron availability in iron balance, *Am. J. Clinical Nutr.,* 54(4), 717, 1991.

54. Cook, C. I. and Yu, B. P., Iron accumulation in aging: modulation by dietary restric-tion, *Mech. Ageing Dev.,* 102(1), 1, 1998.

55. Bothwell, T., Hallberg, L., Clydesdale, F., et al., The effects of cereals and legumes on iron availability, International Anemia Consultative Group, The Nutrition Foun-dation, Washington, D.C., 1982, 23.

56. Minutes of the sixth annual meeting of the International Anemia Consultative Group, Santiago, 1981.

57. Stekel, A. et al., Deficiencia de hierro y enriquecimiento de alimentos, *Rev. Chilean Pediatr.,* 44, 447, 1973.

58. Stekel, A. et al., Leche fortificada con hierro y acido ascorbico en la alimentacion del lactante, *Apartado Cuadernos Medico-Sociales,* 21, 74, 1980.

59. Stekel, A., Mardones-Santander, F., and Hertrampf, E., Breast feeding practices and use of supplemental foods, *Malnutrition: Determinants Consequences,* 139, 1984.

60. Stekel, A. et al., The role of ascorbic acid in the bioavailability of iron from infant foods, *Int. J. Vitam. Nutr. Res.,* 27, 167, 1985.

61. Hertrampf, E. et al., Bioavailability of iron in soy-based formula and its effect on iron nutrition in infancy, *Pediatrics,* 78, 640, 1986.

62. Stekel, A., Olivares, M., and Pizarro, F., Absorption of fortification iron from milk formulas in infants, *Am. J. Clinical Nutr.,* 43, 917, 1986.

63. Stekel, A. et al., Prevencion de la carencia de hierro en lactantes, mediante la fortificacion de la leche. I. Estudio sobre el terreno de una leche semidescremada, *Arch. Latin. Nutr.,* 36, 654, 1986.

64. Pizarro, F. and Stekel, A., Efecto de la acidificacion sobre la biodisponibilidad del hierro de fortificacion de una formula lactea, *Rev. Chilean Tecnol. Med.,* 9, 445, 1986.

65. Franco, E. et al., Prevalencia de anemia por deficit de hierrro en lactantes mapuches alimentados con leche materna, *Rev. Chilean Pediatr.,* 58, 361, 1987.

66. Martinez, H. et al., Anemia en mujeres en edad reproductiva. Resultados de una encuesta probabilistica nacional, *Salud Publica. Mex.,* 37, 108, 1995.

67. Chavez, A., Martinez, C., and Yaschine, T., Nutrition, behavioral development, and mother-child interaction in young rural children, *Fed. Proc.,* 34, 1574, 1975.

68. Bjorn-Rasmussen, E. and Hallberg, L., Iron absorption from maize. Effect of ascorbic acid on iron absorption from maize supplemented with ferrous sulfate, *Nutr. Metab.,* 23, 192, 1974.

69. Hallberg, L. and Rossander, L., Improvement of iron nutrition in developing countries: comparison of adding meat, soy protein, ascorbic acid, citric acid, and ferrous sulphate on iron absorption from a simple Latin American-type of meal, *Am. J. Clinical Nutr.,* 39(4), 577, 1984.

70. Rivero, F. et al., Fortification of precooked maize flour with coarse defatted maize germ, *Arch. Latin. Nutr.,* 44(2), 129, 1994.

71. Karyadi, D. and Bloem, M. W., The role of vitamin A in iron deficiency anemia and implications for interventions, *Biomed. Environ. Sci.,* 9(2-3), 316, 1996.

72. Mejia, L. A., Vitamin A deficiency as a factor in nutritional anemia, *Int. J. Vitam. Nutr. Res. Suppl.,* 27, 75, 1985.

73. Northrop-Clewes, C. A. et al., Effect of improved vitamin A status on response to iron supplementation in Pakistani infants, *Am. J. Clinical Nutr.,* 64(5), 694, 1996.

74. Ribaya-Mercado, J. D., Importance of adequate vitamin A status during iron supplementation, *Nutr. Rev.,* 55(8), 306, 1997.

75. Staab, D. B. et al., Relationship between vitamin A and iron in the liver, *J. Nutr.,* 114(5), 840, 1984.

76. Garcia-Casal, M. N. and Layrisse, M., Dietary iron absorption. Role of vitamin A, *Arch. Latin. Nutr.,* 48(3), 191, 1998.

77. Garcia-Casal, M. N. et al., Vitamin A and beta-carotene can improve nonheme iron absorption from rice, wheat and corn by humans, *J. Nutr.,* 128(3), 646, 1998.

78. Ashmead, H. D., Bioavailability of iron glycine, *Am. J. Clinical Nutr.,* 69(4), 737, 1999.

79. Galdi, M. et al., Ferric glycinate iron bioavailability determined by hemoglobin regeneration method, *Nutr. Rep. Int.,* 38, 729, 1988.

80. Galdi, M., Carbone, N., and Valencia, M. E., Comparison of ferric glycinate to ferrous sulfate in model infant formulas: kinetics of vitamin losses, *J. Food Sci.,* 54, 1530, 1989.

81. Pineda, O. et al., Effectiveness of iron amino acid chelate on the treatment of iron deficiency anemia in adolescents, *J. Appl. Nutr.,* 46, 2, 1994.

82. Olivares, M. et al., Milk inhibits and ascorbic acid favors ferrous bis-glycine chelate bioavailability in humans, *J. Nutr.,* 127(7), 1407, 1997.

83. Pizarro, F. et al., Iron absorption of ferric glycinate is controlled by iron stores, *Nutr. Res.,* 18, 3, 1998.

84. Queiroz, S. and Torres, M., Anemia carencial ferropriva: aspectos fisiopatológicos e experiência com a utilizãçao do leite fortificado com ferro, *Pediatria Moderna,* 32, 441, 1995.

85. Lost, C. et al., Repleting hemoglobin in iron deficiency anemia in young children through liquid milk fortification with bioavailable iron amino acid chelate, *J. Am. Coll. Nutr.,* 17, 187, 1988.

86. Fisberg, M. et al., Ulilizãçao de queijo petit suisse na prevençao da anemia carencial em pré-escolares, *Clinical Pediatr.,* (Brazil) 19, 14, 1995.

87. Allen, L., Bioavailability and efficacy of iron amino acid chelates as iron fortificants for maize, in Proc. of the Int. Conf. on Human Nutrition, Salt Lake City, 1998.

88. Fox, T. E., Eagles, J., and Fairweather-Tait, S. J., Bioavailability of iron glycine as a fortificant in infant foods, *Am. J. Clinical Nutr.,* 67(4), 664, 1998.

89. Ashmead, H., Graff, D., and Ashmead, H., *Intestinal Absorption of Metal Ions and Chelates,* Charles C. Thomas, Springfield, IL, 1985, 1.

90. Iron EDTA for food fortification, Lynch, S. et al., Eds., International Anemia Consultative Group, The Nutrition Foundation, Washington, D.C., 1993.

91. Garby, L. and Areekul, S., Iron supplementation in thai fish-sauce, *Annu. Trop. Med. and Paras,* 68, 467, 1974.

92. Viteri, F. E. et al., Fortification of sugar with iron sodium ethylenediaminotetraacetate (FeNaEDTA) improves iron status in semirural Guatemalan populations, *Am. J. Clinical Nutr.,* 61(5), 1153, 1995.

93. Ballot, D. et al., Fortification of curry powder with NaFe(III)EDTA: report of a controlled iron fortification trial, *Am. J. Clinical Nutr.,* 49, 162, 1989.

94. Lamparelli, R. D. et al., Curry powder as a vehicle for iron fortification: effects on iron absorption, *Am. J. Clinical Nutr.,* 46, 335, 1987.

95. Use of common salt fortified with iron in the control and prevention of anaemic: a collaborative study, Report of the Working Group on Fortification of Salt with Iron, *Am. J. Clinical Nutr.,* 35, 1142, 1982.

96. Narasinga Rao, B., Salt in *Iron Fortification of Foods,* Clydesdale, F. and Wiemer, K., Eds., Academic Press, Orlando, 1985, 155.

97. Foy, H., Fortification of salt with iron, *Am. J. Clinical Nutr.,* 29, 935, 1976.

98. Lotfi, M. et al., Micronutrient fortification of foods. Current practices, research and opportunities, International Agriculture Centre, Ottawa, 81, 1996.

10 Food-Based Approaches

Marie T. Ruel and Carol E. Levin

CONTENTS

0-8493-8569-5/01/$0.00+$.50
© 2001 by CRC Press LLC

10.1   INTRODUCTION

Food based strategies — also referred to as dietary modifications — encompass a wide variety of interventions that aim at: (1) increasing the production, availability, and access to food — in the present case, micronutrient rich foods; (2) increasing the consumption of micronutrient rich foods; and/or (3) increasing the bioavailability of micronutrients in the diet. Examples of interventions used to achieve these goals include the following:

1. Strategies to increase the production of micronutrient rich foods. These strategies include agricultural programs and policies to increase commercial production as well as programs to promote home production of fruits and vegetables (home gardens), small livestock production, and aquaculture (fish ponds).
2. Strategies to increase the intake of micronutrient rich foods. These approaches refer to nutrition education, communication, social marketing, and behavior change programs to guide consumer food choices and to increase the demand for micronutrient rich foods. They also include education interventions targeted at specific age groups such as the promotion of optimal breastfeeding and complementary feeding practices for infants and young children.*
3. Strategies to increase the bioavailability of micronutrients. These include home processing techniques such as fermentation or germination to increase the bioavailability of micronutrients; food combinations that increase the bioavailability of certain micronutrients (also called food-to-food fortification strategies); and preservation and conservation techniques such as solar drying or production of leaf concentrates to extend the availability of seasonal fruits and vegetables throughout the year.
4. Plant breeding strategies. These are technologies currently available through plant breeding to either increase the concentration of certain trace minerals and vitamins or to increase their bioavailability by reducing the

---

* Breastfeeding promotion programs and education interventions to improve complementary feeding practices, although they are important for the control of micronutrient deficiencies, are not reviewed in this chapter.

concentration of antinutrient factors (inhibitors of absorption), or by increasing the concentration of promoters of absorption.*

Most food based strategies use some combination of interventions from these four groups. As an example, nutrition education and communication strategies are often used to complement production interventions in order to ensure that the increased supply of food or the income generated through the sale of products will translate into increased intake by targeted groups.

Food-based strategies are regarded as potentially sustainable approaches because their overall goal is to empower individuals and households to take ultimate responsibility over the quality of their diets.[1] A particularly attractive aspect of food based strategies is that they can address multiple nutrients simultaneously, including calories, proteins, and various micronutrients, without the risk of antagonistic nutrient interactions or overload. This makes these strategies appealing for nutritional anemias, which result from multiple micronutrient deficiencies. In addition, it is well recognized that populations deficient in iron are most likely to also suffer from various other deficiencies, zinc, vitamin A, and B_{12}, in particular. Therefore, a global strategy that aims at achieving long term sustained dietary modifications would seem to be most appropriate for the control of nutritional anemias.

This chapter reviews current knowledge and experience with food based approaches, it discusses some of the lessons learned and the current gaps in knowledge, and it identifies research priorities. The chapter focuses mainly on vitamin A and iron because experience with food based approaches for vitamin B_{12}, folic acid, and copper is practically nonexistent.

The chapter is structured as follows: the next section discusses strategies to increase production and/or intake of micronutrient rich foods; Section 10.3 reviews experience with strategies to improve bioavailability; and Section 10.4 summarizes progress in plant breeding research. The final section summarizes lessons learned and priorities for future research.

10.2 STRATEGIES TO INCREASE PRODUCTION AND/OR INTAKE OF MICRONUTRIENT RICH FOODS

10.2.1 Vitamin A

Home gardens have been by far the most popular food based strategy used to address vitamin A deficiency. Various reviews of home gardening interventions have been published over the past 10 to 20 years. The Vitamin A Support Project VITAL reviewed over 40 publications to look at the impact of home gardens on consumption, nutritional status, and in some cases income.[2-4] The ACC/SCN reviewed 13 evaluations related to dietary modification programs to control vitamin A deficiency, covering work published between 1989 and 1993.[5] We updated this work and reviewed 10 new projects published between 1995 and 1999 (see Table 10.1 for references and summary of the studies reviewed).

---

* Food fortification is also a food-based strategy, but a separate chapter of this book is dedicated to this subject.

TABLE 10.1
Summary of Intervention and Evaluation Designs of Recent Studies Reviewed (1995–1999)[1]

Country	Reference/Year	Target Nutrients	Intervention: Production	Intervention: Nutrition Education (NED)	Target groups	Evaluation: Design	Evaluation: Methods	Findings: Production	Findings: Income	Findings: KAP + Dietary Intake	Findings: Nutritional Status
Nepal	CARE/Nepal 1995	Vitamin A	Home gardening Irrigation Agriculture extension Seed distribution	—	HH Chidren 6–60 mo	Before (1992) After (1995)	HH survey	Increase in % hh producing vegetables	—	Diet shows insufficient vitamin A intake by mothers and children	Deterioration of nutritional status of children (no control)
Bangladesh	Greiner and Mitra 1995	Vitamin A	Home gardening Seeds Farming education	NED	Women Children	Treatment/control Before/after	HH survey Clinical assessment 24-recall	Increase in % hh growing vegetables and fruits in both treatment/control	—	Increased knowledge of function of vitamin A	Slight decrease in night blindness
Vietnam	English et al. 1997 English and Badcock 1999	Vitamin A Vitamin C Iron Iodine Proteins, calories Fat	Home gardens Fish ponds Animals	NED	Mothers Children < 6 y	Treatment/control After	HH survey Morbidity recall KAP Anthropometry Food intake	Increased production of vegetables, fruits, fish, eggs	—	Increased KAP Greater intake of vegetables, fruits, energy, proteins, vitamin A, C, iron in children, compared to control	Reduced severity in incidence of ARI Improved growth of children
Peru	Sanez et al. 1999	Vitamin A Vitamin C Iron	—	NED in community kitchen Capacity building	Nonpregnant women of reproductive age	Treatment/control Before/after	Interviews Focus groups Biochemical assessment	—	—	Increased quality of meals (vitamin C, A) Increased intake of foods rich in iron, vitamin C Increased intake of vitamin C, heme iron, proportion absorbable iron	Reduction in prevalence of anemia

TABLE 10.1 (continued)
Summary of Intervention and Evaluation Designs of Recent Studies Reviewed (1995–1999)[1]

			Intervention			Evaluation		Findings				
Country	Reference/ Year	Target Nutrients	Production	Nutrition Education (NED)	Target groups	Design	Methods	Production	Income	KAP + Dietary Intake	Nutritional Status
Indonesia	dePee et al. 1998	Vitamin A	—	Social marketing campaign, including mass media, face-to-face communication to increase intake of DGLV and eggs	Mothers Children <36 mo	Before/after	HH survey 24-h recall Biochemical analysis	—	—	Increased % children and mothers who ate at least 1 egg in past week Increased amount of vegetables prepared/ person/day Increased vitamin intake of children and mothers Increased vitamin A intake from eggs and plants	Serum retinol increased (associated with egg consumption) Dose response relationship
Bangladesh	IFPRI et al. 1998	Vitamin A Iron	Vegetable production Fish ponds Credit and agricultural training	—	Women Their household and children	3 groups: Fish ponds Vegetables Control Before/after	HH survey Anthropometry Biochemical analysis	Increased production of vegetables and fish	Slight increase in income from adoption of fish or vegetables technology	No increase in consumption of fish among fish pond group Increased vegetable intake among vegetable group	No effect on hemoglobin from fish ponds or vegetable production
Kenya	Hagenimana et al, 1999	Vitamin A	Introduction of new variety of sweet potatoes Training in food processing techniques	NED to increase intake and use processing techniques	Women's groups Children 0–5 y	Treatment/control Before/after	HH survey HKI vitamin A food frequency questionnaire	—	—	Greater HKI score for frequency of intake on vitamin A rich foods in children (control group had decreased intake)	

TABLE 10.1 (continued)
Summary of Intervention and Evaluation Designs of Recent Studies Reviewed (1995–1999)[1]

Country	Reference/ Year	Intervention			Target groups	Evaluation		Findings			
		Target Nutrients	Production	Nutrition Education (NED)		Design	Methods	Production	Income	KAP + Dietary Intake	Nutritional Status
Thailand	Smitasiri and Dhanamitta 1999 Smitasiri et al. 1999	Vitamin A Vitamin C Iron Iodine	Seeds distribution Farmer women training Promotion of gardens, fish ponds, chicken	Education Social marketing	Pregnant, lactating women 2–5 y old School girls	Treatment/control Before/after	HH survey 24-h recall Biochemical assessment (in school girls)	—	—	Increased KAP about vitamin A, iron Increased intake of vitamin A in all target groups No increase in fat intake Increased iron intake in 2–56 y old, in 10–13 y old, in lactating women Increased intake of vitamin C in lactating women	Blood samples in school girls: increased serum retinol reduction in vitamin A deficiency increased mean hb (not significant) reduced anemia prevalence (not significant) reduction in low serum ferritin
Bangladesh	Marsh 1999	Vitamin A	Vegetable home garden Agricultural training Seeds	NED	Women Children	Treatment/control Before/after	HH survey Vegetable production Size of cultivated plot Income Intake of vegetables	Increase in vegetable production Increase in size of plot cultivated Increase in year round availability of vegetables	Increase in income Increase in women's control of income	Increased vegetable consumption per capita Increased vegetable consumption of children	

TABLE 10.1 (continued)
Summary of Intervention and Evaluation Designs of Recent Studies Reviewed (1995–1999)[1]

Country	Reference/Year	Target Nutrients	Intervention		Target groups	Evaluation		Findings			
			Production	Nutrition Education (NED)		Design	Methods	Production	Income	KAP + Dietary Intake	Nutritional Status
Ethiopia	Ayalew et al. 1999	Vitamin A	Agicultural training Food preparation Seeds	Health education NED	Women Children	Treatment/control After	HH survey Qualitative research KHI vitamin A food frequency questionnaire	—	—	Increased KAP about vitamin A, night blindness More diversified diet Higher HKI vitamin A food frequency scores	Reduced prevalence of night blindness and Bitot's spots

[1] Abbreviations: ARI = Acute Respiratory Infeciton; DGLV = Dark Green Leafy Vegetable; HH = Household; HKI = Helen Keller International; NED = Nutrition Education; KAP = Knowledge, Attitude and Practices

By contrast with previous interventions, most recent home production projects included a strong education and communication component. Some of the projects reviewed did not include production activities, but focussed on social marketing and communication activities to increase the intake of micronutrient rich foods, often emphasizing the needs of small children, pregnant, and lactating women. Another important change in the designs of more recent projects is the fact that many now address multiple micronutrients as opposed to as in the past emphasizing vitamin A alone. Below we summarize the evidence of impact of these interventions on three main outcomes: (1) production and income, (2) knowledge, attitude and practices (KAP), intake of targeted foods and nutrients, and (3) nutritional status indicators.

10.2.1.1 Impact on Production and Income

The literature indicates that most home gardens are implemented to increase house-hold production of fruits and vegetables to supplement the grain based diets of rural agricultural households.[6-11] In Nepal and Bangladesh, increases in the proportion of households producing vegetables and fruits were documented as a result of home gardening and farming education interventions.[7-8] The projects reviewed by Marsh[12] in Bangladesh show an increase in the year round availability of vegetables. Only a few studies looked at the impact on income, farmer profits, or household market sales, but those who did, showed modest increases in household income.[12-14]

10.2.1.2 Impact on Knowledge, Attitude, and Practices (KAP) on Dietary Intakes of Vitamin A Rich Foods

Notable in many of the earlier studies reviewed was the absence of integrated behavior change intervention with the home gardening strategy. Not surprisingly, most of those that looked at the impact on food intake or nutritional status failed to demonstrate any significant change.[7,14-15] By 1994, things started to change. Gillespie and Mason's[5] review highlighted two successful nutrition education and social mar-keting interventions using mass-media that showed a positive change in knowledge, attitude, and practices; one study was carried out in Indonesia[16] and the other in Thailand.[17] In Indonesia, among mothers who had heard the radio spots (42%), considerable positive attitudinal changes occurred regarding vitamin A; consumption of dark green leafy vegetables had increased from 10 to 33% after two years, in the targeted group. The coverage of the vitamin A capsules supplementation had increased from 35 to 58%.[16] In Thailand, increased knowledge and awareness about vitamin A resulted in increased intake of ivy gourd and fat (both of which were promoted by the social marketing campaign) among pregnant and lactating women and preschool children.[17] In 1996, a follow-up to this project was implemented.[18-19] It showed a cumulative improvement in KAP with respect to vitamin A and fat, which was accompanied by an increased intake of vitamin A among preschool children and pregnant and lactating women.

Another social marketing campaign promoting intake of dark green leafy veg-etables and eggs in Indonesia documented an increase in the percentage of children who had consumed at least one egg during the previous week, the quantity of dark green leafy vegetables prepared at home, and the total vitamin A intake of both mothers and young children.[20]

A unique educational and behavioral change project in Peru to increase the quality of the meals offered in community kitchens of Lima (*comedores populares*) showed a significant increase in the vitamin A and C content of the meals provided. The resulting increase in the intake of foods rich in iron and vitamin C by women using the community kitchen became apparent.[21]

Home gardening interventions that had a strong educational and behavioral change component reflected an increase in consumption that was attributed to the project. Among these was the HKI/AVRDC project in Bangladesh that demonstrated an increase in average weekly vegetable consumption per capita among target households.[12] Intra-household consumption data showed a higher consumption of dark green leafy vegetables by infants and very young children. In Vietnam, a community nutrition project combining household garden production of carotene-rich fruits and vegetables, fish ponds, and animal husbandry with nutrition education,[9-10] showed that participating mothers had a better understanding of vitamin A compared to mothers from the control commune. In addition, children from participating households consumed significantly more vegetables and fruits, and had greater intakes of energy, protein, vitamin A, and iron. In Kenya, new varieties of beta-carotene rich sweet potatoes were introduced to women's groups,[22] along with nutrition education, lessons on food processing, and technical assistance. The frequency of consumption of vitamin A rich foods increased in the intervention group, whereas it decreased among a control group. In Ethiopia, a home gardening and health and nutrition education intervention building on a previous dairy goat project increased participants' KAP related to vitamin A, child feeding practices, and the prevention of night blindness.[23] These changes were accompanied by increases in frequency of intake of vitamin A rich foods.

10.2.1.3 Impact on Nutritional Status

The question of whether home gardens have a positive impact on vitamin A status has been examined in prior reviews and in some of the more recent studies, but evidence is still scant. In the set of earlier studies, home gardens were found to be positively associated with decreased risk of vitamin A deficiency[24] and reduced clinical eye signs of vitamin A deficiency.[6] Gillespie and Mason[5] also conclude from their review that there is evidence that food-based approaches can be effective in the control of vitamin A deficiency. In our review of recent works, still only a few of the home garden and nutrition education studies measured their impact on vitamin A status indicators. In Bangladesh, Greiner and Mitra[8] documented a slight reduction in night blindness associated with an increase in intake of dark green leafy vegetables in young children. Also in Bangladesh, increased intake of eggs and dark green leafy vegetables among children and mothers was associated with greater serum retinol.[20] In Thailand, serum retinol was measured only among school girls, but significant increases of serum retinol were observed among the treatment group as well as reductions in the prevalence of vitamin A.[19] In addition to the social marketing intervention, this project included a strong school component, which aimed at improving nutrient content of school lunches. In Vietnam, serum retinol was not measured, but the home production of vegetables, fish, and animal husbandry combined with nutrition education were associated with increased growth among preschool children and reductions in the severity and incidence of acute respiratory infections.[9-10] In Ethiopia, the prevalence of night blindness and Bitot's spots was lower among participants in the home gardening and nutrition education intervention, compared to a control group.[23]

10.2.2 IRON

Production and education interventions to increase the supply and intake of iron from plant foods have not been as popular as vitamin A interventions. This is not surprising considering that the potential for plant sources to make a major contribution to the control of iron deficiency in developing countries has been questioned for some time.[25-26] Although many nonanimal foods contain relatively large amounts of iron, the nonheme form of iron present in these foods has poor bioavailability. In addition, plant foods often contain a variety of inhibitors of nonheme iron such as tannins, phytates, and polyphenols. It is believed that to increase the household supply of bioavailable iron, promotional efforts may have to support the production of animal products such as small animal husbandry or fish ponds, which would increase the supply of more bioavailable heme iron. Several examples are included in Table 10.1. The 10 new studies reviewed showed that all of those that targeted increases in iron intake or iron status included the promotion of animal products intake and/or production. The study in Vietnam promoted fish ponds and animal husbandry,[9] the Peru intervention promoted low cost sources of heme iron such as organ meats,[21] the study in Bangladesh included fish ponds,[13] and the study in Thailand promoted fish ponds and chicken production in addition to home gardening.[18]

10.2.2.1 Impact on Iron Intake and Iron Status

The Vietnam project documented an increase in the intake of iron among children of households in the intervention communities (home gardens, fish ponds, and animal husbandry) compared with control communities.[9-10] No mention was made, however, of whether the increased iron was from vegetable or animal sources; iron status was not measured. In Peru, the promotional efforts to improve the quality of the meals offered at the community kitchens showed significant impact on the intake of foods rich in iron and vitamin C, the total daily intake of vitamin C and heme iron, and the proportion of absorbable iron by the targeted group of women of reproductive age.[21] The prevalence of anemia was also reduced significantly as a result of the intervention. In Bangladesh, preliminary results from the evaluation of adoption of fish ponds or commercial vegetable production suggest that there was no increase in intake of fish or vegetables among adopting households.[13] There was also no evidence of improved iron status among members of adopting households. The evaluation is continuing and longer term impacts will be assessed.

In Thailand, increased intake of iron among preschoolers, school children, and lactating women was documented as well as an increase in vitamin C (promoter of nonheme iron absorption) among lactating women.[18-19] Biochemical indicators of iron status were measured only among school girls, but significant improvements in serum ferritin were observed. Unfortunately, the effects of the food-based intervention could not be separated from the effects of the overall strategy targeted to school girls, which included the weekly distribution of iron tablets for 12 weeks and improved dietary quality of school lunches.[19] Preliminary results of a study in Ethiopia of the effects of commercialization of crossbred cows found a 72% increase in household income among adopters, while their food expenditure increased by only 20%.[27] Vitamin A and iron intakes were higher among adopters compared to nonadopters, but the authors did not differentiate between animal and plant sources of the micronutrients. Forthcoming analyses of the data will assess the impact on children's nutritional status.

10.2.3 CONCLUSIONS ABOUT STRATEGIES TO INCREASE PRODUCTION AND/OR INTAKE OF VITAMIN A AND IRON RICH FOODS

The findings are consistent in showing the success of well-designed promotional activities including nutrition education, social marketing, and the use of mass media campaigns (with or without home gardening) in achieving significant increases in the consumption of micronutrient rich foods, particularly vitamin A. Compared to the home gardening interventions carried out in the 1980s, which often did not include educational activities, the new generation of integrated production and education projects seem to have been successful in improving knowledge, awareness, attitude, and practices related to vitamin A. Evidence of impact on nutritional status is still scant. Poor evaluation designs and inadequate statistical analysis of findings have slowed down progress in understanding the real potential of production and education interventions for the control of vitamin A deficiency.

Experience with food-based approaches for iron is even more limited and the situation is more complex due to the high cost of foods rich in bioavailable iron. Experience with the production of animal products raises the issue of the trade-offs farmers face between increasing their income through the sale of produce, versus enriching their diet through consumption of self produced goods. Evidence from Bangladesh and Ethiopia suggests that households tend to raise their income rather than improving their diet, and that promotion of animal products without a strong education component may not translate into greater dietary diversity. The question of what exactly can be achieved through well designed integrated production/education interventions to promote increased intake of animal products and to improve iron status remains largely unanswered.

10.3 STRATEGIES TO INCREASE THE BIOAVAILABILITY OF MICRONUTRIENTS AND THEIR RETENTION DURING PROCESSING

Various home processing techniques are available to either increase the bioavailability of micronutrients or to ensure their retention during preparation, cooking, or other processing techniques. For provitamin A compounds, the two main issues are: (1) to ensure the retention of provitamin A during home preparation, cooking, and preserving; and (2) to increase the availability of the highly seasonal fruits and vegetables rich in provitamins A throughout the year by home preservation techniques. For nonheme iron, the most crucial issue is to increase its bioavailability and this can be achieved through: (1) home processes such as fermentation or germination; and (2) food-to-food fortification (or the selection of food combinations that promote nonheme iron bioavailability by increasing the amount of enhancers of absorption or decreasing the amount of inhibitors of absorption). Cooking in iron pots is another way to increase the iron content of foods.

10.3.1 VITAMIN A

10.3.1.1 Effect of Cooking and Processing on the Bioavailability of Provitamins A

A recent review of the effects of cooking and processing techniques on the bioavailability of provitamin A indicates that due to insufficient and often conflicting information, it is currently impossible to derive a clear estimate of the effect of processing and storage on the bioavailability of provitamins A in food.[28] It is clear that heat treatments such as deep frying, prolonged cooking and baking, and a combination of several preparation and processing methods result in substantial losses of provitamins A. Retention through processing can be improved by simple modifications such as cooking with the lid on, reducing the time lag between peeling or cutting and cooking, and limiting the cooking, processing, and storage time.[28]

10.3.1.2 Preservation Techniques to Increase Availability Throughout the Year

The main rationale for developing techniques to preserve provitamins A rich foods is to make them available for consumption through seasons or periods of lower availability. Another reason is to compact food, reduce its volume, and increase the concentration of provitamins A, as seen in the production of leaf concentrates.[29]

Solar drying is one of the most popular preservation methods for fruits and vegetables rich in provitamins A and has been promoted in many countries in recent years. Solar drying is an improved alternative to the traditional sun drying method widely used in tropical countries, which results in significant losses of beta-carotene due to direct exposure to sunlight. Although the rate of retention of beta-carotene in different products varies with solar drying, the range of retention is estimated to be between 50% and 80%.[1] Efforts to promote solar drying have been reported in Mali, Tanzania, Senegal, Haiti, and the Dominican Republic.[30] These studies focussed primarily on testing the feasibility of implementing solar dryers in various settings using locally available products and on testing the retention of provitamins A. We are also aware of a project carried out by the International Center for Research on Women and Opportunities for Micronutrients Intervention (OMNI) in Tanzania to determine the extent to which women's use of solar dryers could decrease seasonal variations in the availability of vitamin A rich foods and could contribute to household economic security. The results are not yet available.

To our knowledge, the nutritional impact of solar drying interventions on dietary intake or on the micronutrient status of vulnerable groups has not been documented. The same is true for similar initiatives such as the sweet potato buds in Guatemala[29] and the leaf concentrates production in Sri Lanka[31] and India[30] that have pursued the same objectives of processing provitamins A rich foods to concentrate and preserve their content during storage. Although promising, these approaches have remained largely at the pilot project level and have not been evaluated for their impact on nutrition.

10.3.2   IRON

10.3.2.1   Home Processing Techniques to Reduce Inhibitors of Nonheme Iron Absorption

As indicated earlier, nonheme iron from cereals or other plants is poorly absorbed because of the presence of inhibitors of iron absorption, such as phytic acid, tannins, and selected dietary fibers. Phytic acid is considered the most potent inhibitor of nonheme iron and is present in large concentrations in cereals, legumes, and vegetables. Various food processing techniques exist to reduce the phytic acid content of plant based staples. Some techniques such as fermentation, germination, or malting involve enzymatic hydrolysis of phytic acid, whereas other nonenzymatic methods such as thermal processing, soaking, or milling can also reduce the concentration of phytic acid in some plant staples. Detailed information about these methods and their effect on improving nonheme iron bioavailability is available in the literature.[32-35]

10.3.2.1.1   Enzymatic Hydrolysis of Phytic Acid

Enzymatic hydrolysis of phytic acid in whole grain cereals and legumes can be achieved by soaking, germination, or fermentation. These processes enhance the activity of endogenous or exogenous phytase.[36-37]

Germination is a process that consists of soaking seeds in water in the dark, usually for up to 3 days, to promote sprouting. During the germination process, phytase activity increases which breaks down phytic acid. Other antinutrients, including polyphenols and tannins, are also reduced with germination. The amount of certain vitamins, including riboflavin, B_6 and vitamin C increases during germination as well as the bioavailability of calcium, iron, and zinc.[38]

Malting is a technique that involves the grinding and softening of grains by soaking them in water until sprouting occurs. Malting is typically followed by drying and milling. Many cereal based porridges are prepared by malting, a process that increases bioavailability of iron and zinc by reducing phytic acid levels.

Fermentation: Acid and alcoholic fermentation can be used for cereals, legumes, or vegetables, to increase their nutritional value and improve their physical characteristics. Fermentation can be spontaneous (using the microorganisms that are naturally present in food), or started with an inoculation. The main nutritional advantage of fermentation is that it improves the bioavailability of minerals, such as iron and zinc, as a result of phytic acid hydrolysis. Other advantages are the increase in riboflavin and the fact that some microorganisms can produce vitamin B_{12}, thus making the vitamin available in plant derived foods where it is normally not present. There is also some evidence that fermented foods have antidiarrheal effects in children. Additionally, fermentation can be a time saving device for mothers because fermented foods can be used safely throughout the day without being cooked.

Soaking is another technique to increase the amount of soluble iron. Soaking of flour for 24 hours has been shown to increase the amount of soluble iron up to 10-fold.[35] Soaking of wheat or rye flour for 2 hours under optimal pH conditions resulted in complete hydrolysis of phytic acid.[39]

Experiences with combinations of fermentation, soaking, and germination techniques have also been shown to be highly efficient in activating endogenous phytase enzymes to degrade phytic acid and to reduce the amounts of polyphenols, which also inhibit nonheme iron absorption.[35] Sour dough leavening is thought to result in almost complete degradation of phytic acid.

10.3.2.1.2 Nonenzymatic Methods for Reducing Phytic Acid Content

Nonenzymatic methods such as thermal processing, soaking, and/or milling can be used to reduce the phytic acid content of plant based staples. Mild heat treatment is said to reduce the phytic acid content of tubers but not cereals and legumes.[40] Soaking can reduce the phytic acid content of certain legumes and cereals that contain water soluble sodium or potassium phytate.[41] Milling can also help reduce the phytic acid content of certain cereals if their phytic acid is localized within a specific part of the grain such as the germ (corn) or aleurone layer (wheat, triticale, rice, sorghum, rye).[42] This strategy will also result in significant losses of vitamins and minerals (iron among others), which are also found in the aleurone layer or germ.

10.3.2.1.3 Experience with Home Processing Techniques

Several studies have been carried out to develop complementary food mixtures using germination and malting, also referred to as the amylase rich food technology.[32,43-47] This method consists of sprouting cereal grains, drying them, and then grinding into flour. Amylase — an enzyme that breaks down starch and reduces its water holding capacity — is activated during germination. Hence only small amounts of the flour are needed to reduce the viscosity of thick porridges. Interest in this technology has been driven by the need to reduce the viscosity, while maintaining the nutrient density of complementary food mixtures, to benefit young infants who have limited gastric capacity.[43,48] Various studies have documented the resulting reductions in viscosity and the nutrient composition of foods prepared with amylase and others looked at preparation time, cost and organoleptic properties.[43-47] Only a few community trials have tested the acceptability of the products by mothers and children, and the impact of promotional efforts on behavior change, adoption rates, and sustainability over time.[49-52] No information was found on the impact of these interventions on the nutrient intake or the nutritional status of weaning age infants, the main target group of these interventions.

Gibson and collaborators initiated a community trial in Malawi using an integrated approach that combines a variety of the strategies described previously to increase production, intake and bioavailability of iron, zinc, and vitamin A in the diets of mothers and children.[53] The evaluation of this project will contribute immensely to our understanding of the potential of integrated food based strategies to alleviate micronutrient malnutrition in young children and mothers.

10.3.2.2   Food-to-Food Fortification (or Dietary Combinations)

Food-to-food fortification strategies to improve iron nutrition consist of dietary modifications to either include foods that can promote the absorption of nonheme iron in meals or to exclude foods that inhibit nonheme iron absorption.

10.3.2.2.1   Increasing the Intake of Enhancers of Nonheme Iron Absorption

Food-to-food fortification strategies involve increasing the intake of foods that enhance nonheme iron absorption such as ascorbic acid rich fruits and vegetables consumed at the same meal as nonheme iron food sources.[54] Meat and fish consumed even in small amounts are also known to markedly increase nonheme iron absorption. The iron bioavailability of a typical Latin American diet based on maize and beans, for example, can be improved by the same magnitude with either 75 g of meat or 50 mg of ascorbic acid.[35] The addition of small amounts of meat or fish to the diet would seem like one of the most desirable and effective approaches to increase the bioavailability of nonheme iron, but economic, cultural, or religious factors among at-risk populations in developing countries often hamper the feasibility of this approach. We are unaware of any community trial that has tested either the efficacy or the feasibility of this strategy in developing countries.

The effect of ascorbic acid to improve body iron stores has been tested in a few prospective studies summarized by Svanberg.[35] These experiments all used vitamin C supplements, as opposed to food sources of vitamin C, and thus are not considered food based approaches. A recent community trial carried out in rural Mexico tested the efficacy of adding lime juice (as a source of ascorbic acid) to a maize, beans, and salsa meal to improve iron bioavailability from the diet of nonanemic iron deficient women. The study showed that 25 mg of ascorbic acid (in the form of lemonade) consumed 2 meals a day for 8 months doubled iron absorption from the typical meal and improved iron status of the participating women, compared to a control group.[55] Effectiveness trials are needed to test whether this type of dietary modification can be sustained over time.

10.3.2.2.2   Reducing the Intake of Inhibitors of Nonheme Iron

The other dietary modification that can improve nonheme iron absorption is to reduce the intake of foods and beverages with meals that inhibit nonheme iron absorption. For instance, consumption of only one cup of tea of normal strength has been shown to reduce iron absorption by as much as 60%.[56] In Costa Rica, coffee consumption among pregnant women was associated with a lower iron status (hemoglobin) of their infants, one month after birth.[57] Foods such as oregano, red sorghum, spinach, and cocoa, which all contain galloyl phenolic groups and are known to inhibit nonheme iron absorption, should be avoided with meals containing foods of vegetable origin.[58] Again, very little experience is available to determine whether such approaches could be effective in improving iron status among poor populations in the developing world. A recent study carried out in Guatemala tested the effects of reducing coffee intake on growth, morbidity, and iron status of iron deficient toddlers.[59] Reducing coffee consumption had no impact on the iron status of young children, and only mild effects on the growth of children who previously consumed more than 100 ml of coffee per day. Evidence of the efficacy of this type of interventions in other population groups is urgently needed.

10.3.2.3   Cooking in Iron Pots

Cooking in iron pots has long been recognized as a potential way to increase the iron content of food.[60] Two recent studies, one in Brazil and one in Ethiopia, conducted experimental trials testing the effectiveness of promoting the use of iron cooking pots on the iron status of young children.[61-62] Both studies showed statistically significant improvements in hematologic values, including iron stores, over periods of 8 and 12 months in the Brazil and Ethiopia studies, respectively. The iron added to food cooked in iron pots was found to be bioavailable,[61] and the laboratory segment of the Ethiopian study found five times more available iron in meat and vegetables cooked in an iron pot compared to the same meal cooked in an aluminum pot. Iron pots appear to be a relatively low cost and possibly sustainable approach to increase the iron intake and status of deficient populations (at least of young children).

10.3.3   CONCLUSIONS ABOUT STRATEGIES TO INCREASE THE BIOAVAILABILITY AND RETENTION OF MICRONUTRIENTS DURING PROCESSING

This review highlights two contrasting facts. On the one hand, it is clear that the technologies exist to address some of the main concerns about the bioavailability of vitamin A and iron. Many of these technologies seem to involve simple and probably low cost home processing techniques, which in some cases are even part of the traditional background of the target populations. On the other hand, it is striking to see how little has actually been done to promote, implement, or evaluate the available technologies in community trials or in large scale interventions. It is not clear why this is the case, but surely, the scarcity of funding for research and implementation in this area has been a main constraint.

10.4   PLANT BREEDING STRATEGIES

The possibilities of improving micronutrient nutrition through plant breeding are numerous. They range from: (1) increasing the concentration of minerals (iron or zinc) or vitamins (beta-carotene), (2) reducing the amount of antinutrients such as phytic acid; and (3) raising the levels of sulfur containing acids, which are believed to promote the absorption of zinc. The potential nutritional benefits of each of these approaches are summarized below and a brief update on progress is presented. More detailed information can be found in the literature.[63-65]

10.4.1   INCREASING THE MINERAL OR VITAMIN CONCENTRATION OF STAPLE CROPS

Staple crops provide a large proportion of the daily intake of energy and other nutrients, including micronutrients, among poor populations who have limited access to animal foods.[66-67] The main sources of iron in these populations are staple cereals, starchy roots, tubers, and legumes and are in nonheme iron form and have low bioavailability.[68] Estimates indicate that cereals contribute up to 50% of iron intakes among households from lower socioeconomic groups.[65] For zinc, the contribution from nonanimal sources was found to be as high as 80% among preschoolers in Malawi.[67] This means that doubling the iron or zinc density of food staples could increase total intakes by at least 50% assuming that the percent absorption remains constant. This, however, may not be the case because of the large amounts of phytic acid contained in diets based on nonanimal staples. Human bioavailablility studies are urgently needed to determine the net increase in absorbed minerals that can be achieved from mineral dense staple foods.

To date, most of the progress in developing mineral dense staple crops has been in the screening for genetic variability in concentration of trace minerals. All crops tested (wheat, maize, rice, and beans) have shown significant genotypic variation, up to twice that of common cultivars for minerals (zinc and iron, in particular), and even greater variation was found for beta-carotene in cassava (a plant often used as source for tapioca). Positive correlations between mineral concentrations were found, which means that varieties with greater iron concentration were most likely to contain greater concentrations of zinc. Increasing seed ferritin is another plant breeding approach that is currently being investigated to increase the content of bioavailable iron in plants.[69] The approach seems promising because ferritin is the common source of stored iron in seeds and developing plants; ferritin iron appears to be highly bioavailable.[69] Genetic engineering experiments are being conducted with rice to simultaneously increase its concentration of vitamin A and iron.[70] Although encouraging, this area of research is still at early stages of development.

10.4.2 REDUCING THE PHYTIC ACID CONCENTRATION IN THE PLANT

A complementary approach to increasing the concentration of minerals in plants is to act directly on their main inhibitor of absorption, phytic acid. Research has shown that minimal amounts of phytic acid added to meals can produce a severe inhibition of nonheme iron absorption.[71] Although studies do not agree on the exact cut-off point where nonheme iron is significantly improved by removal of phytic acid, some found that almost complete removal (<10 mg/meal) was necessary,[72] or that levels as low as 50 mg of phytic acid caused a 78 to 92% reduction in nonheme iron absorption.[73] A key issue is whether plant breeding can achieve the magnitude of reduction in phytic acid that may be necessary to obtain significant improvements in absorption of both zinc and nonheme iron. If, as suggested by Raboy,[74] phytic acid in staple foods can be reduced by a factor of two-thirds, and if dietary phytic acid comes mainly from staple foods, it is likely that this strategy would impact bioavailability of zinc and iron simultaneously, and potentially calcium, manganese, magnesium, and other trace minerals.

A small pilot study measured iron absorption from a low phytate maize that contained approximately 35% of the phytic acid content of regular varieties. The concentration of macronutrients and minerals in the low phytate mutant remained unchanged compared to traditional varieties.[75] Iron absorption among 14 nonanemic men was almost 50% greater from the low phytic maize compared to the traditional maize. These results are encouraging for populations that consume maize based diets, efforts to reduce even further the phytic acid content of staple cereals are under way.

10.4.3   INCREASING THE CONCENTRATION OF PROMOTER COMPOUNDS (SULFUR CONTAINING AMINO ACIDS)

Another potentially complementary approach to increase the bioavailability of minerals in staple crops is to increase the concentrations of specific amino acids that are thought to promote their absorption. These are sulfur containing amino acids, namely methionine, lysine, and cysteine. There is little information about the agronomic advantages or disadvantages to increasing the concentration of sulfur containing amino acids in staple foods. In terms of nutrition, it seems that the magnitude of the increase in amino acid concentration needed to positively affect the bioavailability of iron or zinc may be small, and therefore, unlikely to affect plant functions significantly.[76]

10.4.4   CONCLUSIONS ABOUT PLANT BREEDING APPROACHES

The involvement of agricultural research in the fight against micronutrient malnutrition holds great promise. Because trace minerals are important not only for human nutrition, but for plant nutrition as well, plant breeding has the potential to make a significant, low cost,[64] and sustainable contribution to reducing micronutrient, particularly mineral deficiencies, in humans and may have important spin-off effects for increasing farm productivity in developing countries. There is increasing evidence that because iron, zinc, and provitamins A have such important synergies in absorption, transport, and function in the human body, maximum impact could be achieved by enhancing all three nutrients simultaneously.[77-78] The genetic resources needed to meet this challenge are available and research is ongoing to unveil the most promising alternatives.

10.5   CONCLUSIONS AND RECOMMENDATIONS FOR FUTURE RESEARCH

Probably the most recurrent question raised throughout this review is what can be achieved through food based approaches for reducing micronutrient malnutrition. This is true for both iron and vitamin A and would most likely be true for other micronutrients as well. It is clear that the various strategies reviewed are at different stages of development, and that experience and progress with vitamin A and iron for reduction of micronutrient malnutrition differs. The question of the efficacy and of the effectiveness of food based approaches remains largely unanswered, despite that some strategies such as home gardening for vitamin A deficiency have been extremely popular and have been implemented in a large number of countries for decades. A summary of current knowledge relative to the efficacy and the effectiveness of the food based strategies reviewed is presented in Tables 10.2 and 10.3 for vitamin A and iron, respectively. The research needed to improve our understanding of the potential of food based approaches for the alleviation of vitamin A and iron deficiency is summarized in this table (in italic).

It is clear from Table 10.2 that plant breeding strategies are still at a very early stage compared to other approaches. Information is not yet available on their potential efficacy and effectiveness and human bioavailability studies are needed to understand their full potential. Research in this area, however is well justified, because plant breeding strategies have a great potential to improve the dietary quality of populations relying mainly on cereal staples. The main benefit of these approaches is that they may not require any behavioral change on the part of the consumer if new varieties are similar to traditional varieties in organoleptic characteristics. This eases one of the main constraints of most food-based approaches.

Until a few years ago, the potential for plant sources to control vitamin A deficiency was assumed, based on calculations made using the conventional bioconversion factor that was applied to all beta-carotene sources.[79] It was estimated that families needed to cultivate only a small plot to grow enough vegetables to meet their daily requirements.[12] It was assumed that increasing provitamin A intake through home gardening would be both efficacious and feasible. The recent controversy suggesting that carotenes have much lower bioavailability than previously assumed[26,80-82] however challenges these estimates and raises fundamental questions regarding the potential efficacy of all plant based strategies to control vitamin A deficiency. Research needs to be initiated to revise the bioconversion factors and the concentration of bioavailable vitamin A in different foods. Epidemiological well controlled trials are also needed to establish what can be achieved by dietary modifications and how to maximize impact. For example, which products should be promoted, in what amounts, for how long, and what are the roles of various factors at the host level (such as age, health, nutritional status, and parasites) and at the food level (food matrix, food processing, and composition of the diet) that affect the bioavailability of provitamin A?

At the same time, evidence continues to accumulate about the effectiveness of well designed and carefully implemented strategies promoting the intake and/or production of provitamin A rich foods using social marketing and behavioral change approaches. Although evaluation designs are often weak and, thus, do not allow firm conclusions about impact, there is certainly a consistent trend indicating a positive association between these interventions and vitamin A intake and status. It may be that publication bias is playing a role, in the sense that only positive studies make it to the published literature, but there are also some examples of nonconclusive results in studies that have weaker designs. Information about the efficacy of food based approaches is lacking, but we believe that well designed food based approaches play an important role in the control of vitamin A deficiency.

A similar gap in information exists for iron relative to the potential efficacy of food based approaches relying on plant foods to improve iron status. For nonheme iron, however, there is a lot more pessimism than for provitamin A, because the bioavailability of nonheme iron is low and plant based diets have such high concentrations of inhibitors of absorption. Relative to the efficacy of animal foods, these

TABLE 10.2
Summary of Information Gaps and Research Needs (in italic) Relative to the Efficacy and Effectiveness of Food-Based Approaches to Improve Vitamin A Intakes and Status

Strategy/Efficacy-Effectiveness	Production/Education Strategies to Increase Supply and Intake	Processing Techniques to Increase Bioavailability	Plant Breeding Strategies
	Efficacy		
1. Under ideal conditions, can it improve vitamin A status?	Previous calculations using conventional bioconversion factors established amounts of vegetables/fruits needed to meet daily requirements. Recent efficacy trials challenge these estimates, showing smaller effects than expected and suggesting that beta-carotene in plants is less bioavailable than previously thought.	Same questions as for production/education interventions.	No information available.
	Continued research is needed to revise bioconversion factors for different foods; new efficacy trials are needed to re-establish efficacy of plant foods in improving vitamin A status of different vulnerable groups.	*Same research needs as production/education strategies.*	*More plant breeding research needed. Human bioavailability trials needed.*
2. What are the ideal conditions necessary to improve vitamin A status? How much is needed? Of which product? For how long? Which other factors need to be taken into account?	Research is currently being done in this area. Current information suggest that: A) Bioavailability may be different in children and mothers B) Parasites need to be controlled C) Fat needs to be present in the diet D) Bioavailability may be greater in fruits than in dark green leafy vegetables	Same questions as for production/education interventions.	No information available.
A) At the host level (parasites, age, nutrition, health status) B) At the food level (food matrix, food preparation, composition of the diet)	*Continued research is needed to determine how various host and food factors affect bioavailability of carotenoids and what are the conditions that can maximize efficacy of interventions based on plant food sources.*	*Same research needs as production/education strategies.*	*Same as above.*

TABLE 10.2 (continued)
Summary of Information Gaps and Research Needs (in italic) Relative to the Efficacy and Effectiveness of Food-Based Approaches to Improve Vitamin A Intakes and Status

Strategy/Efficacy-Effectiveness	Production/Education Strategies to Increase Supply and Intake	Processing Techniques to Increase Bioavailability	Plant Breeding Strategies
	Effectiveness		
1. What impact do these interventions have in real life conditions?	Although evaluation designs are often weak, various production/education strategies have demonstrated an impact on a variety of outcomes, including vitamin A intake and status.	No information was found on effectiveness of these types of interventions to improve vitamin A status.	No information available.
	Well-designed, prospective evaluation studies are needed to look at the impact of different intervention approaches on all outcomes that may be affected. Evaluations need to carefully monitor mechanisms, long-term impacts, cost and sustainability.	*Research is needed to understand potential effectiveness of techniques such as solar drying, leaf concentrates.*	*Research in this area is still premature.*
2. What elements of these interventions are necessary to achieve impact?	Strong education components seem to be essential for interventions to increase production or intake, although this has not been tested formally.	No information	No information available.
	Many strategies use integrated approaches, that seem to be successful, but this does not allow us to disentangle the effects of specific components.		
	Research is needed to evaluate the contribution of various components of the intervention packages to the impact and to establish best intervention packages for particular situations.	*Same as above*	*Same as above.*

TABLE 10.3
Summary of Information Gaps and Research Needs (in italic) Relative to the Efficacy and Effectiveness of Food-Based Approaches to Improve Iron Intakes and Status

Strategy/Efficacy-Effectiveness	Production/Education Strategies to Increase Supply and Intake	Processing Strategies to Increase Bioavailability	Plant Breeding Strategies
		Efficacy	
1. Under ideal conditions, can it improve iron status?	Plant foods: There are serious doubts about the potential efficacy of improving iron status through the promotion of plant based foods only. *The potential to improve iron status through plant based strategies needs to be assessed. Perphaps a combination of production, education, and methods to increase bioavailability would be efficacious.* Animal foods: Evidence exists from developed countries that animal food consumption improves and can maintain adequate iron status.	Food processing: Information exists on their impact on the bioavailability of iron in food. Their potential impact on iron status is not known. Food-to-food fortification: There is some evidence of efficacy of lemon juice to improve iron status. *More research is needed on the efficacy of these strategies to improve iron status.*	Small efficacy trial tested the impact of low phytate maize on iron absorption. Efficacy trial the impact of iron dense rice on iron status of women is about to start in the Philippines. *More plant breeding research is needed as well as human bioavailability trials.*
2. What are the ideal conditions necessary to improve iron status? How much is needed? Of which product? For how long? Which other factors need to be taken into account? A) At the host level (parasites, age, nutrition, health status)	Plant foods: None of these questions has been formally addressed. Animal foods: It is not clear how much of different animal products would be needed to improve iron status of different groups.	Food processing strategies: No information. Food-to-food fortification: One pilot study shows amount of lime juice and duration of intervention that could improve ferritin levels of women.	No information available.

TABLE 10.3 (continued)
Summary of Information Gaps and Research Needs (in italic) Relative to the Efficacy and Effectiveness of Food-Based Approaches to Improve Iron Intakes and Status

Strategy/Efficacy-Effectiveness	Production/Education Strategies to Increase Supply and Intake	Processing Strategies to Increase Bioavailability	Plant Breeding Strategies
B) At the food level (food preparation, diet composition (absorption inhibitors, promotors)	*Efficacy trials are needed to answer these questions for plant and animal foods and for different age and physiological status groups. For animal foods, minimal requirements to improve and/or maintain iron status should be established because of issue of cost.*	*Research is needed on doses, levels, specific aspects of these strategies that will provide 'ideal' conditions for efficacy*	*Same as above.*
Effectiveness			
1. What impact do these interventions have under real life conditions?	Plant foods: No evidence of impact on iron of any plant based strategies only production/education interventions. *Effectiveness trials of plant based strategies should be carried out once efficacy trials have established their potential for impact.* Animal foods: Although evaluation designs are often weak, a few recent production/education strategies have demonstrated an impact on iron status.	Food processing: Some community trials show feasibility of implementing these interventions, but no information on impact on iron status. Food-to-food fortification: No information available.	No information available.

TABLE 10.3 (continued)
Summary of Information Gaps and Research Needs (in italic) Relative to the Efficacy and Effectiveness of Food-Based Approaches to Improve Iron Intakes and Status

Strategy/Efficacy-Effectiveness	Production/Education Strategies to Increase Supply and Intake	Processing Strategies to Increase Bioavailability	Plant Breeding Strategies
	Well designed, prospective evaluation studies are needed to look at the impact of different intervention approaches on all outcomes that may be affected. Evaluation should monitor mechanisms, long term impacts, cost, and sustainability.	*Need effectiveness trials to determine potential of these approaches to achieve impact and to be sustainable.*	*Research in this area would be premature until efficacy is demonstrated.*
2. What elements of these interventions are necessary to achieve impact?	Animal foods: A strong education component will be necessary to promote increased intake of animal products. Production alone is not sufficient to achieve greater dietary diversity and it remains to be seen whether education can overcome economic constraints related to consumption of animal products	No information.	No information available.
	Evaluation research should specifically address the issue of affordability of animal products, the trade-offs between increased income from the production and sale of products, and improved household dietary quality.		*Research in this area would be premature until efficacy is established.*

products can improve absorption of nonheme iron and maintain iron status at least among certain population groups. The exact amounts of different foods required and the frequency of intake needed, however, are not well documented. Efficacy trials to determine the minimum requirements of animal products to control iron deficiency among different age and physiological status groups are needed to determine whether this is an area that should be pursued. The main concern about promoting animal products to improve iron status is their prohibitive cost for most of the populations affected by the deficiency. More information about the minimum amounts of animal products required to complement a plant based diet to achieve a net amount of absorbed iron would be the first step in assessing the chances of success of such approaches. The few studies that have looked at the effectiveness of promoting the production of animal products have encountered the predictable problem that increased income resulting from adoption may not result in improved dietary quality.[13,27] The promotion of increased intake of lower cost sources of animal foods such as liver and entrails has been successful in Lima with the community kitchen project[21] and the approach should be considered in other contexts. Additional limitations of interventions that promote animal products, are that cultural and religious factors often prohibit their inclusion in the diet of the most at-risk populations.

Although much is known about various processing techniques and food combinations and their effects on increasing the bioavailability of nonheme iron, little information exists in the literature on the efficacy of these approaches for the control of iron deficiency. Very little has been done to look at the feasibility and effectiveness of promoting the necessary behavioral changes to reduce the intake of inhibitor compounds or to increase the intake of promoters with meals. Some of these approaches may not be successful, especially long term, because they often require behavioral changes of strongly entrenched cultural practices. Research should address both the feasibility of modifying specific practices and what changes are necessary to achieve improvement in iron bioavailability that will make a difference for iron status.

In conclusion, our review suggests that food-based approaches have been increasingly active over the past few decades and have led to significant improvements relative to the design and implementation of strategies. This work has been largely driven by nongovernmental organizations and other local institutions, and has mainly targeted vitamin A deficiency. The area, however, has been dramatically neglected by the research community and by donor agencies interested in nutrition, communication, and agriculture research. This gap prevents further progress because even the most basic information is lacking for advocacy purposes, to stimulate interest, or to generate funds for research and implementation programs. Without the fundamental demonstration of efficacy, it will be difficult to motivate investment in sophisticated effectiveness and evaluation trials. Another problem is the complexity of food based approaches, which often involve a set of integrated strategies and a variety of inputs and outcomes to be measured. This makes evaluation designs complex and costly. Food-based approaches need to be revisited and they need to be treated with scientific rigor. They represent an essential part of the long term global strategy for the fight against micronutrient malnutrition and their real potential needs to be explored.

REFERENCES

1. Food Agriculture Organization of the United Nations) and International Life Sciences Institute, *Preventing Micronutrient Malnutrition: A Guide to Food-Based Approaches, A Manual for Policy Makers and Programme Players*, Washington, D.C., 1997.
2. Peduzzi, C., *Home and Community Gardens Assessment Program Implementation Experience: The Tip of the Iceberg,* Vitamin A Field Support Project, Rep. No. TA-2, ISTI, Washington, D.C., 1990.
3. Soleri, D., Cleveland, D. A., and Wood, A., Vitamin A Nutrition and Gardens Bibliography, Vitamin A Field Support Project, Rep. No. IN-1, ISTI, Washington, D.C., 1991.
4. Soleri, D., Cleveland, D. A., and Frankenberger, T. R., *Gardens and Vitamin A: A review of Recent Literature,* Vitamin A Field Support Project, Rep. No. IN-2, ISTI, Washington, D.C., 1991.
5. Gillespie, S. and Mason, J., Controlling vitamin A deficiency, Nutrition Policy Discussion Paper No. 14, United Nations/Administrative Committee on Coordination/Subcommittee on Nutrition, Geneva, 1994.
6. Solon, F., Fernández, T. L., Latham, M. C., and Popkin, B. M., An evaluation of strategies to control vitamin A deficiency in the Philippines, *Am. J. Clinical Nutr.,* 32, 1445, 1979.
7. *A Study on Evaluation of Home Gardening Program in Bajura and Mahottari Districts,* Cooperative for Assistance and Relief Everywhere (CARE), Katmandu, Nepal, September 1995.
8. Greiner, T. and Mitra, S. N., Evaluation of the impact of a food-based approach to solving vitamin A deficiency in Bangladesh, *Food Nutr. Bull.,* 16 (3), 1995.
9. English, R., Badcock, J., Giay, Tu, Ngu, Tu, Waters, A-M., and Bennett, S. A., Effect of nutrition improvement project on morbidity from infectious diseases in preschool children in Vietnam: comparison with control commune, *Br. Med. J.,* 315 (7116), 122, 1997.
10. English, R. and Badcock, J., A community nutrition project in Viet Nam: Effects on child morbidity, *Food Nutr. Agric.,* 22, 15, 1998.
11. Home Gardening in Bangladesh: Evaluation report, Helen Keller International/Asian Vegetable Research and Development Center, Bangladesh, 1993.
12. Marsh, R., Building on traditional gardening to improve household food security, *Food Nutr. Agric.,* 22, 4, 1998.
13. International Food Policy Research Institute, *Commercial Vegetable and Polyculture Fish Production in Bangladesh: Their Impacts on Income, Household Resource Allocation, and Nutrition,* Rep., Vol. 1, Royal Veterinary and Agricultural University, Bangladesh, November 1998.
14. Brun, T., Reynaud, J., and Chevassus-Agnes, S., Food and nutritional impact of one home garden project in Senegal, *Ecol. Food Nutr.,* 23, 91, 1989.
15. Ensing, B. and Sangers, S., Home Gardening in a Sri Lankan Wet Zone Village: Can It Contribute to Improved Nutrition, manuscript, Wageningen, The Netherlands, 1986, 41.
16. Pollard, R., *The West Sumatra Vitamin A Social Marketing Project,* Department of Health Indonesia and HKI Rep., 1989.
17. Smitasiri, S., Attg, G. A., Valyasevi, A., Dhanmitta, S., and Tontisirin, K., *Social Marketing Vitamin A Rich Foods in Thailand, a Model Nutrition Communication for Behavior Change Process,* Salaya, Thailand, Institute of Nutrition, Mahidol University, Thailand, 1993.

18. Smitasiri, S. and Dhanamitta, S., *Sustaining Behavior Change to Enhance Micronutrient Status: Community- and Women-Based Interventions in Thailand,* Opportunities for Micronutrients Intervention (OMNI) Research Rep. Series No. 2, International Center for Research on Women, Washington, D.C., 1999.

19. Smitasiri, S., Sa-ngobwarchar, K., Kongpunya, P., Subsuwan, C., Banjong, O., Chitchumroonechokchai, C., Rusami-Sopaporn, W., Veeravong, S., and Dhanamitta, S., Sustaining behavioral change to enhance micronutrient status through community- and women-based interventions in north-east Thailand: Vitamin A, *Food Nutr. Bull.,* 20 (2), 243, 1999.

20. de Pee, S., Bloem, M. W., Satoto, Yip, R., Sukaton, A., Tjiong, R., Shrimpton, R., Muhilal, and Kodyat, B., Impact of a social marketing campaign promoting darkgreen leafy vegetables and eggs in Central Java, Indonesia, *Int. J. Vitam. Nutr. Res.,* 68, 389, 1998.

21. Carrasco-Sanez, N. C., deUbillas, R. M. D., Guillén, I. S., and Ferreira, S. M., *Increasing Women's Involvement in Community Decision-Making, A Means to Improve Iron Status,* OMNI Research Rep. Series No. 1, International Center for Research on Women, Washington, D.C., 1998.

22. Hagenimana, V., Anyango Oyunga, M., Low, J., Njoroge, S. M., Gichuki, S. T., and Kabira, J., *Testing the Effects of Women Farmers' Adoption and Production of Orange-Fleshed Sweet Potatoes on Dietary Vitamin A Intake in Kenya,* OMNI Research Rep. Series No. 3, International Center for Research on Women, Washington, D.C., 1999.

23. Ayalew, W. Z., Wolde, G., and Kassa, H., *Reducing Vitamin A Deficiency in Ethiopia: Linkages with a Women-Focused Dairy Goat Farming Project,* OMNI Research Rep. Series No. 4, International Center for Research on Women, Washington, D.C., 1999.

24. Cohen, N., Jalil, M. A., Rahman, H., Matin, M. A., Sprague, J., Islam, J., Davidson, J., Leemhuis de Regt, E., and Mitra, M., Landholding, wealth and risk of blinding malnutrition in rural Bangladeshi households, *Soc. Science Med.,* 21(11), 1269, 1985.

25. Yip, R., Iron Deficiency: contemporary scientific issues and international programmatic approaches, *J. Nutr.,* 125, 1479S, 1994.

26. de Pee, S. and West, C. E., Dietary carotenoids and their role in combating vitamin A deficiency: a review of the literature, *Eur. J. Clinical Nutr.,* 50 (Suppl.), S38, 1996.

27. Ahmed, M. M., Ehui, S., and Jabbar, M., Household level economic and nutritional impact of market-oriented dairy production in the Ethiopian highlands, presented at the IRRI/IFPRI Workshop on: Improving Human Nutrition through Agriculture: the Role of International Agricultural Research, Los Baños, Philippines, October 5 to 7, 1999.

28. Rodríguez-Amaya, D. B., *Carotenoids and Food Preparation: the Retention of Provitamin A Carotenoids in Prepared, Processed, and Stored Foods,* OMNI Project, John Snow, Inc., Washington, D.C., 1997.

29. Solomons, N. W. and Bulux, J., Identification and production of local carotene-rich foods to combat vitamin A malnutrition, *Eur. J. Clinical Nutr.,* 51 (Suppl. 4), S39, 1997.

30. International Vitamin A Consultative Group, Toward Comprehensive Programs to Reduce Vitamin A Deficiency, XV International Vitamin A Consultative Group Meeting, Arusha, Tanzania, March 8 to 12, 1993.

31. Cox, D. N., Rajasuriya, S. V., Soysa, P. E., Gladwin, J., and Ashworth, A., Problems encountered in the community-based production of leaf concentrate as a supplement for pre-school children in Sri Lanka, *Int. J. Food Sci. Nutr.,* 44, 123, 1993.

32. Allen, L. H. and Ahluwalia, N., *Improving Iron Status through Diet. The Application of Knowledge Concerning Dietary Iron Bioavailability in Human Populations,* OMNI Project, John Snow, Inc., Washington, D.C., 1997.

33. Miller, D. D., Effects of cooking and food processing on the content of bioavailable iron in foods, in *Micronutrient Interactions: Impact on Child Health and Nutrition*, International Life Sciences Institute Press, Washington, D.C., 1996, 58.

34. Gibson, R. S. and Ferguson, E. L., Food processing methods for improving the zinc content and bioavailability of home-based and commercially available complementary foods, in *Micronutrient Interactions: Impact on Child Health and Nutrition*, International Life Sciences Institute Press, Washington, D.C., 1996, 50.

35. Svanberg, U., Dietary interventions to prevent iron deficiency in preschool children, in *Iron Interventions for Child Survival*, Nestel, P., Ed., USAID, OMNI, and ICH, London, 1995.

36. Lorenz, K., Cereal sprouts: composition, nutritive value, food applications, *CRC Crit. Rev. Food Sci. Nutr.*, 13, 353, 1980.

37. Chavan, J. K. and Kadam, S. S., Nutritional improvement of cereals by fermentation, *CRC Crit. Rev. Food Sci. Nutr.*, 28 (5), 349, 1989.

38. Camacho, L., Sierra, C., Campos, R., Guzmán, E., and Marcus, D., Nutritional changes caused by germination of legumes commonly eaten in Chile, *Arch. Latinoam. Nutr.*, 42, 283, 1992.

39. Sandberg, A. S. and Svanberg, U., Phytate hydrolysis in cereals: effects on *In Vitro* estimation of iron availability, *J. Food Sci.*, 56, 1330, 1991.

40. Marfo, E. K., Simpson, B. K., Idowu, J. S., and Oke, O. L., Effect of local food processing on phytate levels in cassava, cocoyam, yam, maize, sorghum, rice, cowpea, and soybean, *J. Agric. Food Chem.*, 38, 1580, 1990.

41. Cheryan, M., Phytic acid interactions in food systems, *CRC Crit. Rev. Food Sci. Nutr.*, 13, 297, 1990.

42. O'Dell, B. L. O., de Bowland, A. R., and Koirtyohann, S. R., Distribution of phytate and nutritionally important elements among the morphological components of cereal grains, *J. Agric. Food Chem.*, 20, 718, 1972.

43. Gopaldas, T., Mehta, P., Patil, A., and Gandhi, H., Studies on reduction in viscosity of thick rice gruels with small quantities of an amylase-rich cereal malt, *Food Nutr. Bull.*, 8, 42, 1986.

44. Mosha, A. C. and Svanberg, U., Preparation of weaning foods with high nutrient density using flour of germinated cereals, *Food Nutr. Bull.*, 5(2), 10, 1990.

45. Hansen, M., Pedersen, B., Munck, L., and Eggum, B. O., Weaning foods with improved energy and nutrient density prepared from germinated cereals. 1. Preparation and dietary bulk of gruels based on barley, *Food Nutr. Bull.*, 11(2), 40, 1989.

46. Pedersen, B., Hansen, M., Munck, L., and Eggum, B. O., Weaning foods with improved energy and nutrient density prepared from germinated cereals, 2. Nutritional evaluation of gruels based on barley, *Food Nutr. Bull.*, 11(2), 46, 1989.

47. Singhavanich, C., Jittinandana, S., Kriengsinyos, W., and Dhanamitta, S., Improvement of dietary density by the use of germinated cereals and legumes, *Food Nutr. Bull.*, 20(2), 261, 1999.

48 Brown, K. H. and Bégin, F., Malnutrition among weanlings of developing countries: still a problem begging for solutions, *J. Pediatric Gastroenterol. Nutr.*, 17, 132, 1993.

49. Vaidya, Y., Weaning foods in Nepal, in *Improving Young Child Feeding in Eastern and Southern Africa*, Alnwick, D., Moses, S., and Schmidt, O. G., Eds., International Development Research Center, Ottawa, 1988.

50. Gopaldas, T., Deshpande, S., Vaishnav, U., Shah, N., Mehta, P., Tuteja, S., Kanani, S., and Lalani, K., Transferring a simple technology for reducing the dietary bulk of weaning gruels by an amylase-rich food from laboratory to urban slum, *Food Nutr. Bull.*, 13(4), 318, 1991.

51. Guptil, K. S., Esrey, S. A., Oni, G. A., and Brown, K. H., Evaluation of a face-to-face weaning food intervention in Kwara State, Nigeria: knowledge, trial, and adoption of a home prepared weaning food, *Soc. Sci. Med.*, 36, 665, 1993.

52. Kibona, N., Doland, C., Watson, F. E., Alnwick, D., and Tomkins, A., An evaluation of a project to improve child nutrition in Tanzania, *Int. J. Food Sci. Nutr.*, 46, 233, 1995.

53. Gibson, R. S., Yeudall, F., Drost, N., Mtitimuni, B., and Cullinan, T., Dietary interventions to prevent zinc deficiency, *Am. J. Clinical Nutr.*, 68 (Suppl.), 484S, 1998.

54. Monsen, E. R., Iron nutrition and absorption: dietary factors which impact iron bioavailability, *J. Am. Diet. Assoc.*, 88, 786, 1988.

55. García, O. P., Díaz, M., Rosado, J. L., and Allen, L. H., Community trial of the efficacy of lime juice for improving iron status of iron deficient Mexican women, *FASEB J.*, 12 (5), A647, 1998.

56. Disler, P. B., Lynch, S. R., Charlton, R. W., Torrance, J. D., and Bothwell, T. H., The effect of tea on iron absorption, *Gut*, 16,193, 1975.

57. Muñoz, L. M., Lönnerdal, B., Keen, C. L., and Dewey, I. G., Coffee consumption as a factor in iron deficiency anemia among pregnant woman and their infants in Costa Rica, *Am. J. Clinical Nutr.* 48, 645, 1988.

58. Gibson, R. S., Technological approaches to combating iron deficiency, *Eur. J. Clinical Nutr.*, 51, (Suppl. 4), S25, 1997.

59. Dewey, K. G., Romero-Abal, M. E., Quan de Serrano, J., Bulux, J., Peerson, J. M., Engle, P., and Solomons, N., A randomized intervention study of the effects of discontinuing coffee intake on growth and morbidity of iron-deficient Guatemalan toddlers, *J. Nutr.*, 127, 306-313, 1997.

60. Brittin, H. C. and Nossaman, C. E., Iron content of food cooked in iron utensils, *J. Am. Diet. Assoc.*, 86, 897, 1986.

61. Borigato, E. V. M. and Martínez, F. E., Iron nutritional status is improved in Brazilian preterm infants fed food cooked in iron pots, *J. Nutr.*, 128, 855, 1998.

62. Adish, A. A., Esrey, S. A., Gyorkos, T. W., Jean-Baptiste, J., and Rojhani, A., Effect of consumption of food cooked in iron pots on iron status and growth of young children: a randomised trial, *Lancet*, 353, February, 1999.

63. Graham, R. D. and Welch, R. M., Breeding for Staple Food Crops with High Micronutrient Density, Working Papers on Agricultural Strategies for Micronutrients No. 3, International Food Policy Research Institute, Washington, D.C., April 1996.

64. Ruel, M. I. T. and Bouis, H. E., Plant breeding: a long-term strategy for the control of zinc deficiency in vulnerable populations, *Am. J. Clinical Nutr.*, 68(2-S), 1998.

65. Bouis, H., Enrichment of food staples through plant breeding: a new strategy for fighting micronutrient malnutrition, *Nutr. Rev.*, 54,131, 1996.

66. Allen, L. H., Backstrand, J. R., Chávez, A., and Pelto, G. H., Functional Implications of Malnutrition, Final Report, Mexico Project, Mexico, 1992.

67. Ferguson, E. L., Gibson, R. S., Thompson, L. U., and Ounpuu, S., Dietary calcium, phytate, and zinc intakes and the calcium, phytate, and zinc molar ratios of the diets of a selected group of East African children, *Am. J. Clinical Nutr.*, 50, 1450, 1989.

68. Gibson, R., Zinc nutrition in developing countries, *Nutr. Res. Rev.*, 7, 151, 1994.

69. Theil, E. C., Burton, J. W., and Beard, J. L., A Sustainable solution for dietary iron deficiency through plant biotechnology and breeding to increase seed ferritin control, *Eur. J. Clinical Nutr.*, 51, S28, 1997.

70. Ye, X., Al-Bbili, S., Kloti, A., Zhang, J., Lucca, P., Beyer, P., Potrykus, I., Engineering the provitamin A (beta-carotene) biosynthetic pathway into (carotenoid-free) rice endosperm, *Science*, January 14; 287:303, 2000.

71. Sandström, B. and Lönnerdal, B., Promoters and antagonists of zinc absorption, in *Zinc in Human Biology. Human Nutrition Reviews,* Mills, C. F., Ed., Springer-Verlag, U.K., 1989, 57.

72. Hurrell, R. G., Juillerat, M.-A., Reddy, M. B., Lynch, S. R., Dassenko, S. A., and Cook, J. D., Soy protein, phytate, and iron absorption in humans, *Am. J. Clinical Nutr.,* 56, 573, 1992.

73. Reddy, M. B., Hurrell, R. F., Juillerat, M. A., and Cook, J. D., The influence of different protein sources on phytate inhibition of nonheme-iron absorption in humans, *Am. J. Clinical Nutr.,* 63, 203, 1996.

74. Raboy, V., Cereal low phytic mutants: a global approach to improving mineral nutritional quality, *Micronutrients Agric.,* 2, 15, 1996.

75. Mendoza, C., Viteri, F. E., Lönnerdal, B., Young, K. A., Raboy, V., and Brown, K. H., Effect of genetically modified, low-phytic acid maize on absorption of iron from tortillas, *Am. J. Clinical Nutr.,* 68, 1123, 1998.

76. Welch, R. M., The optimal breeding strategy is to increase the density of promoter compounds and micronutrient minerals in seeds; caution should be used in reducing anti-nutrients in staple food crops, *Micronutrients Agric.,* 1, 20, 1996.

77. Graham, R. D. and Rossner, J. M., Carotenoids in staple foods: Their potential to improve human nutrition, presented at the IRRI/IFPRI Workshop on: Improving Human Nutrition through Agriculture: the Role of International Agricultural Research, Los Baños, Philippines, October 5 to 7, 1999.

78. García-Casal, M. N., Layrisse, M., Solano, L., Barón, M. A., Arguello, F., Llovera, D., Ramírez, J., Leets, I., and Tropper, E., Vitamin A and β-carotene can improve nonheme iron absorption from rice, wheat and corn by humans, *J. Nutr.,* 128: 646, 1998.

79. Florentino, R. F., Pedro, M. R. A., Candelaria, L. V., Ungson, B. D., Zarate, R. U. Jr., et al., *An Evaluation of the Impact of Home Gardening on the Consumption of Vitamin A and Iron Among Preschool Children,* Vitamin A Field Support Project, Rep. No. IN-17, ISTI, Washington, D.C., 1993, 52.

80. de Pee, S., West, C. E., Muhilal, Karyadi, D., and Hautvast, G. A. J., Can increased vegetable consumption improve iron status? *Food Nutr. Bull.,* 17 (1), 34, 1996.

81. de Pee, S., Bloem, M. W., Gorstein, J., Sari, M., Satoto, Yip, R., Shrimpton, R., and Muhilal, Reappraisal of the role of vegetables in the vitamin A status of mothers in Central Java, *Am. J. Clinical Nutr.,* 68, 1068, 1998.

82. Jalal, F., Nesheim, M. C., Agus, Z., Sanjur, D., and Habicht, J. P., Serum retinol concentrations in children are affected by food sources of β-carotene, fat intake, and anthelminthic drug treatment, *Am. J. Clinical Nutr.,* 68, 623, 1998.

11 Public Health Measures to Control Helminth Infections

Andrew Hall, Lesley Drake, and Don Bundy

CONTENTS

11.1 INTRODUCTION

Iron deficiency anemia is probably the most widespread and intractable micronutrient deficiency in the world today and is a major public health problem for people living in developing countries. The cause of iron deficiency anemia is usually complex and multifactorial but several types of parasitic worms can make a significant contribution, usually by causing a loss of blood. This review will concentrate on these parasitic worms, usually called parasitic helminths by parasitologists, or simply helminths. The first section will describe the most important features of the biology and life cycles of these helminths and show how they can contribute to anemia. The second section will discuss the epidemiology of helminth infections and identify characteristics that influence whether and to what degree they contribute to anemia. The final section will describe the short and long term measures that can help to prevent the transmission of helminths, as well as provide guidance on how control measures can be assessed.

11.2   THE WORMS AND THEIR CONTRIBUTION TO ANEMIA

Over 300 species of worms have been recorded as being associated with human beings but only about 20 are common enough to infect more than 5 million people.[1] Several of these species cause the most common infectious diseases in the world today;[2] six of them cause losses of blood. The names and characteristics of these helminths are summarized in Table 11.1.

11.2.1   Hookworms

The first major group comprises the hookworms, *Ancylostoma duodenale* and *Necator americanus*, which are typically dealt with together because they have similar life cycles and habits, and because the eggs of the two species cannot be distinguished when examining feces under a microscope. For this reason, it is necessary to culture stools and identify the characteristic larvae or to expel worms from the gut using an anthelminthic drug and then recover them from the feces. Both methods are time consuming, difficult, and impractical.

Hookworms are soil transmitted nematode worms and it is estimated that 1.3 billion people are infected by them.[2] When a mature female is fertilized by a male, she produces 3000 to 6000 eggs per day by *N. americanus* and 10 to 20,000 eggs per day by *A. duodenale*,[3] a difference which adds complexity to examining the association between fecal egg counts and hemoglobin concentration. Hookworm eggs are excreted in the feces and take a minimum of 5 days to develop into infectious larvae. This means that freshly passed feces are not immediately infectious to humans. This is important when considering control measures.

The number of hookworm eggs excreted by an infected individual is typically proportional to the number of worms in the burden, although the fecundity of worms may be reduced by the presence of other worms (density dependent fecundity). The eggs mature and hatch in warm and humid conditions and can live for several weeks if the environmental conditions are right.[4] When a mature larva on the ground comes into contact with human skin, it penetrates the skin and makes its way through the blood stream to the lungs, where it is coughed up and swallowed. The worm attaches itself to wall of the duodenum or jejunum and uses sharp plates or teeth in its buccal cavity to cut into tissues. The worms' powerful pharynx then sucks up blood and tissue fluids. Hookworms have a requirement for blood, or at least find blood to be an ideal food, because they secrete an anticoagulant.[5] When the worm detaches from the gut wall and moves to a new site, which it may do several times a day, the anticoagulant causes the site to continue bleeding, thereby exacerbating the blood lost during its feeding.[6]

It has been estimated that a single *A. duodenale* worm is responsible for the loss of 0.15 ml/day of blood and for *N. americanus*, a loss of 0.03 ml/day,[7] a five-fold difference. This means that 25 *A. duodenale* worms or 110 *N. americanus* worms

TABLE 11.1
The Important Characteristics of the Parasitic Worms that Contribute to Iron Deficiency Anemia in Humans

	Ancylostoma duodenale and Necator americanus	Trichuris trichiura	Schistosoma mansoni	Schistosoma japonicum	Schistosoma haematobium
Common name	Hookworm	Whipworm			
Name of disease	Hookworm disease	Trichuriasis	Bilharzia or schistosomiasis	Bilharzia or schistosomiasis	Bilharzia or schistosomiasis
Distribution	Global but largely in tropics and subtropics	Global but largely in tropics and subtropics	Africa, Middle East, South America	Asia	Africa and Middle East
Estimated number of people infected (millions)	1277[a]	902[a]	69[b]	95[b]	100[b]
Intermediate host	None	None	Freshwater snails	Freshwater snails	Freshwater snails
Infective stage	Larva in soil	Mature egg on soil	Miracidium in water for snails; cercaria in water for humans	Miracidium in water for snails; cercaria in water for humans	Miracidium in water for snails; cercaria in water for humans
Means of infection	Through skin[c]	Orally	Through skin when bathing or wading	Through skin when bathing or wading	Through skin when bathing or wading
Site of adult worm	Attached by mouth to small intestine	Head embedded in large intestine	In blood vessels around intestine	In blood vessels around intestine	In blood vessels around urinary bladder
Cause of blood lost	Worm feeding and bleeding from site of attachment	Worm feeding, inflammation, and dysentery	Bleeding into small intestine caused by passage of eggs; dysentery	Bleeding into small intestine caused by passage of eggs; dysentery	Bleeding into bladder by passage of spined eggs
Diagnosis	Eggs in feces[d]	Eggs in feces	Eggs in feces	Eggs in feces	Eggs in urine; blood in urine

[a] Source: Chan, M.-S., The global burden of intestinal nematode infections — fifty years on, Parasitology Today, 13, 438, 1997.

[b] Source: Warren, K.S., Bundy, D. A. P., Anderson, R. M., Davis, A. R., Jamison, D. T., Prescott, N., and Senft, A., Helminth infection, Disease Control Priorities in Developing Countries, Jamison, D. T., Moseley, W. H., Measham, A. R., and Bobadilla, J. L., Eds., Oxford Medical Publications, Oxford, 1993, 131.

[c] It is thought that the larvae of Ancylostoma duodenale can also infect humans when swallowed.

[d] The eggs of the two species cannot be distinguished under a microscope.

would cause a loss of about 5 ml/day of blood containing 1.85 mg iron.[7] The differences between species in the volume of blood loss suggests that the distribution of each hookworm may influence the prevalence of anemia. A study in schools in Zanzibar has provided epidemiological evidence for this: the percentage of school children with anemia was about 20% higher in schools where the prevalence of *A. duodenale* was higher than *N. americanus*.[8] Such an effect is likely to be site specific.

In general, both hookworm species are said to occur together although *N. americanus* may prevail in the tropics and subtropics while *A. duodenale* tends to occur in cooler and drier climates.[7] Hookworm can also occur in warm places in cold climates, such as mines and tunnels. When the St. Gotthard Tunnel was dug under the Swiss alps in 1879, indiscriminate defecation by miners underground led to an epidemic of hookworm disease. Hundreds of men died and there were thousands of cases of severe anemia.[9]

Hookworms contribute to such anemia by several mechanisms. The first is by feeding on blood, probably very wastefully, because like most intestinal parasites they are in contact with unlimited supplies of food and do not need to use an aerobic metabolism.[10] Second, as already mentioned, the sites where the worms were attached to the gut continue to bleed after the worms have moved, as a result of the persistent effects of the anticoagulants they secrete. Third, hookworms live and feed in the duodenum and jejunum, the same sites where most iron is absorbed[11] and may thus impair uptake. Fourth, moderate to heavy burdens may impair the appetite.[12,13] And finally, in a vicious cycle, the anemia to which hookworms contribute may reduce human productivity which may in turn affect the quality and quantity of nutrients such as iron in the diet.

Several studies have looked at the association between hookworm infections and anemia and many of them have been reviewed periodically over the last 30 years.[14-16] Most age groups are affected. Studies have shown a significant association between hookworm and anemia among school age children, adolescents, and adults.[17-19] Hookworm is, however, not usually a cause of iron deficiency anemia among children under 5 years of age because they tend to be lightly infected. Nevertheless, moderately to heavily infected preschool children on the coast of Kenya (among whom the prevalence of infection was only 29%) have been found to have significantly lower hemoglobin concentrations than uninfected children.[20] Such cross-sectional data cannot reliably be interpreted in terms of cause and effect, however, and both worms and anemia are associated with poverty.

An analysis of several studies of the relationship between hookworm egg counts and hemoglobin concentrations has provided more convincing evidence of the strength of an association. The analysis has used the relationship to try to determine where hookworm anemia is a public health problem in East Africa.[21] The relationship between the concentration of hookworm eggs in feces (an indicator of the number of worms in the intestine) and the hemoglobin concentration varies among study sites.[21,22] This suggests that other factors influence the relationship, indicating that it is site specific.

Hookworm anemia is characterized by hypochromic microcytic erythrocytes and is typically of the iron deficiency type.[14] This has been shown by a number of studies in which subjects infected with hookworms were treated only with iron and their hemoglobin concentrations were shown to recover to normal within a few weeks. The response to deworming alone was much slower and took 12 to 18 months to achieve the same improvement in hemoglobin as seen with iron alone, indicating the important role of dietary iron in recovery.[14] When supplementary iron is given, other diseases or dietary deficiencies may influence recovery. A study in Tanzania in which ferrous sulphate was given to children after anthelminthic treatment, showed that hemoglobin concentrations were simply sustained rather than improved. Children who received no treatment showed declines in their hemoglobin concentrations.[22] Sustaining hemoglobin concentration can be an important achievement, especially during pregnancy. In a randomized trial in Sierra Leone, women infected with hookworms who were given anthelminthics at the end of the first trimester of their pregnancies had hemoglobin concentrations nearly 7 g/L higher on average than untreated controls. Women who were given ferrous sulphate had hemoglobin concentrations that were nearly 14 g/L higher than the controls.[23] Although the effects were additive for the group which received both albendazole and iron, the treatments only sustained the initial hemoglobin concentration while the hemoglobin concentrations of women who were not treated fell significantly during the study.

When compared with cross-sectional investigations, there have been relatively few studies on the impact of anthelminthic treatment on anemia or its effects on physical fitness and productivity. A study of schoolchildren on the coast of Kenya showed that treating hookworm infections led in 7 weeks to an improvement in scores on the Harvard Step test.[24] A school based program in Zanzibar showed that the risk of moderate to severe anemia was associated with moderate to severe hookworm infections,[25] that 73% of severe anemia was attributable to hookworm,[26] and that mass treatment reduced the risk of severe cases of anemia, although it had no effect on the overall prevalence of anemia. These studies used a relatively low threshold of 110 g/L to define anemia but reported a very high prevalence of anemia of 62%.[26] Although an attributable fraction analysis indicated that hookworms contributed to this anemia, it is also likely that the very low iron content of the diet of people living along the East African coast is a major factor contributing to the anemia.[18] The study which looked at the impact of iron supplements after albendazole and praziquantel treatment of schoolchildren and found negligible improvement[22] also suggests that other factors may be limiting hemopoiesis, such as malaria or other micronutrient deficiencies. Giving vitamin A in addition to iron to pregnant women in Indonesia, led to a one-third greater improvement in hemoglobin response of 3.7 g/L than giving daily iron doses alone.[27]

These studies indicate that although hookworm infection can cause significant blood loss that contributes to anemia, removing hookworms or giving ferrous sulphate does not automatically lead to a rapid recovery. Multiple micronutrient supplements may be required to achieve recovery.

11.2.2 *Trichuris trichiura*

The other ubiquitous species of intestinal nematode associated with anemia is *Trichuris trichiura*, the whipworm. It is estimated that 900 million people in the world are infected.[2] Like hookworms the whipworm also has a direct, soil transmitted life cycle but, in this case, the eggs transmitted in human feces simply develop in warm and humid conditions and become infectious in 2 to 3 weeks.[3] When a mature egg is swallowed, perhaps in contaminated food or from dirty fingers, the larva hatches in the gut and then penetrates the wall of the large intestine. After several stages of maturation, the worm develops a filamentous anterior end, which remains embedded in the gut wall, while the thicker posterior end is eventually pushed into the intestinal lumen. The worm secretes a pore forming protein that is believed to create a syncitial tunnel that serves two purposes, to help anchor the worm and provide lysed cells to consume.[28] The damage to the mucosa and its blood vessels in heavy infections is reflected by chronic colitis, mucosal hemorrhaging, dysentery and, occasionally, rectal prolapse.[29]

It is possible that worms consume blood as a part of their food intake but it seems more likely that the greatest loss of blood occurs as a result of dysentery and damage to the mucosal epithelium.[29] Because the blood is lost into the large bowel, it is probable that none of the iron in hemoglobin can be reabsorbed from the gut. It has been estimated that the blood loss is of the order of 0.005ml per worm per day[30] and therefore only heavy infections will contribute to anemia. For example, a study in Jamaica found that only children with >10,000 *T. trichiura* eggs/g of feces had significantly lower hemoglobin concentrations than uninfected children.[31] A similar cross-sectional study in Panama found that low hemoglobin concentrations in children were associated with >5000 *T. trichiura* eggs/g of feces and that children concurrently infected with moderate to heavy hookworm were even more anemic.[32] These two studies illustrate that there may not be a consistent relationship between the intensity of a single helminth species and lowered hemoglobin concentrations, and that it is typical to find that more than one helminth contributes to anemia in a population.

11.2.3   SCHISTOSOMA SPECIES

Three major species of trematode blood flukes of the genus *Schistosoma* are associated with blood loss: *Schistosoma mansoni*, *S. japonicum*, and *S. haematobium*. The distribution of these worms has been quite well mapped and shows that *S. mansoni* and *S. haematobium* occur in Africa and the Middle East; *S. mansoni* has a similar distribution to *S. haematobium* but also occurs in eastern South America; and *S. japonicum* occurs mostly in China and the Philippines (Table 11.1).[33] Two other species are also parasites of humans but they are uncommon and highly focal in their geographical distribution: *S. mekongi*, found on the borders of Laos and Thailand, and *S. intercalatum*, found in Central Africa.[33] It is estimated that 100 million people are infected with *S. haematobium* and that 70% of the cases occur in sub-Saharan Africa. Some 70 million people are infected with *S. mansoni*, and 95 million with *S. japonicum*.[34]

All species of schistosomes have an indirect life cycle in which an infective egg excreted from the human host hatches when it comes into contact with fresh water, and the larva, called a miracidium, penetrates a particular species of snail.[3] It is the specificity of the parasite for the snail intermediate host that largely governs the distribution of this genus of helminths, not the distribution of the definitive human host. The larva multiplies asexually within the snail's digestive gland and eventually releases thousands of infective stages into fresh water. These cercariae are typically released in greatest numbers around midday, the period when humans are most likely to be in contact with water. When a cercaria comes into contact with human skin it attaches and rapidly burrows through the tissue into the blood stream.

The adult male and female worms of *S. mansoni* and *S. japonicum* live in the mesenteric blood vessels around the intestine while *S. haematobium* lives in blood vessels around the bladder.[35] The disease due to these worms and the blood loss they cause is largely due to the parasite's eggs, although the adults in the blood stream feed on blood and erythrocytes. In order to get their eggs into the gut or bladder and to the outside world, depending on the species, female schistosomes release their eggs into the smallest blood vessels they can reach, so that many eggs become wedged there. The presence of sharp spines on the eggs of *S. haematobium* and *S. mansoni* help to cut through tissue, and when an egg is forced into the gut or bladder lumen, the site of penetration then bleeds. The blood lost due to *S. haematobium*, called hematuria, can turn the urine pink or even red, although blood is typically usually seen in the last few drops. Untypically for a helminth, the symptoms of urinary schistosomiasis are specific enough to estimate the prevalence among schoolchildren: a questionnaire has been used to identify schools where the disease is a problem[36] and where mass treatment would be warranted according to WHO recommendations.[37] This questionnaire has also been shown, in Tanzania at least, as a way of providing selective treatment to children. When asked whether they currently had schistosomiasis, around 75% of the children were correct in their self-diagnoses.[38]

Studies of small numbers of people have shown daily blood losses ranging between 0.5 ml and 125 ml per day; patients with severe or persistent hematuria were losing 22 ml per day.[39] Studies of schoolchildren in Niger and Kenya have found associations between the hemoglobin concentration and the intensity of infection with *S. haematobium*.[40,41] The 33 infected children studied in Kenya showed a significant linear correlation between the concentration of eggs in urine and the daily amount of iron lost ($r = 0.4$, P <0.01).[41] The study also found quite a wide variation in iron losses among children with roughly similar egg counts: from about 0.04 mg/24 h to about 1.4 mg/24 h among children who passed around 100 eggs/10 ml urine.[41] Although the bleeding into the bladder due to *S. haematobium* means that the iron is effectively lost from the body, some of the iron lost in bleeding due to *S. mansoni* and *S. japonicum* infections might be reabsorbed from the intestine. The fact that infections with *S. mansoni* are associated with dysentery[42,43] and anemia[44] suggests, however, that little digestion or absorption of blood takes place. A questionnaire about blood in the stools of schoolchildren in Tanzania has been used to try to identify schools where *S. mansoni* occurs, but was much less sensitive or specific than the questionnaire about blood in urine related to *S. haematobium* infections.[45]

11.2.4 OTHER SPECIES

An association between *Ascaris lumbricoides*, the large intestinal roundworm, and anemia has been observed in school age children in Nepal.[46] How this worm causes anemia is uncertain because the worm feeds on the gut contents rather than on blood.

It is possible that *A. lumbricoides* causes anorexia or malabsorption of iron because the worm lives in the duodenum and jejunum, the sites where iron absorption occurs.[11] A study in Indonesia indicated that treating infections from *A. lumbricoides* led to improved appetites.[47] It is also likely that infection with *A. lumbricoides* is simply associated with poverty and poor diet.

Finally, a species of tapeworm named *Diphyllobothrium latum* that can grow up to 20 m in length can cause a pernicious anemia by virtue of the fact that when present in the jejunum it selectively absorbs cyanocobalamin (vitamin B_{12}) from the gut, thus depriving the host.[48] This worm is relatively uncommon and occurs mostly in Scandinavia among people who eat uncooked fish containing an infective plerocercoid larva.

11.3   EPIDEMIOLOGY OF HELMINTHS

In order to understand how and when worms contribute to anemia and, perhaps as importantly, why and when they may not, it is useful to understand how helminth infections are acquired, how they are distributed between hosts, and what factors promote their transmission.

Worm loads are typically accumulated slowly. Each worm in a host is the result of exposure to an infective stage and, as most worms do not multiply within their hosts, moderate to heavy worm burdens typically result from exposure over long periods to many worm eggs or larvae. The disease and debilitation caused by worms tend to be gradual in onset, and chronic in duration rather than rapid and acute like most bacterial, viral, or protozoal diseases. The gradual nature of helminth disease and the fact that the symptoms are also nonspecific may mean that people are not aware of a slow loss of health and insidious debilitation.

The amount of blood lost due to worms is largely dependent on the number of worms present in the human host. Simply being infected is no guarantee of being anemic, and morbidity such as anemia is typically associated with moderate to heavy worm loads. Unless a host is extremely young or malnourished, a few worms are not likely to make a great impact on the hemoglobin concentration. The size of the worm burden is usually estimated indirectly by determining the concentration of eggs in excreta. The concentration of hookworm eggs in feces, for example, can vary from day to day within individuals by amounts that cannot be explained by dilution effects.[49] Egg counts are poor indicators of the intensity of infection for individuals. When averaged for a sample size of more than 30 subjects, egg counts can give an indication of average worm burdens in the group under study; mean egg counts for such groups are typically better predictors of hemoglobin concentration than the prevalence of infection. There may be local variations in the relationship between the hemoglobin concentration and a given concentration of eggs in feces.[21]

Worms are not uniformly or normally distributed (in the statistical sense) between hosts. They tend to be aggregated so that at any one time only a small proportion of people contain a large proportion of worms. Figures of 80% of all worms in 20% of all hosts have been cited to describe this aggregation or overdispersion of worms.[50] Quantitative studies in which burdens of *A. lumbricoides* expelled after treatment have been counted indicate that the degree of aggregation of worms tends to decline exponentially above a prevalence between 50 and 60%, so that above prevalence of 80% for example, 80% of worms may occur in 50% of hosts.[51] The aggregated distribution of worms means that not all infected people will benefit to the same extent from treatment, whether benefits are measured in terms of hemoglobin concentration, weight gain, or any other parameter. The minority of moderately or heavily infected people will probably benefit most.[52]

Over the short term the benefits of treating these people may tend to be lost in the group mean. In the long term, however, evidence from studies of reinfection with *Ascaris lumbricoides* indicates that a larger proportion of people may become heavily reinfected than cross-sectional data would suggest[53] so that any benefit is likely to be cumulative. This has important consequences for studies that attempt to evaluate the effectiveness of measures to control helminths. Long term follow up is likely to be required to detect an impact on a public health scale. It also means that repeated treatment is needed in helminth control programs to sustain low worm burdens.

The scale of the public health problem due to worms such as hookworm and *Trichuris trichiura* is worth considering. Even if only 1% of infections caused disease, 13 million people infected with hookworm and 9 million people infected with *T. trichiura* would experience morbidity. In 1995, the WHO estimated that hookworm caused clinical symptoms in 96 million people and *T. trichiura* in 133 million, while hookworm killed 90,000 people.[54] Although the proportion of infected people who experience disease may be small, the absolute numbers are large.

It is difficult to predict from the prevalence of infection how many people may be moderately to heavily infected. Figure 11.1 shows how the relationship between the prevalence of infection with hookworm and the mean concentration of hookworm eggs in feces varies among samples of about 50 children studied in each of 39 primary schools in Tanzania. The fitted curve is exponential ($y = 41.963e^{0.0394x}$, $r = 0.86$, $P < 0.001$) and shows how above a 50% prevalence egg counts rise steeply, but the vertical scatter of points above this threshold is quite large. This increase is typical of most intestinal nematodes. Theoretical studies using different thresholds of worm burden have shown that morbidity is also likely to increase exponentially above a prevalence around 50%.[55] Even though a prevalence of infection up to 50% may seem to be quite high, prevalences lower than this are associated with low average worm burdens, although a few individuals might be moderately to heavily infected. A large impact on the population as a whole of measures to control intestinal helminths is much less likely when the prevalence is <50% than when the prevalence is >50%, or unless control measures are implemented for a long enough period for the impact to be detected.

The prevalence and intensity of infections vary with age and occupational risks and may thus have a greater impact on specific groups. For example, school age children tend to harbor the heaviest infections with species of schistosomes, *A. lumbricoides* and *Trichuris trichiura*. Figure 11.2A shows that the prevalence of infection with *T. trichiura* rises rapidly with age in a poor urban community in Bangladesh so that around 90% of people aged 3 years and above are infected. In contrast, the intensity of infection estimated by the concentration of eggs in feces shown in Figure 11.2B has a distinct peak among children aged 5 to 15 years old.

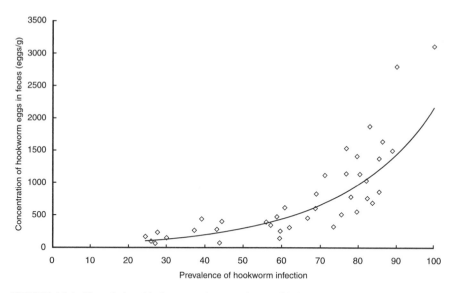

FIGURE 11.1 The relationship between the prevalence of infection with hookworms and the concentration of eggs and feces of samples of about 50 children per school in 39 schools in Tanga Region, Tanzania.

The fact that school age children have the heaviest infections could occur because it takes until late adolescence to develop a degree of immunity which protects them against heavy infections; and/or their behavior puts them at particular risk of infection. School age children are particularly vulnerable to the effects of such moderate to heavy burdens of helminths because infections occur at a time when the chidren are growing and learning rapidly and have an increasing physiological demand for iron. The heaviest infections with hookworms, in contrast, tend to occur in adolescents and adults, and therefore may make an important contribution to anemia among women of reproductive age. Very young children tend to be lightly infected with hookworm if the worm is endemic but may acquire infections with *A. lumbricoides* and *Trichuris trichiura* at a very early age, so treating them is often justified, anyway.

Some occupational risks, particularly those involving contact with water in sub-Saharan Africa, expose people to infection with schistosomes. For example, adolescent fisherboys in Ghana have been found to be more heavily infected with *Schistosoma haematobium* and consequently more anemic than boys of the same age who are enrolled in school.[56]

The duration of infection is likely to be an important factor in determining the severity of anemia, in addition to the intensity of infection. Worms can live for several years: the life expectancy of *T. trichiura* is 1 to 2 years, hookworms live for 2 to 3 years, and *S. haematobium* and *S. mansoni* for 3 to 5 years.[50] Although Figure 2A presents cross-sectional data it also suggests that most people are chronically infected for their entire lives. The duration of infection and its contribution to a disease such as iron deficiency anemia is difficult to quantify but, if nothing

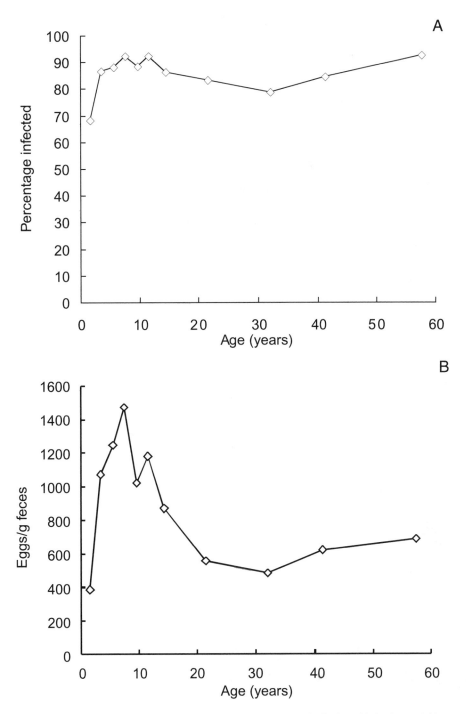

FIGURE 11.2 (A) The relationship between age and the prevalence of infection with *Trichuris trichiura* in people living in Dhaka, Bangladesh. (B) The relationship between age and the concentration of *T. trichiura* eggs in feces, an indicator of the intensity of infection in the same subjects.

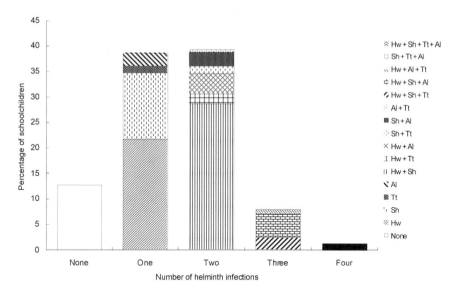

FIGURE 11.3 The percentage of children uninfected or infected with one or more helminth infections among 1900 children in schools in Tanga Region, Tanzania. Hw = hookworm; Sh = *Schistosoma haematobium*; Tt = *Trichuris trichiura*; Al = *Ascaris lumbricoides*.

else changes, it seems reasonable to assume that moderate infections can contribute to anemia.

It is important to appreciate that polyparasitism is the rule rather than the exception. In many parts of the world, people may be concurrently infected with hookworms, other nematodes, and perhaps one or both species of *Schistosoma* as well. For example, Figure 11.3 shows the percentage of nearly 2000 schoolchildren in rural Tanzania who had zero to four infections with either hookworm (overall prevalence = 65%), *S. haematobium* (54%), *A. lumbricoides* (17%), and *T. trichiura* (10%). Nearly half of all subjects were infected with two or more parasites; 37% had hookworm and *S. haematobium*, both of which contribute to anemia; and 83% had hookworm or *S. haematobium*. These children also lived in an area where malaria was holoendemic, and chronic *Plasmodium* infections can also contribute to anemia.

This complex mixture of epidemiological factors creates a situation in which it is difficult to predict for individuals, let alone for the community as a whole, the contribution that helminths make to iron deficiency anemia without trying to account for the influence of iron stores and dietary iron intake. A considerable body of evidence indicates that helminths contribute to iron deficiency anemia in a number of ways and with varying consequences.

11.4   PUBLIC HEALTH STRATEGIES TO CONTROL THE HELMINTHS THAT CONTRIBUTE TO ANEMIA

The target of many 20th century disease control programs has been to eradicate infectious agents. The successful campaign to eradicate smallpox, the unsuccessful malaria eradication program of the 1960s, and the current annual efforts in all developing countries to vaccinate young children against polio are good examples of this target. Such a target may, however, have created something of an unreasonable expectation as far as many parasitic worms are concerned. This has led to pessimism about the prospects of eradication in the face of a number of other factors including the lack of naturally acquired protective immunity to helminth infections, the failure to develop protective vaccines against helminths for humans, the rapidity of rein-fection after treatment, and the general persistence of infections in the community. This pessimism is probably unwarranted because, where parasitic worms are con-cerned, it is largely a result of the failure to distinguish between the infection and disease, or the failure to understand how targeted control measures can contribute to preventing transmission as well as disease. As noted earlier, light infections with helminths are rarely very harmful, and *it is* the moderate to heavy infections *that* cause disease and probably contribute most to sustaining the transmission of the parasite. There is a growing realization, based on the practical experience of large scale programs, that measures directed at communities where moderate to heavy infections are most common can make a significant impact on health and reduce transmission. The target of helminth control programs is thus becoming the control of disease rather than eradicating the worms. This section will describe various strategies to control helminth disease and discuss how to evaluate these programs.

The strategies to control helminth infections can be divided into two types: short to medium term interventions such as periodic chemotherapy that can bring direct relief from disease, promote child development, and help slow transmission; and long term programs such as vector control, water and sanitation measures, or health education to change behavior that will help to prevent transmission. Table 11.2 summarizes the relevance of these options related to the major species of helminths that contribute to anemia.

11.4.1   Short Term to Medium Term Measures

To a great extent, the success of measures to control anemia caused by helminths will depend on having the tools to do so and developing simple and effective mechanisms to use them. The development of safe and highly effective single dose drugs to treat helminths has provided such tools so that the emphasis over the last few years has been to promote policies that encourage control efforts and to foster research to develop strategies to deliver those treatments effectively to communities at the lowest possible cost. A description of the drugs — usually called anthelminthics — may be useful.

Controlling diseases caused by helminths, such as iron deficiency anemia, has been greatly facilitated by the development of effective and safe single dose treat-ments. Two benzimidazole drugs, albendazole and mebendazole, are effective against all the major intestinal nematodes including *A. lumbricoides*, *T. trichiura*, and the hookworms; praziquantel is effective against all three major species of schistosomes. The fact that these drugs can be given as a single dose is a boon for compliance with treatment, and the safety of the drugs means that mass treatment — treatment without prior diagnosis — is now recommend by the WHO as the best strategy for helminth control programs.[57]

TABLE 11.2
A Summary of Measures to Control Parasitic Helminth Infections that Contribute to Iron Deficiency Anemia

Category and Type of Control Measure	Species of Helminths			
	Hookworms[a]	*Trichuris trichiura*	*Schistosoma mansoni* or *S. japonicum*	*Schistosoma haematobium*
Vector Control				
Killing snails	X	X	✔	✔
Sanitation and Hygiene				
Safe disposal of feces	✔	✔	✔	X
Safe disposal of urine	X	X	X	✔
Clean water for bathing	X	X	✔	✔
Behavior Change/Education				
Wearing shoes	✔	X	X	X
Handwashing before eating	X	✔	X	X
Bathing in clean water	X	X	✔	✔
Chemotherapy				
Single dose drugs	Benzimidazoles[b]	Benzimidazoles[b]	Praziquantel	Praziquantel
Priority target groups	Adolescents and women	School age children	School age children	School age children
Frequency of treatment	6–12 months	6–12 months	12–24 months	12–24 months

[a] *Necator americanus* and *Ancylostoma duodenale*
[b] Albendazole and mebendazole are the most common.[58]

Note: ✔ = Appropriate; X = Not appropriate.

The two benzimidazole drugs are given as a standard dose to everyone aged 1 year or older[58,59] and can be formulated as chewable tablets or emulsions, which makes them easy for young children to take. A large trial comparing the standard dose of albendazole (400 mg) with mebendazole (500 mg) found that both drugs were highly effective against *A. lumbricoides* and cured >97% of infections; both drugs were very effective against hookworms and reduced egg counts by >80%. Albendazole was significantly more effective (97.7% vs. 82.4%, *P* <0.001) and may be preferred where hookworms occur. Both drugs were moderately effective against *T. trichiura* and reduced egg counts by 81.6% and 73.3%, respectively (*P* <0.001).[60] There is some evidence that both these benzimidazoles may be less effective against *T. trichiura* in Asia,[61] so more than one dose may be needed.[62,63] Two other drugs — levamisole and pyrantel pamoate — have also been quite widely used but, because they are less effective than the benzimidazoles against hookworm, or ineffective against *T. trichiura*, they are gradually being superseded by albendazole and mebendazole. The cost of albendazole or medendazole can be less than $0.05 (U.S.) per treatment.

All three main species of *Schistosoma* can be treated very effectively by a single dose of praziquantel but dosage has to be adjusted according to body weight with a target of 40 mg/kg body weight.[58,59] This dosage can achieve a cure rate of 60 to 90% with a reduction in egg counts of >90%.[64] The administration of praziquantel is also more complicated than treatment with benzimidazole drugs as the tablets have to be swallowed. Giving praziquantel has been made simpler for mass treatment programs in poor developing countries, by determining the dose on the basis of height rather than weight. An analysis of the relationship between the weight and height of schoolchildren in Ghana, Tanzania, and Malawi has indicated that the correlation is good enough to give the drug on the basis of height rather than weight, something that has been done for with ivermectin, a drug used to treat river blindness caused by the worm *Onchocerca volvulus*.[65] The analysis has indicated that if tablets of praziquantel weighing 600 mg are cut into quarters, then 70 to 80% of children can be given dosages to treat schistosomiasis that is within the same range that is normally given on the basis of body weight.[66] This relationship has been used during large scale school health programs in several districts of Ghana and Tanzania. Tablet poles were devised so that teachers could work out the doses of praziquantel tablets required to treat their pupils. In Mozambique, where 600 mg tablets could only be cut in half were used in a school based health program, analysis showed that over 90% of children would have received dosages within the same range normally given on the basis of body weight.

The simplicity and safety of these drugs have provided powerful tools for use in controlling disease due to helminths. A program in Tanzania in which mass treatment with albendazole and praziquantel was given by teachers to their pupils in about 150 primary schools in 3 districts, recorded an increase in hemoglobin concentrations of around 5 g/L, without iron supplementation, 15 months after treatment.[67] Large scale programs in which albendazole or praziquantel have been given to schoolchildren have also shown that treating this age group can serve to reduce the prevalence of infections among untreated members of the community.[68,69]

The recommendation by the World Health Organization for mass treatment when the prevalence of intestinal helminths or schistosomes is greater than 50%[57] is very important. This means that when the combined prevalence of *A. lumbricoides*, *T. trichiura,* and hookworms, or any one of these species separately is greater than 50%, then mass treatment without prior diagnosis is warranted. The same applies to the species of schistosomes. From a nutritional perspective, the ACC/SCN recommended that priority be given to deworming programs if parasites are widespread and more than 25% of children are underweight.[70]

The WHO recommendation[57] is based on sound epidemiological principles, such as making schoolchildren the principal targets of control programs.[71] It also recognizes the trade offs between the costs of diagnosis and the costs of mass treatment, and the fact that the benzimidazole drugs and praziquantel are very safe, and can be given to uninfected people without harm. "Mass treatment" means treatment of people without prior diagnosis and can be "universal" by which all members of the community are treated, or "targeted" to specific groups in the community such as schoolchildren.[72]

The WHO has also supported randomized trials in China, Kenya, and the Philippines, which have shown that it is safe to use albendazole and praziquantel together.[73] Consequently, the coadministration of either albendazole or mebendazole and praziquantel is now recommended.[57] This simplifies treatment considerably as these drugs no longer have to be given a week apart. School age children are a particular focus of many programs delivering both these treatments because they tend to be the most heavily infected members of the community. The prevalence of infection in schoolchildren can also be used to estimate the prevalence in adults,[74] so a survey of infections in schoolchildren, an easily accessible group, can be used to assess the prevalence in the whole community.

Because school age children bear a large burden of disease due to helminths and because in many countries they are accessible while they attend schools, there has been considerable interest in providing periodic anthelminthic treatment in schools. In 1993, the World Bank identified such school health services as one of five potentially cost effective public health interventions,[75] a theoretical analysis that has since been confirmed by cost analyses of school based programs in Ghana and Tanzania.[76,77] These programs have provided mass treatment with albendazole and praziquantel to children in schools, using a number of strategies to keep the process simple.

First, a parasitological survey in a small sample of schools was done in each district to confirm that the prevalence of intestinal worms was greater than 50% and that mass treatment with a benzimidazole drug was warranted. This is based on the understanding that within the same environment the distribution of intestinal worms is similar and fairly uniform. If several different environments exist within a region or district, schools in each should be sampled. A 5% sample of schools or a minimum of 5 schools and 50 children per school is usually sufficient. The Kato-Katz smear is the recommended diagnostic technique.[78]

Second, a questionnaire can be used to identify schools where mass treatment for urinary schistosomiasis, caused by *Schistosoma haematobium*, is required. The distribution of urinary schistosomiasis can be quite focal because it is dependent on the presence of freshwater for the survival of the snail intermediate host. The symptoms of urinary schistosomiasis are specific and include pain when urinating, lower abdominal pain, and blood visible in urine. Research in several countries in Africa has indicated that the prevalence of disease reported by schoolchildren is highly correlated with the actual prevalence of infection.[36] This means that the questionnaire can be used to identify schools where mass treatment is required. In Tanzania, for example, a prevalence of reported schistosomiasis of 25% was found to be equivalent to a 50% prevalence of infection.[79]

The questionnaire approach has also been evaluated for *Schistosoma mansoni* in Tanzania but with less success in terms of the sensitivity and specificity of diagnosis. Blood in urine reported by schoolchildren was strongly associated with infection with *S. haematobium* (odds ratio 7.71, P ≤0.001) whereas the association between reported blood in stools and infection with *S. mansoni* was only weakly significant (OR 1.62, P = 0.045).[45] The difference is probably because blood is only seen in the feces when infections are very heavy, whereas blood is seen in urine in moderate to heavy infections and is associated with symptoms, such as pain when urinating, that are more specific.

By these simple techniques, a small survey of intestinal worms in schoolchildren and a questionnaire survey in schoolchildren about the symptoms of urinary schistosomiasis, decisions can be made about the need for mass treatment with a benzimidazole drug that can be co-administered with praziquantel. School based health programs in Tanzania and Ghana have used the educational infrastructure to deliver anthelminthics to children in several hundred schools in each country. Teachers have administered the drugs with technical supervision from local health center staff, using poles marked with the number of tablets to determine the dosage of praziquantel. An analysis of the costs of these programs has shown that albendazole and praziquantel can be given at a cost per child of around $1.00 to $1.50 (U.S.), and that the use of proprietary drugs constituted about 70% of these amounts, so there are considerable possibilities for savings.[76,77] Several other countries in sub-Saharan Africa including Malawi, Mozambique, and Guinea, are establishing similar programs to treat intestinal helminths and schistosomiasis. In Indonesia and Viet Nam, teachers have given albendazole alone to children.

There is less practical research on control programs delivering anthelminthics to other groups such as pregnant women and young children, but these groups are targets for treatment according to UNICEF[80,81] and the WHO.[82] The findings of the study in Sierra Leone described earlier (Section 11.1)[23] and in Sri Lanka in an area where hookworm was common, suggested that giving mebendazole in addition to iron to pregnant women after the first trimester of pregnancy[83] can have a significant effect in reducing anemia. Although a large scale cross-sectional study did not show any evidence of congenital birth defects among mothers who had taken mebendazole during or after the first trimester of pregnancy,[84] anthelminthic treatment is still not recommended before the end of the first trimester.[58] Treating children aged 1 to 5 years, or until the age when they enter school, is also recommended.[80] The WHO/UNICEF program on the integrated management of childhood illness (IMCI) recommends giving children anthelminthics if hookworm or whipworm are problems in the locality and if the children are 2 years old and have not received treatment in the last 6 months.

11.4.2 LONG TERM MEASURES

Because the infective stages of all the major helminths that contribute to anemia (see Table 2) are expelled from the infected host in feces or urine, the disposal of human waste is a crucial point at which transmission could be broken.[85] Latrines are expensive to construct and difficult to maintain in such a manner that children will always use them. In some Asian countries human feces is a valuable resource and is used as a fertilizer — known euphemistically as "night soil." Hookworm infection in farmers is associated with the use of night soil as a fertilizer in Viet Nam,[86] another example of an occupational risk of helminth infection. Unless the feces are left to stand for at least 6 months, the eggs of some parasites will not be killed. This is typically done in double pit latrines. One pit is filled with feces over time, treated with lime, and then left to ferment — a process that kills helminth eggs.[85] Sanitation programs have shown variable successes in reducing the transmission of *A. lumbricoides*, but the evidence according to a review by Esrey and colleagues[87] is generally positive. No significant benefit was noted for hookworm, although many of the studies reviewed were deemed inadequate.[87]

Providing clean water to communities is, in theory, the ideal way to prevent people from coming into contact with schistosome cercariae, but it is very costly. The largest experiment to provide clean water was conducted in St. Lucia in the West Indies. Household water supplies, communal washing facilities, and pools for children were provided to some communities, and the incidence of new infections with *S. mansoni* was compared with communities served only by standpipes. A 75% reduction was observed.[88]

Because all species of schistosomes have an obligatory stage of development in a freshwater snail, killing snails or destroying their food or habitat can also contribute to controlling the transmission of the parasites. Snails can be killed using molluscicides, but the cost, toxicity to harmless species of snails, and the scale of the problem — particularly when snails can survive in puddles of water as well as on the shores of some of the largest lakes in the world — means that there are few successful examples of long term snail control using chemicals.[88] Irrigation schemes have been major contributors to the spread of *Schistosoma* infections and keeping waterways free of the vegetation that the snails feed upon can help prevent transmission. Yet this also has risks. The men who keep canals free of waterweeds face an occupational risk of infection with schistosomes. A study has shown that this risk can be reduced if the cleaners work in the water early in the day, before the peak release of cercariae from snails.[89]

Another component of helminth control programs, especially those that are based in schools, is health education. This is based on the view that if children wear closed shoes to avoid contact with the larvae of hookworm, wash their hands before eating to remove eggs of *T. trichiura*, and do not bathe in freshwater ponds to avoid contact with the cercariae of *Schistosoma* species, they will not be infected with these worms. Although it is axiomatic that these behaviors will prevent infection there is no evidence that such specific health education messages lead to a significant change in infection with helminths because, as far as we aware, no such trials have been published. Some of these behaviors may also be impracticable. For example, schoolteachers have a dilemma if they instruct children about the benefits of using latrines and washing their hands if their schools do not have latrines or running water.

The ideal method of providing long term protection against helminth infections and reducing transmission is an effective vaccine. Although worms stimulate antibody production in humans, the responses do not seem to protect against reinfection. It seems that most helminth infections of humans have developed mechanisms to evade the immune response and there is no evidence of fully protective immunity.[90] It is possible that an immune response develops over time as a result of long term exposure to worms and this response acts to reduce the intensity of reinfection, but it is very hard to disassociate such an effect from differences among people in their exposure to infection.

The development of an immune response that protects against superinfection could explain why the intensity of infection is lower among adults than it is in children (see Figure 11.2B). The lower intensity could also be a result of changes in exposure to infection with age as a result of better personal hygiene. Evidence indicates that treating schistosome infections can accelerate the development of an acquired immune response, perhaps because when worms die in the blood stream after praziquantel treatment, they release antigens that stimulate the production of antibodies.[91] Whether this is protective has not been assessed and assessment will be difficult. Several groups are working on potential vaccines against schistosomes and hookworms but none has yet produced sterilizing immunity.

11.4.3 EVALUATING MEASURES TO CONTROL PARASITIC INFECTIONS

Because the prevalence of infection is a poor and insensitive indicator of the intensity of infection and morbidity, it is also a poor indicator of the impact of a control program. A prevalence of 50% infection to determine need for mass treatment was simply chosen because above this threshold the chance that moderate to heavy infections will occur increases exponentially. Studies of reinfection after mass treatment have shown that the prevalence of infection can rebound rapidly, but that the intensity of infection takes longer to return to the levels that existed before treatment.[53] The prevalence of infection may give a false picture of the lack of impact of a program. It is therefore better to assess the intensity of infection through parameters such as the concentrations of eggs in feces.[92]

The immediate impact of treatment can be measured in terms of the egg reduction rate, which is the concentration of eggs in feces 21 days after treatment expressed as a percentage of the initial concentration.[72] This assessment may not be needed in terms of assessing the efficacy of the drug, except perhaps in the case of *Trichuris trichiura*, because benzimidazole drugs and praziquantel are well known to be highly effective. The egg reduction rate method, however, may be useful to assess the possible development of drug resistance over several rounds of treatment. Based on evidence from theoretical studies, if mass treatment is given only to specific groups such as schoolchildren in a community, then the presence of a population of worms that is not exposed to the drug may help to prevent resistance from developing as rapidly as if universal treatment was given.[93]

Although the threshold at which mass treatment is warranted is straightforward, there is no clear and simple recommendation about how often treatment might be needed in the first few years of a program. If the rate of reinfection is being monitored to help decision making about intervals between treatments, there is also no clear guidance about when treatment should be repeated. Many programs provide annual mass treatment, but in places such as rural Zanzibar[94] and urban Bangladesh[53] where reinfection is very rapid, intestinal helminths may need to be treated twice a year in the first few years of a program. The general aim of a program should be to sustain a prevalence of infection with intestinal nematodes or schistosomes below 50%.

11.5 CONCLUSIONS

Several species of parasitic helminths cause blood losses either directly or indirectly; the hookworms (*Necator americanus* and *Ancylostoma duodenale*) and the schistosomes, particularly *Schistosoma haematobium*, make the largest direct contributions to anemia. If the loss of iron from the body due to helminths means that the net loss is greater than the amount absorbed from the diet, helminths will contribute to the development of anemia after iron stores have been exhausted. The rate at which the hemoglobin concentration falls will depend on the species of worm, the intensity of infection, and the intake and absorption of iron from the diet. A moderate infection over a long period may have the same effect as a heavy infection over a short period. Treating helminth infections can stem blood losses but the rate at which the hemoglobin concentration recovers will depend on the net intake of absorbable iron and its incorporation into hemoglobin and erythrocytes, unless iron supplements are provided and no other nutrient is lacking. The aim of helminth control programs is usually to prevent disease, such as anemia, rather than to eradicate infections; disease is typically associated with prevalences above 50%. Short term control measures such as mass treatment with anthelminthics can bring immediate relief and, if targeted at school age children, can promote child development and reduce transmission in the community as a whole. Measures such as provision of clean water, sanitation, and health education are likely to be required in the long term to sustain low levels of transmission.

ACKNOWLEDGMENTS

We thank the donors to the Partnership for Child Development including the Rockefeller Foundation, the UNDP, the Edna McConnell Clark Foundation, the Wellcome Trust, and the World Bank.

REFERENCES

1. Coombs, I. and Crompton, D. W. T., *A Guide to Human Helminths*, Taylor & Francis, London, 1991.
2. Chan, M-S., The global burden of intestinal nematode infections — fifty years on, *Parasitol. Today,* 13, 438, 1997.
3. Muller, R., *Worms and Disease,* William Heinemann Medical Books, London, 1975.
4. Smith, G., The ecology of the free-living stages: a reappraisal, in *Hookworm Disease. Current Status and New Directions,* Schad, G. A. and Warren, K. S., Eds., Taylor & Francis, London, 1990, 89.
5. Hotez, P. and Cerami, A., Secretion of a proteolytic anticoagulant by *Ancylostoma* hookworms, *J. Exp. Med.,* 157, 594, 1983.
6. Kalkofen, U. P., Intestinal trauma resulting from feeding activities of *Ancylostoma caninum. Am. J. Trop. Medical Hyg.,* 23, 1046, 1974.
7. Pawlowski, Z. S., Schad, G. A., and Stott, G. J., *Hookworm Infection and Anemia. Approaches to Prevention and Control*, World Health Organization, Geneva, 1991.

8. Albonico, M., Stoltzfus, R. J., Savioli, L., Tielsch, J. M., Chwaya, H. M., Ercole, E., and Cancrini, G., Epidemiological evidence for a differential effect of hookworm species, *Ancylostoma duodenale* or *Necator americanus*, on iron status of children, *Int. J. Epidemiol.*, 27, 530, 1998.

9. Chandler, A. C., *Hookworm Disease,* Macmillan, New York, 1929.

10. Bryant, C., Biochemistry, in *Modern Parasitology*, Cox, F. E. G., Ed., Blackwell Scientific Publications, Oxford, 1982.

11. Bothwell, T. H., Iron balance and the capacity of regulatory systems to prevent the development of iron deficiency and overload, in *Iron Nutrition in Health and Disease*, Hallberg, L. and Asp, N-G., Eds., John Libbey & Co, London, 1996.

12. Stephenson, L. S., Latham, M. C., Adams, E. J., Kinoti, S. N., and Pertet, A., Physical fitness, growth and appetite of Kenyan schoolboys with hookworm, *Trichuris trichiura* and *Ascaris lumbricoides* infections are improved 4 months after a single-dose of albendazole, *J. Nutr.*, 123, 1036, 1993.

13. Hadju, V., Stephenson, L. S., Abadi, K., Mohammed, H. O., Bowman, D. D., and Parker, R. S., Improvements in appetite and growth in helminth-infected schoolboys three and seven weeks after a single dose of pyrantel pamoate, *Parasitology,* 113, 497, 1996.

14. Roche, M. and Layrisse, M., The nature and causes of hookworm anemia, *Am. J. Trop. Med. Hyg.*, 15, 1029, 1966.

15. Crompton, D. W. T. and Whitehead, R. R., Hookworm infections and human iron metabolism, *Parasitology,* 107, Suppl. S137, 1993.

16. Stoltzfus, R. J., Dreyfuss, M. L., Chwaya, H. M., and Albonico, M., Hookworm control as a strategy to prevent iron deficiency, *Nutr. Rev.,* 55, 223, 1997.

17. Olsen, A., Magnussen, P., Ouma, J. H., Andreassen, J., and Friis, H., The contribution of hookworm and other parasitic infections to hemoglobin and iron status among children and adults in western Kenya, *Trans. R. Society Trop. Med. Hygiene*, 92, 643, 1998.

18. Tatala, S., Svanberg, U., and Mduma, B., Low dietary iron is a major cause of anemia: a nutrition survey in the Lindi District of Tanzania, *Am. J. Clinical Nutr.*, 68, 171, 1998.

19. Hopkins, R. M., Gracey, M. S., Hobbs, R. P., Spargo, R. M., Yates, M., and Thompson, R. C. A., The prevalence of hookworm infection, iron deficiency and anemia in an aboriginal community in north-west Australia, *Medical J. Aust.*, 166, 241, 1997.

20. Brooker, S., Peshu, N., Warn, P. A., Mosobo, M., Guyatt, H. L., Marsh, K., and Snow, R. W., The epidemiology of hookworm infection and its contribution to anemia among pre-school children on the Kenyan Coast, *Trans. R. Society Trop. Med. Hygiene*, 93, 240, 1999.

21. Lwambo, N. J. S., Bundy, D. A. P, and Medley, G. F. H., A new approach to morbidity risk assessment in hookworm endemic communities, *Epidemiol. Infection*, 108, 469, 1992.

22. Beasley, N. M. R., Tomkins, A. M., Hall, A., Kihamia, Lorri, W., Issae, W., Nokes, C., and Bundy, D. A. P., The impact of population level deworming on the hemoglobin levels of school children in Tanga, Tanzania, *Trop. Med. Int. Health*, 4, 744, 1999.

23. Torlesse, H., Parasitic Infection and Anemia during Pregnancy in Sierra Leone, Ph.D. Dissertation, University of Glasgow, U.K., 1999.

24. Stephenson, L. S., Latham, M. C., Kinoti, S. N., Kurz, K. M., and Brigham, H., Improvements in physical fitness of Kenyan schoolboys infected with hookworm, *Trichuris trichiura* and *Ascaris lumbricoides* following a single dose of albendazole, *Trans. R. Society Trop. Med. Hygiene*, 84, 277, 1990.

25. Stoltzfus, R. J., Albonico, M., Chwaya, H. M., Tielsch, J. M., Schulze, K. J., and Savioli, L., Effects of the Zanzibar school-based deworming program on iron status of children, *Am. J. Clinical Nutr.*, 68, 179, 1998.

26. Stoltzfus, R. J., Chwaya, H. M., Tielsch, J. M., Schulze, K. J., Albonico, M., and Savioli, L., Epidemiology of iron deficiency anemia in Zanzibari schoolchildren: the importance of hookworms, *Am. J. Clinical Nutr.,* 65, 153, 1997.

27. Suharno, D., West, C. E., Muhilal, Karyadi, D., and Hautvast, J. G. A. J., Supplementation with vitamin A and iron for nutritional anemia in pregnant women in West Java, Indonesia, *Lancet,* 342, 1325, 1993.

28. Drake, L., Korchev, Y., Bashford, L., Djamgoz, M., Wakelin, D., Ashall, F., and Bundy, D. A. P., The major secreted product of the whipworm, *Trichuris*, is a pore-forming protein, *Proc. Royal Society of London B, Biological Sciences*, 257, 255, 1994.

29. Bundy D. A. and Cooper, E. S., *Trichuris* and trichuriasis in humans, *Adv. Parasitol.,* 28, 107, 1989.

30. Layrisse, M., Aparcedo, L., Martínez-Torres, C., and Roche, M., Blood loss due to infection with *Trichuris trichiura*. *Am. J. Trop. Med. Hygiene*, 16, 613, 1967.

31. Ramdath, D. D., Simeon, D. T., Wong, M. S, and Grantham McGregor, S. M., Iron status of schoolchildren with varying intensities of *Trichuris trichiura* infection, *Parasitology*, 110, 347, 1995.

32. Robertson, L. J., Crompton, D. W. T., Sanjur, D., and Nesheim, M. C., Hemoglobin concentrations and concomitant infections of hookworm and *Trichuris trichiura* in Panamanian primary schoolchildren, *Trans. R. Society Trop. Hygiene*, 86, 654, 1992.

33. Doumenge, J. P., Mott, K. E., Cheung, C., Villenave, D., Chapuis, O., Perrin, M. F., and Reaud-Thomas, G., *Atlas of the Global Distribution of Schistosomiasis/Atlas de la Répartition Mondiale des Schistosomiases,* World Health Organization, Geneva, 1987.

34. Warren, K. S., Bundy, D. A. P., Anderson, R. M., Davis, A. R., Henderson, D. A., Jamison, D. T., Prescott, N., and Senft, A., Helminth infection, in *Disease Control Priorities in Developing Countries*, Jamison, D. T., Moseley, W. H., Meashem, A. R., and Bobadilla, J. L., Eds., Oxford Medical Publications, Oxford, 1993, 131.

35. Sturrock, R. F., The parasites and their life cycles, in *Human Schistosomiasis*, Jordan, P., Webbe, G., and Sturrock, R. F., Eds., CAB International, Wallingford, U.K., 1993.

36. Red Urine Study Group, *Identification of High-Risk Communities for Schistosomiasis in Africa: a Multi-Country Study*, Social and Economic Research Project Report No. 15, Special Programme for Research and Training in Tropical Diseases, World Health Organization, Geneva, 1995.

37. *Guidelines for the Evaluation of Soil-Transmitted Helminthiasis and Schistosomiasis at Community Level*. World Health Organization, WHO/CTD/SIP/98.1. Geneva, 1998.

38. Partnership for Child Development, Self-diagnosis as a possible basis for treating urinary schistosomiasis: a study of schoolchildren in rural Tanzania, *Bull. World Health Organ.,* 77, 477, 1999.

39. Stephenson, L. S., The impact of schistosomiasis on human nutrition, *Parasitology*, 107, Supplement S107, 1993.

40. Prual, A., Daouda, H., Develoux, M., Sellin, B., Galan, P., and Hercberg, S., Consequences of *Schistosoma haematobium* infection on the iron status of schoolchildren in Niger, *Am. J. Trop. Med. Hygiene*, 47, 291, 1992.

41. Stephenson, L. S., Latham, M. C., Kurz, K. M., Miller, D., Kinoti, S. N., and Oduori, M. L., Urinary iron loss and physical fitness of Kenyan children with urinary schistosomiasis, *Am. J. Trop. Med. Hygiene*, 34, 322, 1985.

42. Ndamba, J., Makaza, N., Kaondera, K. C., and Munjoma, M., Morbidity due to Schistosoma mansoni among sugar-cane cutters in Zimbabwe, *Int. J. Epidemiol.*, 20, 787, 1991.

43. Gryseels, B. and Polderman, A. M., The morbidity of *Schistosomiasis mansoni* in Maniema (Zaire), *Trans. R. Society Trop. Med. Hygiene*, 81, 202, 1987.

44. Sturrock, R. F., Kariuki, H. C., Thiongo, F. W., Gachare, J. W., Omondi, B. G., Ouma, J. H., Mbugua, G., and Butterworth, A. E., Schistosomiasis mansoni in Kenya: relationship between infection and anemia in schoolchildren at the community level, *Trans. R. Society Trop. Med. Hygiene,* 90, 48, 1996.

45. Booth M., Mayombana, C., Machiya, H., Masanja, H., Odermatt, P., Utzinger, J., and Kilima, P., The use of morbidity questionnaires to identify communities with high prevalences of schistosome or geohelminth infections in Tanzania, *Trans. R. Society Trop. Med. Hygiene,* 92, 484, 1998.

46. Curtale, F., Tilden, R., Muhilal, Vaidya, Y., Pokhrel, R. P., and Guerra, R., Intestinal helminths and risk of anemia among Nepalese children, *Panminerva Medica,* 35, 159, 1993.

47. Jalal, F., Effects of Deworming, Dietary Fat Intake, and Carotenoid Rich Diets on Vitamin A Status of Preschool Children Infected with *Ascaris lumbricoides* in West Sumatra Province, Indonesia, Ph.D. Dissertation, Cornell University, Ithaca, 1991.

48. Von Bonsdorff, B. and Gordin, R., Castle's test (with vitamin B_{12} and normal gastric juice) in the ileum in patients with genuine and patients with tapeworm pernicious anemia, *Acta Medica Scandinavica,* 208, 193, 1980.

49. Hall, A., Quantitative variability of nematode egg counts in faeces: a study among rural Kenyans, *Trans. R. Society Trop. Med. Hygiene,* 75, 682, 1981.

50. Anderson, R. M. and May, R. M., *Infectious Diseases of Humans,* Oxford University Press, Oxford, 1991.

51. Hall, A., Anwar, K. S., Tomkins, A., and Rahman, L., The distribution of *Ascaris lumbricoides* in human hosts: a study of 1,765 people in Bangladesh, *Trans. R. Society Trop. Med. Hygiene,* 93, 503, 1999.

52. Hall, A., Intestinal parasitic worms and the growth of children, *Trans. R. Society Trop. Med. Hygiene,* 87, 241, 1993.

53. Hall, A., Anwar, K. S., and Tomkins, A. M., The intensity of reinfection with *Ascaris lumbricoides* and its implications for parasite control, *Lancet,* 339, 1253, 1992.

54. *The World Health Report 1995. Bridging the Gaps,* World Health Organization, Geneva, 1995, p. 28.

55. Guyatt, H. L. and Bundy, D. A. P., Estimating prevalence of community morbidity due to intestinal helminths: prevalence of infection as an indicator of the prevalence of disease, *Trans. R. Society Trop. Med. Hygiene,* 85, 778, 1991.

56. Fentiman, A., Hall, A., and Bundy, D. A. P., Health and cultural factors associated with enrolment in basic education: a study in rural Ghana, *Soc. Science Med.,* in press.

57. *Health of School Children. Treatment of Intestinal Helminths and Schistosomiasis,* WHO/SCHISTO/95.112; WHO/CDS/95.1, World Health Organization, Geneva, 1995.

58. *WHO Model Prescribing Information. Drugs Used in Parasitic Diseases,* 2nd ed., World Health Organization, Geneva, 1995.

59. de Silva, N., Guyatt, H., and Bundy, D. A. P., Anthelmintics. A comparative review of their clinical pharmacology, *Drugs,* 53, 769, 1997.

60. Albonico, M., Smith P. G., Hall, A., Chwaya, H. M., Alawi, K. S., and Savioli, L., A randomised controlled trial comparing mebendazole 500 mg and albendazole 400 mg against *Ascaris, Trichuris* and the hookworms, *Trans. R. Society Trop. Med. Hygiene,* 88, 585, 1994.

61. Bennett, A. and Guyatt, H., Reducing intestinal nematode infection: efficacy of albendazole and mebendazole, *Parasitol. Today,* 16, 71, 2000.

62. Hall, A. and Nahar, Q., Albendazole and infections with Ascaris lumbricoides and Trichuris trichiura in children in Bangladesh, *Trans. R. Society Trop. Med. Hygiene,* 88, 110, 1994.

63. Abdi, Y. A., Gustafsson, L. L., Ericsson, O., and Hellgren, U., *Handbook of Drugs for Tropical Parasitic Infections*, 2nd ed., Taylor & Francis, London, 1995.

64. *The Control of Schistosomiasis*, WHO Technical Report Series 830, World Health Organization, Geneva, 1993.

65. Alexander, N. D. E., Cousens, S. N., Yahaya, H., Abiose, A., and Jones, B. R., Ivermectin dose assessment without weighing scales, *Bull. World Health Organ.*, 71, 361, 1993.

66. Hall, A., Nokes, C., Wen, S-T., Adjei, S., Kihamia, C., Mwanri, L., Bobrow, E. de Graft-Johnson, J., and Bundy, D. A. P., Alternatives to body weight for estimating the dose of praziquantel needed to treat schistosomiasis, *Trans. R. Society Trop. Med. Hygiene*, 93, 653, 1999.

67. The nutritional impact on rural Tanzania schoolchildren of mass anthelmintic treatments and health education given by teachers, Partnership for Child Development, Oxford, 1999.

68. Asaolu, S. O., Holland, C., and Crompton, D. W. T., Community control of *Ascaris lumbricoides* in rural Oyo State, Nigeria: mass, targeted and selective treatment with levamisole, *Parasitology*, 103, 291, 1991.

69. Butterworth, A. E., Sturrock, R. F., Ouma, J. H., Mbugua, G. G., Fulford, A. J., Kariuki, H. C., and Koech, D., Comparison of different chemotherapy strategies against *Schistosoma mansoni* in Machakos District, Kenya: effects on human infection and morbidity, *Parasitology*, 103, 339, 1991.

70. Tomkins, A. and Watson, F., *Malnutrition and Infection: A Review*, State-of-the-Art Series Nutrition Policy Discussion Paper No. 5, ACC/SCN, Geneva, 1989.

71. Partnership for Child Development, Better health, nutrition and education for the school-aged child, *Trans. R. Society Trop. Med. Hygiene*, 91, 1, 1997.

72. *Report of the WHO Informal Consultation on the Use of Chemotherapy for the Control of Morbidity Due to Soil-transmitted Nematodes in Humans*, World Health Organization, Geneva, 1996.

73. Olds, G. R., King, C., Hewlett, J., Olveda, R., Wu, G., Ouma, J., Peters, P., McGarvey, S., Odhiambo, O., Koech, D., Liu, C. Y., Aligui, G., Gachihi, G., Kombe, Y., Parraga, I., Ramirez, B., Whalen, C., Horton, R. J., and Reeve, P., Double-blind placebo-controlled study of concurrent administration of albendazole and praziquantel in schoolchildren with schistosomiasis and geohelminths, *J. Infect. Dis.*, 179, 996, 1999.

74. Guyatt, H. L., Brooker, S., and Donnelly, C. A., Can prevalence of infection in school-aged children be used as an index for assessing community prevalence? *Parasitology*, 118, 257, 1999.

75. World Bank, *World Development Report 1993. Investing in Health*, Oxford University Press, Oxford, 1993.

76. Partnership for Child Development, Cost of school-based drug delivery in Tanzania, *Health Policy Plann.*, 13, 384, 1998.

77. Partnership for Child Development, The cost of large-scale school health programmes which deliver anthelmintics to children in Ghana and Tanzania, *Acta Tropica*, 73, 183, 1999.

78. *Basic Laboratory Methods in Medical Parasitology*, World Health Organization, Geneva, 1991.

79. *The Self-reported Health Problems of Primary School Children in Tanga Region Assessed Using a Questionnaire Administered by Teachers, with Particular Concern for Schistosomiasis*, UKUMTA Report Series No. 6., Dar es Salaam, Tanzania, 1997.

80. *Promoting Child Development through Helminth Control Programmes*, Report of workshop February 24 and 25, 1997, UNICEF, New York, 1997.

81. Hall, A., Orinda, V., Bundy, D. A. P., and Broun, D., Promoting child health through helminth control — A way forward? *Parasitol. Today,* 13, 411, 1997.

82. *Report of the WHO Informal Consultation on Hookworm Infection and Anemia in Girls and Women,* WHO/CTD/SIP/96.1. World Health Organization, Geneva, 1996.

83. Atukorala, T. M., de Silva, L. D., Dechering, W. H., Dassenaeike, T. S., and Perera R. S., Evaluation of effectiveness of iron-folate supplementation and anthelminthic therapy against anemia in pregnancy — a study in the plantation sector of Sri Lanka, *Am. J. Clinical Nutr.,* 60, 286, 1994.

84. de Silva, N. R., Sirisena, J. L., Gunasekera, D. P., Ismail, M. M., and de Silva, H. J., Effect of mebendazole therapy during pregnancy on birth outcome, *Lancet,* 353, 1145, 1999.

85. Feachem, R. G., Bradley, D. J., Garelick, H., and Mara, D. D., *Sanitation and Disease. Health Aspects of Excreta and Wastewater Management,* John Wiley & Sons, London, 1983.

86. Humphries, D. L., Stephenson, L. S., Pearce, E. J., The, P. H., Dan, H. T., and Khanh, L. T., The use of human faeces for fertiliser is associated with increased intensity of hookworm infection in Vietnamese women, *Trans. R. Society Trop. Med. Hygiene,* 91, 518, 1997.

87. Esrey, S. A., Potash, J. B., Roberts, L., and Shiff, C., Effects of improved water supply and sanitation on ascariasis, diarrhoea, dracunculiasis, hookworm infection, schisto-somiasis, and trachoma, *Bull. World Health Organ.,* 69, 609, 1991.

88. Webbe, G. and Jordan, P., Control, in *Human Schistosomiasis*, Jordan, P., Webbe, G., Sturrock, R. F., Eds., CAB International, Wallingford, U.K., 1993.

89. Tameim, O., Abdu, K. M., el Gaddal, A. A., and Jobin, W. R., Protection of Sudanese irrigation workers from schistosome infections by a shift to earlier working hours, *J. Trop. Med. Hygiene,* 88, 125, 1985.

90. Maizels, R. M., Bundy, D. A. P., Selkirk, M. E., Smith, D. F., and Anderson, R. M., Immunological modulation and evasion by helminth parasites in human populations, *Nature,* 365, 797, 1993.

91. Mutapi, F., Ndhlovu, P. D., Hagan, P., Spicer, J. T., Mduluza, T., Turner, C. M., Chandiwana, S. K., and Woolhouse, M. E., Chemotherapy accelerates the development of acquired immune responses to *Schistosoma haematobium* infection, *J. Infect. Dis.,* 178, 289, 1998.

92. Bundy, D. A. P., Hall, A., Medley, G. F., and Savioli, L., Evaluating measures to control intestinal parasitic infections, *World Health Statistics Q.,* 45, 168, 1992.

93. Barnes, E. H., Dobson, R. J., and Barger, I. A., Worm control and anthelmintic resistance. Adventures with a model, *Parasitol. Today,* 11, 56, 1995.

94. Albonico, M., Smith, P. G., Ercole, E., Hall, A., Chwaya, H. M., Alawi, K. A., and Savioli, L., A randomised controlled trial comparing mebendazole 500 mg and albendazole 400 mg against *Ascaris, Trichuris* and the hookworms: 4 and 6 months follow up, *Trans. R. Society Trop. Med. Hygiene,* 89, 538, 1995.

12 Conclusions

Usha Ramakrishnan and Mahshid Lotfi

Nutritional anemia is a grave public health problem affecting the health and well being of millions worldwide. Much progress has been made in our understanding of the causes and consequences of this condition, but more needs to be done in prevention and control. Advances in the assessment of nutritional anemia, especially the use of simple techniques such as the Hemocue™ for hemoglobin estimation and blood spot techniques for indicators of iron and folate status have significantly enhanced our ability to document the magnitude and extent of this condition.[1] While most anemia worldwide is due to iron deficiency, the relative contributions of other factors are not always known in different settings[2] and need to be examined to plan appropriate and effective strategies.

Nutritional anemia affects almost all segments of society and has functional consequences of varying degrees and magnitude throughout the life cycle. Although there remains considerable scientific debate on the exact nature of these adverse consequences, especially for mild and moderate forms of anemia, it is clear that severe anemia is a major threat to the health, survival, and well being of mothers and children.[3,4] Even if anemia is not causally related to outcomes such as low birth weight and delayed child growth,[3] the evidence for impaired intellectual development,[4] poor attention and school performance,[5] and decreased work productivity[6] is very compelling and should prompt policy makers to invest in strategies that will eliminate this condition. Levin[7] estimated that manual work output increased by 1 to 2% for every 1 g/dl increase in hemoglobin levels in anemic subjects. Based on these estimates and the known impact of childhood anemia on cognitive achievement, Ross and Horton[8] estimated that the per capita productivity loss due to iron deficiency anemia (IDA) would amount to 1.9% of Gross Domestic Product (GDP) in a country like Bangladesh. The median value based on several country examples was 0.9%, but the actual losses are staggering for South and Southeast Asia where the prevalence of anemia is extremely high, around 60 and 46%, respectively: the magnitude of such losses >$5 billion annually. In contrast, the per capita cost of interventions such as fortification of flour with iron is minimal (less than 20 cents per person per year).[9] Even supplementation, which is more expensive, would still be cost effective, provided the issues of distribution and compliance are addressed.[10] However, in addition to the economic benefits gained when anemia is prevented or reduced, such interventions will help protect human resources, enhance individuals' well being and allow community members to approach their physical and mental potentials — itself a social value well justifying investments.

It is important to note that although considerable progress has been made towards the virtual elimination of vitamin A deficiency and iodine deficiency disorders in

0-8493-8569-5/01/$0.00+$.50
© 2001 by CRC Press LLC

the past decade, recent examinations of global progress in controlling micronutrient deficiencies[11] show no detectable change in the prevalence of anemia in any region. In fact, prevalences calculated for 1995 are broadly in line with the 1975–1997 averages, and thus with those given by WHO (1997, Table 8).[12]. The goal of reducing the prevalence of IDA by one third in pregnant women and young children that was agreed upon at the World Summit for Children in 1990 and the International Conference on Nutrition in 1992[13] has not been met. Furthermore, despite a wider spread in anemia prevalences among pregnant women subgroups compared to non-pregnant women, "a consistent trend of increased prevalences of anemia is evident in pregnant versus non-pregnant women across all regions and the numbers affected are increasing — the exception being South Asia, perhaps because prevalences have already peaked in this region."[11]

While nutritional anemia persists in developing countries, most industrialized nations have succeeded in addressing this problem in the past century. Clearly, economic growth combined with improvements in sanitation have contributed to some of this; however, widespread fortification of staple foods with key nutrients such as iron and routine consumption of supplements have also contributed to this decline. Recent concerns about iron overload[14] have led several countries to reconsider their fortification policies, especially in parts of Europe. It remains to be seen whether the reversal of policies that mandated fortification of flour with iron, will lead to an increase in anemia among vulnerable groups. Without doubt, ensuring an adequate intake of bioavailable iron in a sustainable and cost effective manner is a key strategy, but remains a major challenge, especially in resource limited settings. A number of technical barriers (perceived and real) in approaches such as fortification and supplementation in the prevention and control of anemia remain, but some progress has been made.[9,10] Nevertheless, to implement highly effective control measures in areas with a high prevalence of anemia, several issues demand attention. For instance, regarding iron supplementation during pregnancy, while most of the iron tablet supply is from domestic sources, evidently the external sources of iron tablets only cover around 3% of the need during pregnancy.[11] This very low level of external supply could be improved as a step toward more effective programs. Expansion of program coverage needs to be linked to identification of better methods to ensure access to and consumption of iron/folate tablets throughout pregnancy. At the same time, since such programs only deal with increased requirement for iron during pregnancy, strategies need to be identified and implemented to improve the iron status of child bearing age women long before they become pregnant.

Fortification of staple foods such as wheat and corn is being adopted widely by several industrialized countries to prevent occurrence of anemia in their general populations. However, implementing the same intervention in developing countries leads to concerns regarding the efficiency of iron absorption from the plant based high phytate diets consumed in many of these countries. Interventions aimed at increasing dietary iron must be accompanied by direction on methods to reduce the phytate content of the final food product to be consumed. This is perhaps more of an issue if iron intake is increased through plant breeding and selection of iron dense plant varieties to be included in daily high phytate diets. Approaches to decrease inhibitors to iron absorption and increase absorption enhancers should be part of any effective dietary modification strategy to improve iron nutrition. Foods rich in absorbable iron must be identified through examination of food intake and meal composition data and their consumption should be encouraged. Attention must also be paid to bioavailability and absorption of other micronutrients such as zinc and copper from the diet, when dietary iron intake from staple foods is increased. No matter what intervention is implemented, a combination of approaches including attention to associated deficiencies (e.g., vitamin A, folate) needs to be considered.

Perhaps real barriers to implementation of effective programs are the lack of (1) awareness at different levels of society, (2) political will, and (3) effective communication. It is in this context that attention should be paid to the changing market economies in many parts of the world which provide unique opportunities for partnerships between the private and public sector to address this problem. The recent dialogue and involvement of international agencies such as the Asian Development Bank, large multinational food and pharmaceutical companies, nongovernment agencies, and governments in several Asian countries serve as excellent examples of such partnerships.[15] There is an urgent need to evaluate and learn from the successful experience in the elimination of iodine deficiency in many parts of the world in the last 20 years. The steward role of the salt industry in this effort[16] is to be applauded and similar challenges can be set for others, such as flour manufacturers, to eliminate nutritional anemia.

Where do we go from here? There is clearly a need to design and monitor better programs that are innovative and combine different approaches. Traditionally, we have tended to focus on one approach which has its proponents and opponents for example, those in favor of supplementation do not interact with those who advocate food fortification. Similarly, researchers and program planners do not meet and address the issues that need to be answered. There is an urgent need to improve the skills of decision makers and program planners in many developing countries to better understand the nature and extent of the problem in their local setting, implement the appropriate mix of strategies that address the needs of different population groups, monitor progress, and measure impact. For example, strategies that work for school age children[5] may not be appropriate for pregnant women and infants. There is a serious scarcity of representative and national data on anemia prevalence in many countries. We need to give priority for repeating surveys in the same country to allow better assessment of progress in reducing anemia through time. Without representative baseline data, it is not possible to know whether efforts to reduce anemia have had any effect.[11] One of the consensus statements of a UNICEF/UNU/WHO/MI Technical Workshop notes: "Plans for any major national or sub-national health and nutrition surveys should add the measurement of hemoglobin to the survey to gain information on the actual levels of iron deficiency anemia in subgroups of the population".[17]

Finally, although the solutions for nutritional anemias lie in providing improved access to better food and nutrition, the importance of other health-based strategies cannot be overlooked. For example, the potential of helminth control especially for school age children has been demonstrated effectively.[18] Similarly, although malaria is not a direct cause of nutritional anemia, and has not been discussed separately in this book, it is an important public health concern that co-occurs with nutritional anemia and has often hampered iron supplementation efforts due to safety concerns.

However, a recent meta-analyses of placebo controlled trials concluded that iron supplementation in malarious areas is unlikely to increase the risk of malarial morbidity and the latest consensus statement by the International Nutrition Anemia Consultative Group (2000) recommends that 1) iron supplementation should continue in malarious areas where IDA is prevalent and 2) since the number of studies were limited, more work is still needed.[19] Examining the effectiveness of strategies that address both the prevention and control of malaria (impregnated bed-nets, chemo-prophylaxis) and nutritional anemia will provide valuable answers. Last but not the least, although food based strategies that utilize resources at the household and/or community level and communication strategies that address behavior change would be more sustainable, more work is needed to demonstrate that these approaches are effective both alone and in combination with other strategies.[20] In conclusion, while there are still many questions to be answered, the challenge is to focus our efforts to reduce nutritional anemia based on current knowledge and experience.

REFERENCES

1. Lynch, S. and Green, R., Assessment of nutritional anemia, Chapter 3, this volume, 2001.
2. Allen, L. and Casterline-Sabel, J., Prevalence and causes of nutritional anemia, Chapter 2, this volume, 2001.
3. Ramakrishnan, U., Functional consequences of nutritional anemia during pregnancy and early childhood, Chapter 4, this volume, 2001.
4. Lozoff, B. and Wachs, T., Functional correlates of nutritional anemia during infancy and early childhood — child development and behavior, Chapter 5, this volume, 2001.
5. Jain, S. P. and Vir, S. C., Functional consequences of nutritional anemia in school age children, Chapter 6, this volume, 2001.
6. Beard, J. L., Functional consequences of nutritional anemia in adults, Chapter 7, this volume, 2001.
7. Levin, H. M., A benefit-cost analysis of nutritional programs for anaemia reduction, *Res. Observer,* 1, 219, 1986.
8. Ross, J. and Horton, S., *Economic Consequences of Iron Deficiency,* The Micronutrient Intiative, Ottawa, 1998.
9. Walter, T., Olivares, M., Pizarro, F., and Hertrampf, E., Fortification, Chapter 9, this volume, 2001.
10. Ekström, E. C., Supplementation, Chapter 8, this volume, 2001.
11. Mason, J., Lotfi, M., Dalmiya, N., et al., Progress in controlling micronutrient deficiencies, *The Micronutrient Initiative,* in press.
12. World Health Organization, Prevalence of anemia among different populations based on national data, Tables from MDIS Group paper number 3, Geneva, 1997.
13. International Conference on Nutrition (ICN), Rome, 1992.
14. Olsson, K. S., Safwenberg, J., and Ritter, B., The effect of iron fortification of the diet on clinical iron overload in the general population, *Ann. N.Y. Acad. of Sci.,* 526, 290–300, 1988.

15. Maberly, G., The potential for protecting populations from minerals and vitamins deficiencies through healthy quality foods in Asian countries, in preparation and planning for *Food Fortification Policy, The Manila Forum,* December 7, 1999.
16. Salt 2000 Symposium, The Hague, Netherlands, May 8–11, 2000.
17. UNICEF/UNU/WHO/MI Technical Workshop. Preventing iron deficiency in women and children. Technical consensus on key issues. 7-9 October 1998. Unicef, New York.
18. Hall, A., Drake, L., and Bundy, D. A. P., Public health measures to control helminth infections, Chapter 11, this volume, 2001.
19. INACG Consensus Statement. Safety of iron supplementation programs in malaria-endemic regions. INACG, Dec 1999.
20. Ruel, M.T. and Levin, C., Food based strategies, Chapter 10, this volume, 2001.

Index

A

Absorption of iron, *see also* Bioavailability of nutrients
  amino chelates and, 174–175
  fortificants in corn meal, 173
  increasing with fortification, 199–200
  main inhibitor of, 12, 174, 201
  physical exertion and, 118
  promotor compounds, 202
  rate during pregnancy, 134
  requirement for children, 12
ACD (anemia of chronic disease), 26, 27
Adolescents and anemia, *see also* Children and anemia
  causes of nutritional anemia
    deficiency risk and growth velocity, 92
    dietary, 92–93
    infections, 93–94
  consequences of nutritional anemia
    clinical symptoms, 98–99
    cycle of, 99
    growth retardation, 94–95
    impaired mental and motor functions, 96–98
    low birth weight, 98
    maternal mortality, 98
    poor physical performance, 95–96
  intervention measures
    address public health problem, 104
    control of infections, 104
    dietary diversification, 100
    fortification of foods, 100–101
    supplementation, 101–104
  iron requirements, 11–12
  prevalence
    age and, 91
    among girls, 91–92
    by country, 90
    predictors of anemia, 90–91
Adults and anemia
  clinical manifestations
    specific symptoms, 112
    tissue depletion, 112–113
  physiological impairments
    immune function, 113–115
    mental function, 115–117

nonspecific immunity and iron deficiency, 114–115
physical performance, 117–120
relationship to iron, 114
thermoregulation, 120–122
prevalence of IDA, 111
Africa
  anemia prevalence in, 9
  folic acid deficiency in, 15
  maternal deaths from anemia, 46–49
  rice consumption, 156
Agricultural research and anemia reduction, 202
Albendazole
  effectiveness of, 219, 227, 228
  treatment programs using, 229
Alzheimer's disease, 116
Amenorrhea and iron requirements, 10
Amino acids and iron bioavailability, 202
Amino chelates and iron absorption, 174–175
Amylase rich food technology, 198
Amyotrophic lateral sclerosis, 115
Ancylostoma duodenale, see Hookworms
Anemia of chronic disease (ACD), 26, 27
Angular stomatitis, 112
Animal products and bioavailability of iron, 194
Anorexia, 112
Anthelminthics
  dosage and effectiveness, 228–229
  mass treatment recommendation, 229
  types of, 227
  use during pregnancy, 219, 231
Argentina, 156
Ascaris lumbricoides, 13–14, 221–222, 223
Ascorbic acid and iron absorption, 12
Asia
  anemia prevalence in, 9
  maternal deaths from anemia, 46–49
  prevalence of anemia in children, 90
  rice consumption, 156
  wheat imports/exports, 156
Asian Development Bank, 243
Atherothrombosis, 36
Athletes, *see also* Muscles; Physical performance
  iron absorption, 118
  performance and iron status, 117–118
  red cell turnover, 118–119

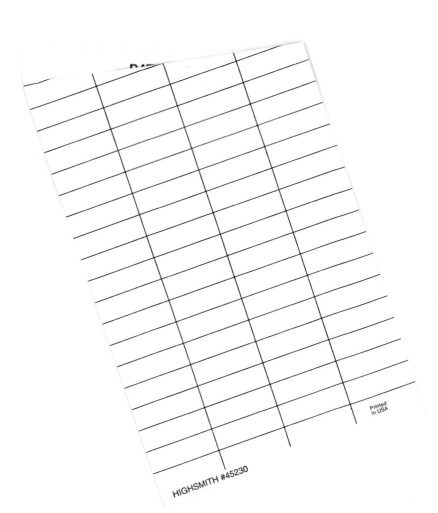

HIGHSMITH #45230

Printed
in USA